THE PSYCHOLOGY
OF VISION

THE PSYCHOLOGY OF VISION

A ROYAL SOCIETY DISCUSSION
ORGANIZED BY H. C. LONGUET-HIGGINS, F.R.S.,
AND N. S. SUTHERLAND

HELD ON 7 AND 8 MARCH 1979

LONDON
THE ROYAL SOCIETY
1980

Printed in Great Britain for the Royal Society
at the
University Press, Cambridge

ISBN 0 85403 141 3

First published in *Philosophical Transactions of the Royal Society of London*,
series B, volume 290 (no. 1038), pages 1–218

Published by the Royal Society
6 Carlton House Terrace, London SW1Y 5AG

CONTENTS

[1]

CONTENTS

Phil. Trans. R. Soc. Lond. B **290**, 3–4 (1980)
Printed in Great Britain

Introduction

By N. S. Sutherland and H. C. Longuet-Higgins, F.R.S.

*Centre for Research on Perception and Cognition, Laboratory of Experimental Psychology
University of Sussex, Brighton BN1 9QG, U.K.*

There is a long-standing tradition of research on vision in Great Britain that goes back at least as far as Newton. The Royal Society is therefore a most suitable venue for a conference on the Psychology of Vision, and it is no accident that two of our distinguished guests from North America are British subjects.

In the first 30 years of this century the Gestalt movement brought about a revolution in our ways of thinking about vision, but the subject then remained rather stagnant for two decades. In more recent years, dramatic discoveries and radical new insights have been forthcoming from three different directions. First, neurophysiologists have laid bare some of the highly systematic wiring that subserves the early stages of the processing of the visual input. Secondly, psychologists and psychophysiologists have uncovered some of the intricacies of the mechanisms that underlie such functions as acuity, contrast discrimination, motion detection and stereopsis. It is becoming possible to put together results from these two directions and to show how mechanisms inferred from psychophysical observations are instantiated in known neurophysiological circuits. The two sets of results indicate that visual processing is both more complex and more elegant than had been suspected 50 years ago. Thirdly, the advent of the digital computer has made it possible to build rigorous computational models of the visual system, to explore and to specify more adequately the nature of the task that the visual system must perform, and to demonstrate precisely how the constraints imposed by the nature of the physical world and of its optics make it possible for the brain to use the patterns of light impinging on the retinae to form a useful representation of the external world. Although this last enterprise may strike some as speculative, it has already led to insights into the nature of vision that have changed our ways of looking at the problems and have made the theories of shape recognition put forward in the 1950s and 1970s, including those of one of us, look extremely superficial.

The study of vision may ultimately prove to be one of the best routes into an even larger and as yet more intractable subject, the study of human intelligence. The human visual system has evolved over tens of millions of years into a very subtle and efficient information processing instrument. It conducts elaborate calculations in parallel and appears to use and to synthesize every single cue to depth that is present in the retinal image; it computes size and brightness constancy effortlessly and with incredible rapidity; and from the tessellated and fragmentary information produced by brightness differences on the retina it recovers with deceptive ease the real disposition of three-dimensional shapes in the world around us. The inferential processes that underlie everyday acts of seeing may be deeper and more subtle than are those exercised by an Einstein in the prosecution of his scientific work, but because we have all evolved to be brilliant at seeing, but not alas at physics, we tend to marvel only at the latter capacity. If recent work on vision had done nothing else, it would still be worth while because it evokes a sense of wonderment at the subtlety and perfection of the visual system. But it has done much else. It has even begun to adumbrate the inferential mechanisms involved in vision, and it may be that these very mechanisms will ultimately provide the key to our understanding of the highest flights of human thought. The role of the visual imagination in scientific thinking has often been stressed and it is well established that there is a high correlation between scientific ability and spatial intelligence. It is perhaps not surprising that when we seek to obtain a scientific understanding of the Universe we should put to new use the structures that have evolved for processing purely visual information, and recast the ideas we are trying to manipulate in a form in which they can be represented and manipulated by existing and well tried structures in the brain.

The psychology of vision is such a vast topic that it would have been impossible to deal with all its aspects in a Discussion Meeting of this length. For example, there are no papers on colour vision since that is a subject in itself. Moreover, although the conference is on the psychology of vision, we have included some papers on visual neurophysiology since, as already pointed out, the psychologist must often draw on the neurophysiological results to interpret his own data. The organization of the proceedings should be obvious. We start with work that can be more or less directly related to neurophysiological findings and move progressively to phenomena that demand explanatory mechanisms that are less and less related to known neurophysiological structures.

Phil. Trans. R. Soc. Lond. B **290**, 5–9 (1980)
Printed in Great Britain

The physics of visual perception

By F. W. CAMPBELL, F.R.S.

The Physiological Laboratory, Cambridge, CB2 3EG, U.K.

By measuring the contrast threshold for gratings of different waveform and spatial frequency, Campbell & Robson suggested in 1968 that there may be 'channels' tuned to different spatial frequencies. By using the technique of adapting to a high contrast grating, it was possible to measure the band-pass characteristics of these channels. Similar techniques were used to establish the orientational tuning of the channels. Reasons are put forward why it is advantageous to organize the visual system in this manner.

Any temporal or spatial stimulus can be characterized by its Fourier transform (Taylor 1965). By varying the contrast and spatial frequency (fineness) of a grating, kept at constant mean luminance, it is possible to measure quantitatively those Fourier components of a visual scene that are available to our eye–brain. This technique, and the results obtained in man and in the cat are described by Campbell & Maffei (1974). The results are summarized in figure 1. (The shaded area is the invisible world of ectoplasm, fairies and ghosts.) How does this approach help us to understand the visual world that we can see (the unshaded area)? Why are we not aware of the undetectable portions of the scene? These problems troubled Helmholtz and Mach (Ratliff 1965).

When we examine a standard optometrist's eye test chart, lines that are too small for us to resolve still seem to be composed of high contrast black letters. Thus, there seems to be some mechanism to ensure contrast constancy, so that as we move about the world, the contrast of objects does not change (Georgeson & Sullivan 1975).

Campbell & Robson (1968) showed that the contrast threshold for gratings with a sinusoidal profile was different from those with a square-wave profile. These observations were extended into the suprathreshold domain by Campbell *et al.* (1978). For gratings with spatial frequency greater than 1 cycle/deg, the square-wave grating is perceived slightly better by a factor of $4/\pi$. If we accept that in this spatial frequency range the visual system performs a quasi-Fourier analysis on the image, this is precisely the expected result, for this is the relative amplitude of the fundamental in a square wave. Indeed, it is difficult to see what other mechanism could account for this finding.

For frequencies less than 1 cycle/deg, the visual system behaves quite differently. At any of these low frequencies, square waves of all spatial frequencies have a constant low (0.25 %) contrast threshold. Even at a spatial frequency of 1 cycle per 180° (i.e. a single edge) this remains valid. As the spatial frequency is clearly irrelevant in this instance, it seems that the square wave is detected by virtue of its individual edges rather than as a gestalt grating. Sinusoidal gratings of these low frequencies are greatly attenuated or invisible. Indeed, they can be removed from a square-wave grating, altering its luminance profile dramatically, but without affecting its appearance or detectability. This effect is analogous to the phenomenon of the missing fundamental in audition (Goldstein 1973), and has a neurophysiological interpretation (Maffei *et al.* 1979).

A sinusoidal grating is physically infinitely blurred, while a square wave is infinitely sharp. A sine wave has only a single frequency component in its Fourier spectrum containing all the wave's power. A square wave has, in addition, a shower of higher odd harmonics of linearly

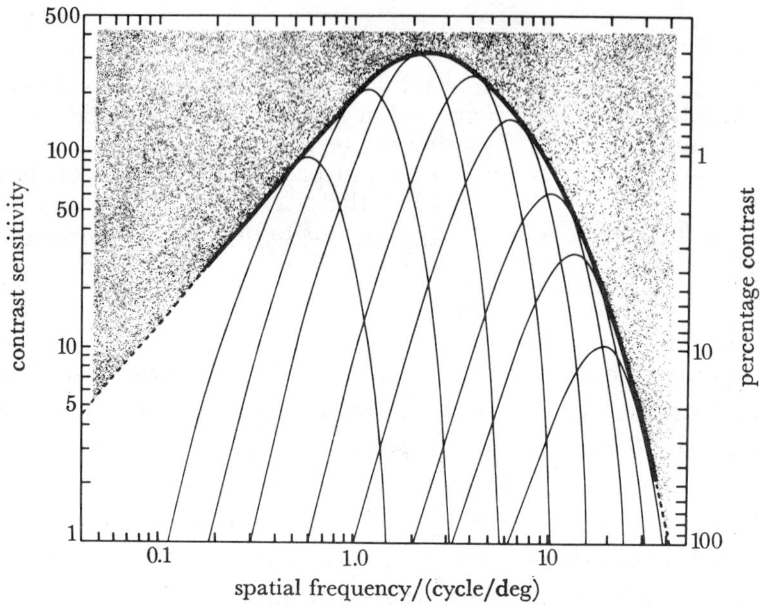

FIGURE 1. The thick curve represents the contrast sensitivity (defined as reciprocal threshold contrast) of the human visual system to a sinusoidal grating, plotted against spatial frequency. The shaded area must always remain invisible to us unless the spatial frequency content of the image is shifted into the visible domain by optical means, such as the microscope. The lighter curves represent channels sensitive to a narrow range of spatial frequencies.

decreasing amplitude. Campbell *et al.* (1978) have shown that low-frequency square gratings are perceived as true square waves, provided that they possess the first few higher harmonics (in appropriate phase). The auditory analogue of this is that the click of a metronome is detected by the neurons tuned to high temporal frequencies. Similar neurons tuned to a band of spatial frequencies approximately one octave wide exist in the visual cortex of the cat (review by Maffei 1978), and the elegant work of De Valois *et al.* (1978) has shown that the monkey visual cortex is similarly organized. Indeed, the important discovery by Hubel & Wiesel (1962) that cells in the visual cortex are sensitive only to a narrow range of stimulus orientations is immediately suggestive of a Fourier analytical process. The existence of channels sensitive to particular bands of spatial frequencies of particular orientation can be demonstrated psychophysically in man by adaptation experiments (review by Braddick *et al.* 1978). Indeed the first evidence for these channels was found psychophysically by Campbell & Robson (1968), who stated that 'a picture emerges of functionally separate mechanisms in the visual nervous system each responding maximally at some particular spatial frequency and hardly at all at spatial frequencies differing by a factor of two. The frequency selectivity of these mechanisms must be determined by integrative processes in the nervous system and they appear to be a first approximation at least, to operate linearly.'

Figure 2 illustrates a picture of a tank that has been analysed by three broad-band channels, respectively sensitive to the low-, medium- and high-frequency components of the original image. An enemy soldier would be most interested in the low-frequency components, and having established that a tank is approaching him, will turn his attention to survival in the undergrowth. The tank troop commander, however, will be most interested in the intermediate frequency components, which reveal the tank type and number, while the sergeant of the maintenance wing will examine the high-frequency components for signs of damage to the trackwork.

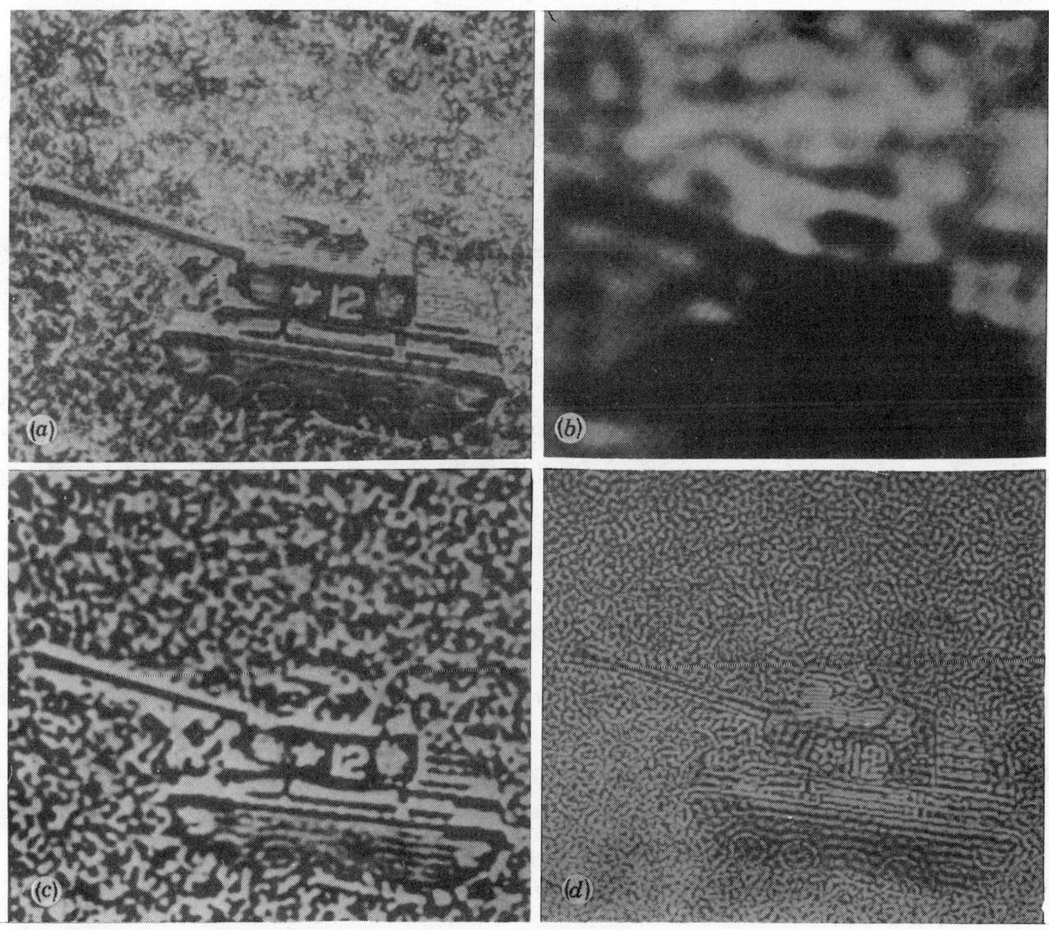

FIGURE 2. (*a*) Original photographic image. (*b*) Same image filtered to pass low spatial frequencies only. (*c*) As (*b*) but with only medium spatial frequencies passed. (*d*) As (*b*) but with only high spatial frequencies passed. (Courtesy of H. C. Andrews.)

The channel model of the visual system raises many interesting questions. For example, Pirenne (1967) has raised an important question when he writes, 'It is a familiar fact that on a moonless night, our vision not only is very blurred, but is also colourless.' If a myope removes his spectacles, high spatial frequencies suffer greater attenuation than do low spatial frequencies. In this case, the visual scene does indeed look very blurred. As the illumination of a scene is reduced, high spatial frequencies are again attenuated much more than low, owing to the shortage of photons available to the visual system, over the eye's integration time (*ca.* 0.1 s), and we might expect Pirenne's prediction of blur to be verified. However, our own observations have led us to the conclusion that at night the visual scene, though devoid of fine detail, is quite definitely not blurred.

A low-frequency sine-wave grating (less than 1 cycle/deg) is always discriminably different from a square-wave grating, even near threshold. This holds to the lowest luminance level. This must mean that some of the higher harmonics of the square wave are being detected. It can also be shown readily that if the eye is defocused by as little as $\pm$ 0.5 dioptres, the resulting optical blur can be detected (night myopia).

Owing to photon shortage at these dim illuminations, the neurons that normally respond to high frequencies and which can function under photopic conditions fail to operate, yet we do not notice their absence. The visual system must be aware that these neurons can never fire at low levels, and assumes, if the question arises (as in the perception of an edge or square wave), that the undetectable frequencies are present. Campbell *et al.* (1978) concluded that 'the visual input appears to be analyzed into its Fourier components and if these constitute a square sequence with no above-threshold components missing, then the perception of a square-wave results. This solves the problem, considered by Helmholtz and Mach (Ratliff 1965, p. 265), of why aberrations of the emmetropic eye do not result in all edges appearing blurred. Only when the blurring is great enough to remove independently detectable high frequency components does the blur become detectable.' Likewise, under scotopic conditions, a square-wave grating always appears to be square because any undetectable missing higher harmonics are not noticed as absent.

Another feature of a moonless night is that the sky is full of stars. It is our opinion that all stars, whether seen in the fovea or on the periphery, look like point sources. This raises an interesting question, for the acuity of vision falls off markedly as eccentricity from the fovea increases. One might expect that when regarding the 'inverted bowl they call the sky' (Fitzgerald 1859) we would see the stars as point sources in the fovea, but as broader and broader smudges as their images fall upon peripheral retinal locations of lower and lower acuity. The fact that we do not suggests that the visual system perceives a small stimulus as a point source, until that stimulus reaches a size great enough for its true size to be signalled by the available channel mechanisms. Thereafter, of course, the true size is perceived, and the objects retain the same apparent size, wherever upon the retina their image falls. The channel system is organized in such a way that where its limited sensitivity intrudes, the stimulus is perceived in its most probable form, be that as a sharp edge or square wave, or as a star.

I acknowledge the help of Mark Lawden in the preparation of this manuscript.

References (Campbell)

Andrews, H. C. 1972 Digital computers and image processing. *Endeavour* **31**, 88–94.

Braddick, O., Campbell, F. W. & Atkinson, J. 1978 Channels in vision: basic aspects. In *Handbook of sensory physiology*, vol. 8, ch. 1, pp. 3–38. Springer-Verlag.

Campbell, F. W. & Maffei, L. 1974 Contrast and spatial frequency. *Scient. Am.* **231** (5), 106–115.

Campbell, F. W. & Robson, J. G. 1968 Application of Fourier analysis to the visibility of gratings. *J. Physiol., Lond.* **197**, 551–566.

Campbell, F. W., Howell, E. R. & Johnstone, J. R. 1978 A comparison of threshold and suprathreshold appearance of gratings with components in the low and high spatial frequency range. *J. Physiol., Lond.* **284**, 193–201.

De Valois, K. K., De Valois, R. L. & Yund, E. W. 1979 Responses of striate cortex cells to grating and checkerboard patterns. *J. Physiol., Lond.* **291**, 483–505.

Fitzgerald, E. 1859 *Rubaiyat of Omar Khayyam*.

Georgeson, M. A. & Sullivan, G. D. 1975 Contrast constancy: deblurring in human vision by spatial frequency channels. *J. Physiol., Lond.* **252**, 627–656.

Goldstein, J. L. 1973 An optimum process theory for the central information of the pitch of complex tones *J. acoust. Soc. Am.* **54**, 1496–1516.

Hubel, D. H. & Wiesel, T. N. 1962 Receptive fields, binocular interaction and functional architecture in the cat's visual cortex. *J. Physiol., Lond.* **160**, 106–154.

Maffei, L. 1978 Spatial frequency channels: neural mechanisms. In *Handbook of sensory physiology*, vol. 8, ch. 1, pp. 39–66. Springer-Verlag.

Maffei, L., Morrone, C., Pirchio, M. & Sandini, G. 1979 Responses of visual cortical cells to periodic and non-periodic stimuli. *J. Physiol., Lond.* **296**, 27–47.

Pirenne, M. 1967 *Vision and the eye*, p. 36. Chapman & Hall.

Ratliff, F. 1965 *Mach bands: quantitative studies on neural networks in the retina.* San Francisco: Holden-Day.

Taylor, C. A. 1965 *The physics of musical sounds.* London: English Universities Press.

Discussion

D. Marr (*The Artificial Intelligence Laboratory, Cambridge, Massachusetts* 02139, *U.S.A.*). Dr Campbell cannot have it both ways! Either one can inspect his tank independently at different spatial frequencies, in which case one should be able to recognize Abraham Lincoln in L. D. Harmon's coarsely sampled and quantized picture of him, or one should be able to do neither. Since one cannot see Lincoln without effectively blurring the image, presumably one cannot inspect the tank in the way that Dr Campbell suggests. Marr & Hildreth (1979) show how information from the different spatial frequency channels may be combined, by using the spatial coincidence assumption. According to this, when zero-crossings from different channels coincide spatially, they are combined into a descriptive unit (an 'edge') and it is this, not the individual channel outputs, that is available to later processes (see Marr 1976; Marr & Hildreth 1979).

References

Marr, D. 1976 Early processing of visual information. *Phil. Trans. R. Soc. Lond.* B **275**, 483–519.

Marr, D. & Hildreth, E. 1980 Theory of edge detection. *Proc. R. Soc. Lond.* B **207**, 187–217.

F. W. Campbell, F.R.S. A suprathreshold edge situated within a hypercolumn's receptive field contains all spatial frequencies and may excite any and all of the neurons within the hypercolumn that have the correct orientation tuning. Such edges, therefore, would be excellent masking stimuli for all spatial frequencies. In the Lincoln's-head picture it is not surprising that the introduction of spurious sharp edges masks the perception of the pattern defined by medium-to-low spatial frequencies. The edge pattern is foreign to the head and is, therefore, a good mask.

The three filtered images of the tank, however, all arise from the same original picture and cooperate to produce a consistent percept. Certainly, one may pay attention selectively to the information contained in any particular waveband of spatial frequencies, but this does not imply that other wavebands disappear – they do not.

For Lincoln's head the masking edges cannot be made to disappear by feats of concentration, and as the information that they contain is not relevant to the perception of Lincoln they continue to act as a mask.

Phil. Trans. R. Soc. Lond. B **290**, 11–22 (1980)

Printed in Great Britain

Spatial frequency analysis in early visual processing

By M. A. Georgeson

*Department of Psychology, University of Bristol, 8-10 Berkeley Square,
Bristol BS8 1HH, U.K.*

The existence of multiple channels, or multiple receptive field sizes, in the visual system does not commit us to any particular theory of spatial encoding in vision. However, distortions of apparent spatial frequency and width in a wide variety of conditions favour the idea that each channel carries a width- or frequency-related code or 'label' rather than a 'local sign' or positional label. When distortions of spatial frequency occur without prior adaptation (e.g. at low contrast or low luminance) they are associated with lowered sensitivity, and may be due to a mismatch between the perceptual labels and the actual tuning of the channels. A low-level representation of retinal space could be constructed from the spatial information encoded by the channels, rather than being projected intact from the retina.

1. The visual representation of retinal space

(a) Channels, features and neural images

When stripped down to its essentials, the multiple spatial frequency channel model of visual analysis – amply reviewed in the previous paper by Campbell – appears to be claiming remarkably little: that for a given retinal location and orientation there exist several visual receptive fields of different sizes (figure 1 a). Such an assertion seems harmless enough, and hardly calculated to split the world forever into Professor Barlow's two camps: the 'frequency freaks', who were for it, and the 'feature creatures', who were against it. Let us therefore dig a little deeper, to see where real disagreement arises.

Assuming linearity, the simple centre-surround receptive field (r.f.) must act as a bandpass spatial filter. Small r.fs respond to high spatial frequencies, large ones to low frequencies, and so on. This is the message from very many studies in neurophysiology and psychophysics. If the topographic projection of the retina onto the cortex were perfectly orderly, then one could literally think of the pattern of cell responses as being a filtered neural image of the stimulus. Restricting the problem to one dimension, that image would be the convolution of the input waveform with the r.f. profile.

Figure 1 (*b*) shows the profiles for four channels computed in response to a single bar of medium width. Small units respond with a characteristic Mach band (peak and trough) pattern at each edge, while the larger units respond with a single peak in the centre of the bar.

In a second example (figure 1 *c*) we see the response to a group of four bars. The smaller units clearly resolve individual bars, while the larger units appear to treat the pattern much as though it were a solid bar.

None of this is the least bit unexpected or controversial, but I have found these computations very instructive in thinking about the problems that the system has to face in interpreting its input. Ironically, the multiple-channel model as stated so far is consistent with almost any theory of spatial representation in what Marr (1976) has called 'early visual processing.'

Emphasis on the spatial profiles of figure 1 could lead to either the traditional image-based, isomorphic projection theories, in which one might include the work of Von Bekesy, Ratliff and Cornsweet, or to more sophisticated feature-map ideas, the most important of which is surely the work of Marr (1976). Marr rightly attacks earlier naïve notions of feature detection, in so far as they assumed a one-to-one correspondence between the firing of a single unit and the detection of a visual feature. Receptive fields are sensitive to a range of stimuli, and therefore 'feature detection' is itself a problem in pattern recognition.

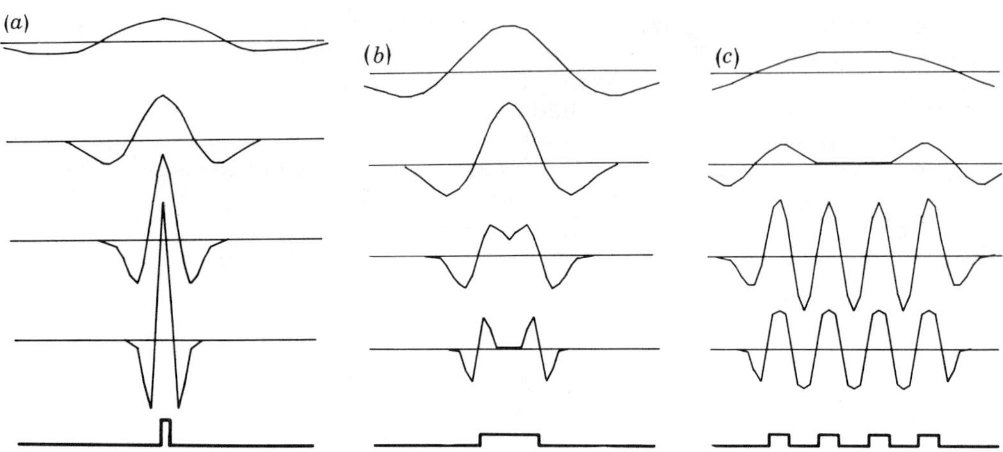

FIGURE 1. Four response profiles ('neural images') computed by convolving four sizes of receptive field weighting function with the stimulus waveform (lowest trace). (*a*) When the input is a narrow pulse, the responses simply illustrate the four weighting functions used. Each is a triple Gaussian function (Macleod & Rosenfeld 1974) and each differs from the next by a factor of two in height and width. (*b*) Responses to an elongated pulse which represents a solid light bar. (*c*) Responses to a cluster of four bars.

(*b*) '*Local signs*' *and Fourier spectra*

Marr's (1976) program analyses the spatial distribution of peaks, troughs and zero crossings in the response profiles to parse or segment the input into a set of visual primitives – EDGE, LINE, SHADING EDGE, etc., each of which is tagged with a list of attributes – orientation, contrast, fuzziness and position. The primal sketch model, of which this is the first stage, is important because it is, as far as I know, the only coherent attempt to solve this theoretical problem in a general way. However, it appears to share with earlier ideas a reliance on the exact preservation of spatial coordinates as a means of determining spatial relations. For example, in a coordinate-based approach, the width of a bar or the separation of two parallel lines could be given by finding the location of each line or edge and then calculating the difference between the two coordinate values. For at least the last two centuries it has been taken as more or less self-evident that the spatial projection of the retina on to the cortex served to set up a spatial coordinate map of this kind (see Boring 1942, p. 78 ff). In the nineteenth century each retinal point had its 'local sign', and in Marr's system each feature ('symbolic assertion') has its positional label.

We can begin to see why the introduction of Fourier ideas had such a shock effect. They appeared to be denying this whole tradition, and replacing the spatial representation of space with its dual: the Fourier transform, in which spatial layout is not represented in an explicit way. Now this never was, or never should have been, the case, since none of the evidence for 'channels' has ever implied that they were anything other than relatively local analysers: receptive fields. The novelty lies in the idea that the pattern of responses across r.f. sizes, rather than across space, might be of primary importance in the encoding of spatial features and spatial relations. Such a pattern could be a neural approximation to the discrete (i.e. spatially limited) Fourier transform.

In short, then, merely discovering the existence of multiple r.f. sizes does not reveal their perceptual roles in representing the visual array. The entire collection of r.f. responses constitutes a data base which could be operated on in a number of ways, and neither single-unit studies nor psychophysical detection experiments give much information about such perceptual operations, since neither approach actually investigates the way that things look.

(c) *Distortions of perceived spatial frequency*

Only one well known phenomenon gives direct support to the frequency-based coding hypothesis. It is Blakemore & Sutton's (1969) after-effect: the spatial frequency shift. Inspection of one spatial frequency makes higher test frequencies seem even higher, lower ones even lower. The result is easily explained as a shift in the balance of frequency channel activity, but is difficult to account for on the spatial coordinate view. There is no reason why altering the sensitivities of the various filters by adaptation should alter the spacing of peaks and troughs in the output profile.

However, the processes of adaptation are not fully understood and there is evidence that Blakemore & Sutton's frequency shift is more complicated than we previously thought (Heeley 1979). Therefore, I have been attempting to devise experiments that can reasonably distinguish between the spatial and the frequency approaches without using adaptation. The subject of the rest of this paper is a class of size and frequency shifts that occur without adaptation, but which also support the frequency coding model. It turns out that a wide range of stimulus manipulations produce variations in apparent width or spatial frequency, and that all the effects conform to a general rule.

2. NATURAL VARIATIONS OF PERCEIVED SIZE

(a) *A possible code for bar width*

To begin with, I chose to look at single bars, because they are simple in the space domain but complex in the frequency domain. The aim was to make apparent width vary in a way predictable from the frequency viewpoint, but not from the spatial one.

On the Fourier view, the width of a bar could be given not by the positions of its edges, but by a computation on the 'neural spectrum' – the distribution of responses across channels. As a concrete example, one effective rule for extracting width is to take a weighted sum of the responses across different sizes of r.f. *centred on the bar*. Thus a possible width index is

$$W = \Sigma \, W_i \, R_i / \Sigma \, R_i,$$

summed across field sizes $i = 1$ to $i = n$, where R_i is response magnitude and W_i is equal to field size. Even with only four channels, W is found to vary monotonically with stimulus width over quite a wide range. In a linear model, dividing by the sum of all R_i makes the index W independent of stimulus strength. The values W_i represent the idea that each r.f. has a size- or frequency-specific label – a 'specific nerve energy' in older terminology – but the final result is a combination of weighted evidence from all r.fs. In fact, here it is the average of the active r.f. sizes, weighted by the amount of their activity.

If now we take a single light bar and add a thin dark bar to its centre, we convert it into a pair of parallel light lines of the same total width. This modification alters the pattern of channel responses, and hence also alters the index W. If the index is taken at the centre of the pattern as before, and only positive responses are included, then an apparent increase in width of about 40 % is predicted. This occurs because responses go negative for small r.fs, but not for large ones. On the other hand, the theory based on location of peaks or edges would predict little or no change in width.

In several experiments similar to those described below I have found that pulse pairs or triplets, or fragments of grating (say 3 or 4 cycles), do look considerably wider than a solid bar of the same physical width, by around 20–40 %. However, there is an obvious difficulty with the assumption that the system applies the same rule for extraction of width to patterns that are so clearly different. The evidence in favour of this particular rule is so far only preliminary. Spatial theories might counter with the older idea of 'contour repulsion' to explain the twin-line experiment, but as a matter of fact neither these computations nor the direct alignment experiment of Rentschler *et al.* (1975) give any support for the existence of contour repulsion.

(b) Perceived bar width as a function of contrast

A second approach, which overcomes the difficulties just described, is to keep the pattern constant throughout, and to vary its contrast. As contrast decreases, the response of relatively high frequency channels should drop below threshold first because they are the less sensitive ones. At low contrasts a bar would be represented only in the lower frequency units, and so should look both wider and more blurred. Subjects fixated midway between two vertical bars on an oscilloscope screen. The left-hand bar varied in contrast from trial to trial, and the subject's task was to adjust the width of the right-hand bar (whose contrast was fixed) to appear to match that of the left.

For all subjects and all bar widths (1.5–24′) the bars looked 1–2′ narrower at the lower contrasts, or equivalently they looked wider at higher contrasts (figure 2). In percentage terms the effects were greatest at the narrower test widths (1.5′, 3′, 6′), and these differences of 30 % or more were perceptually very striking. One immediately thinks of scattered light, or Helmholtz's idea that light regions 'irradiate' into their darker surrounds. This cannot be the explanation, however, because the same result held for dark bars, using two different procedures for blocking and ordering the trials, to control for various possible procedural artefacts. The narrowing effect persisted right down to the threshold of visibility.

(c) Perceived spatial frequency as a function of contrast

Although these results were something of a blow to the hypothesis outlined above, the story took on a new turn with the next experiment: even sinusoidal gratings look finer at low contrast. This result cannot be explained by any of the ideas discussed so far, but along with the bar results it implies an underlying process of some generality. The experiment was similar to that described above, except that the single test and comparison lines were replaced by sinusoidal gratings. To minimize adaptation, the patterns were presented for only 0.5 s every 3.5 s. The subject made the spatial frequency-matching adjustment over a number of presentations until he was satisfied with the match. The results for four subjects are shown in figure 3 for four different spatial frequencies of test grating. Different frequencies were obtained by varying the viewing distance – a procedure deliberately chosen because it kept the number of cycles constant, but varied the target area in a way suitable for each spatial frequency being tested.

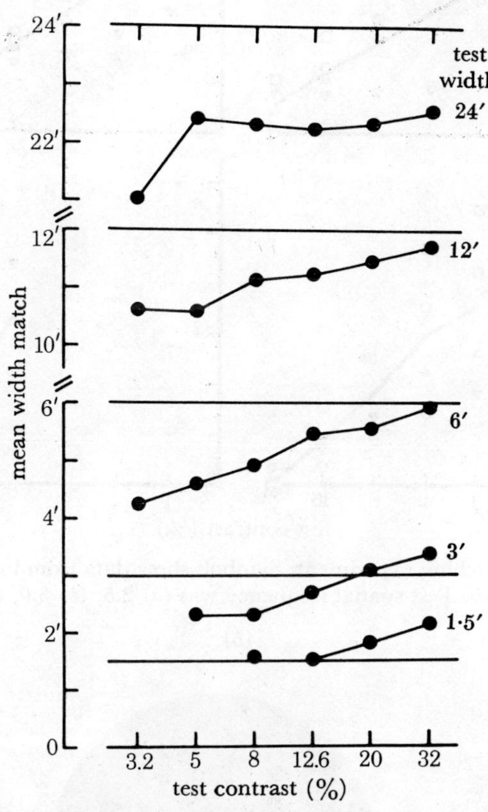

FIGURE 2. Mean results from five subjects who adjusted the width of a comparison bar to match the width of a test bar whose contrast and width are indicated in the figure. Both bars were light increments presented for 1 s every 3 s on a steady luminous background. The bars were vertical and each was $\frac{1}{2}°$ from the fixation point.

The result is surprising but unambiguous: for all subjects and all spatial frequencies, apparent frequency increased linearly as the logarithm of the contrast decreased. The mean shift was very large (30–40 %) at low contrasts, but it is clear from figure 3 that the phenomenon occurs progressively over the whole range of contrasts used, and is not something that arises only when the target is nearly invisible.

The slope of the curves may be steeper for the high frequencies, but unfortunately only two or three contrast levels were visible at 20 cycles/deg, so that any increase in slope must be taken as a tentative result.

It is remarkable that, when the effect is large, not only do the bars seem thinner and more closely packed, but there also appear to be more of them. The difference in appearance between low and high contrast gratings is illustrated in figure 4.

The message to be drawn, I suppose, is that before the frequency-based theory can be tested on bars or other objects with complex spectra, one must know how their individual components would behave. Before attempting an explanation let us consider a few more cases.

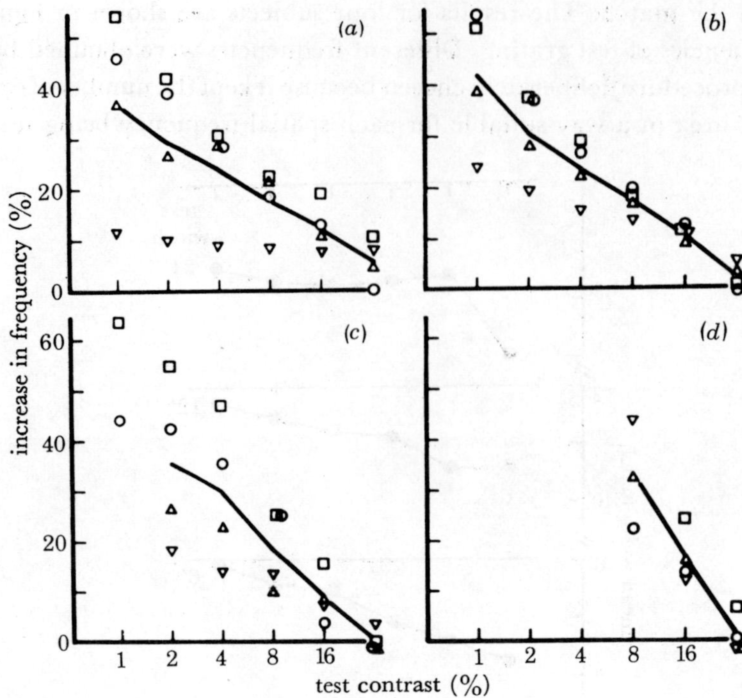

FIGURE 3. Spatial frequency matching experiment. Symbols show data from individual subjects, while solid lines indicate group mean values. Test spatial frequency was (a) 2.5, (b) 5.0, (c) 10.0, (d) 20.0 cycles/deg.

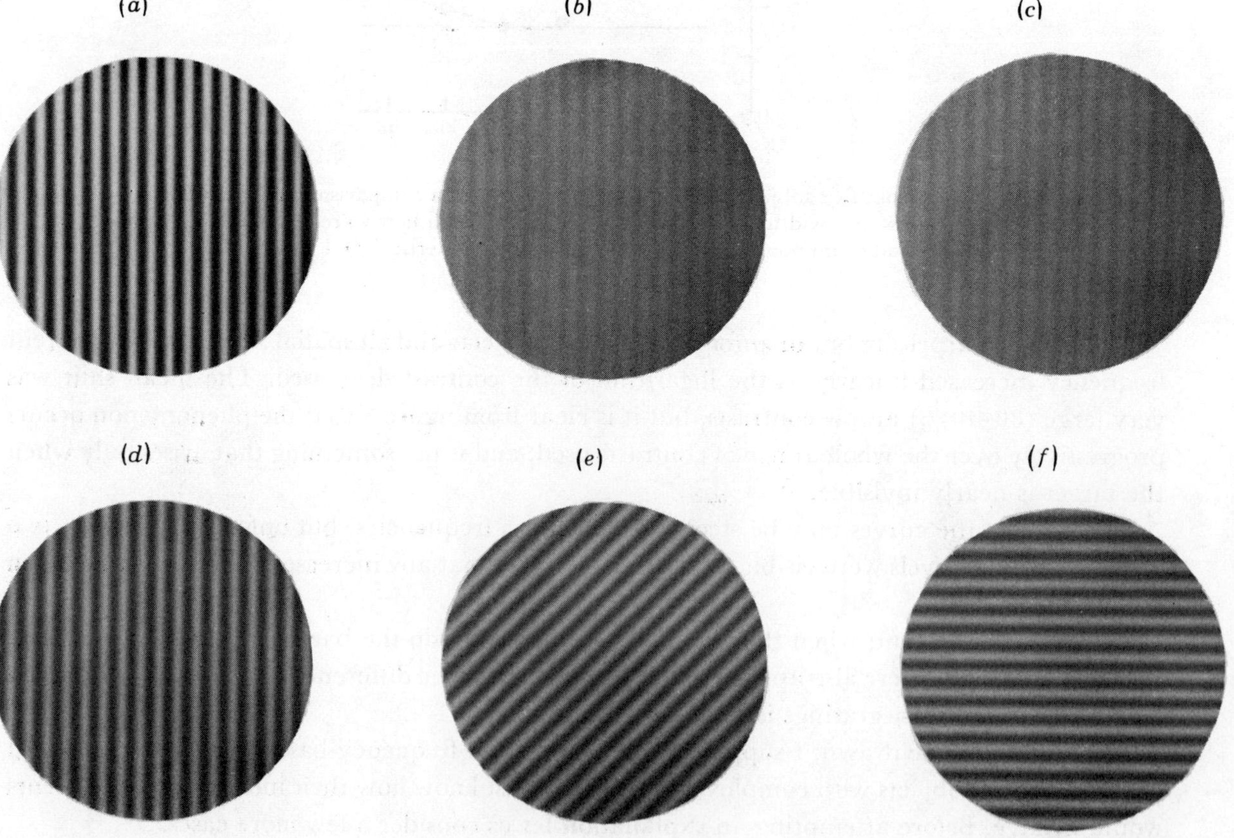

FIGURE 4. Sinusoidal gratings allow the reader to verify for himself the effects reported. All six gratings have the same spatial frequency. Comparison of (a) with (b) should reveal that at low contrast, gratings appear finer than at high. The effect may be enhanced by viewing from several metres away, and by fixating midway between (a) and (b). Alternate fixation of (b) and (c) demonstrates that a peripheral target appears finer than a foveal one. Alternate fixation of (a) and (b) illustrates the interaction between contrast and eccentricity (see text). (d), (e) and (f) demonstrate the effects of orientation. Most observers should see (e) as finer than (d) or (f). Viewing from a distance should again enhance the perceived differences.

(d) *Spatial frequency and retinal eccentricity*

William James (1890, p. 140) noted that objects viewed peripherally looked smaller than those viewed foveally (see also Newsome 1972). It turns out that the apparent spatial frequency of gratings behaves in a similar fashion. Figure 5 illustrates a frequency-matching experiment similar to that of figure 3, except that there were three conditions of fixation. When the observer

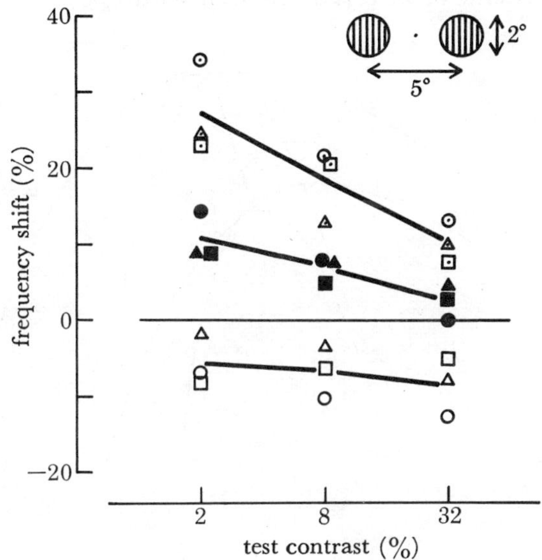

FIGURE 5. Spatial frequency matching as a function of contrast and eccentricity. Symbols show data from three individual subjects; solid lines join group means. Test spatial frequency, 5 cycles/deg. For details see text.

fixated midway between the gratings (solid symbols), apparent frequency increased at low contrast, although with the subjects used the effect was smaller than in figure 3. When fixation was on the right-hand (comparison) grating (open symbols with dot), the test grating, now seen 5° peripherally, seemed to be of an even higher frequency by an extra 10–20%. Correspondingly, a peripheral comparison grating had a higher apparent frequency than a foveal test grating, and so had to be set to a lower frequency for apparent equality (open symbols). Interestingly, the interaction between contrast and fixation position was highly significant: the effect of contrast on apparent frequency was much greater peripherally than foveally. This may explain why the powerful effect of contrast has not previously been reported. Most visual experiments are conducted with foveal viewing, where the influence of contrast is least.

3. EXPLANATORY SCHEME FOR THESE EFFECTS

(a) *Functional similarity in effects of luminance and contrast*

Reduction of mean luminance is a third manipulation that produces an increase of apparent fineness, akin to that produced by reduction of contrast or increase in eccentricity. William James (1890, p. 142) remarked on this phenomenon too, and Virsu (1974) verified it experimentally for gratings and single targets such as letters or spots. Virsu's explanation was that at lower luminances the optimal stimulus size for a receptive field increases, or, equivalently, that the optimal spatial frequency is lower (figure 6). This latter result has recently been established for cat cortical cells by Bisti *et al.* (1977). Virsu's explanation may sound paradoxical, for at low luminance spatial frequencies seem higher, not lower. However, if the significance of a cell's output – its size 'label' – remains unchanged even though its response properties have shifted, then the perceptual result follows. To put it simply, imagine a cell tuned to 5 cycles/deg in bright conditions. If its optimum frequency shifts to 4 cycles/deg in dim conditions, while its label remains at 5, then of course a 4 cycles/deg input is reported as 5 cycles/deg, i.e. higher than it should be. Virsu (1974) found the shift to be greater at high spatial frequencies than low, and the physiological results of Bisti *et al.* fit well with this.

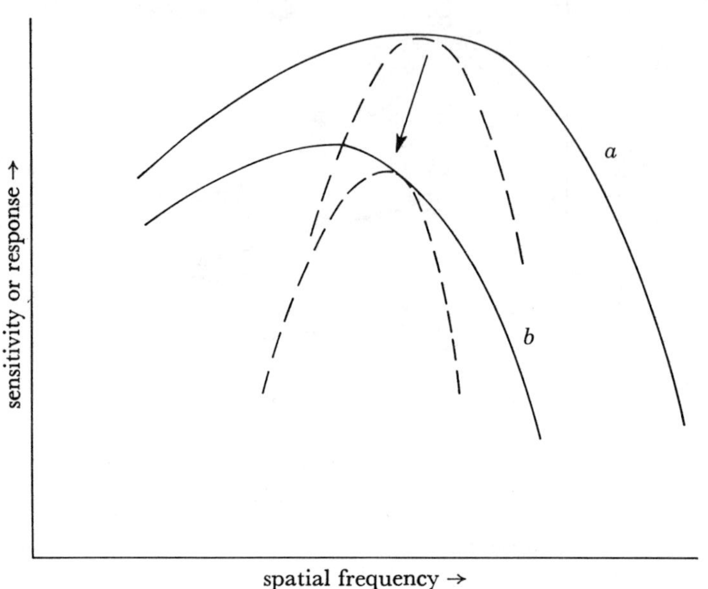

FIGURE 6. Solid curves show schematically the visual system's overall sensitivity in two conditions, (*a*) and (*b*). Broken curves represent the hypothetical shift in spatial frequency tuning of a single channel. Condition (*a*) could be: foveal viewing, high mean luminance, high contrast, vertical orientation or sustained presentation. Condition (*b*) would correspondingly be: peripheral viewing, low luminance, low contrast, oblique orientation or brief presentation.

Therefore I suggest a similar explanation for the effect of contrast, namely that the optimal spatial frequency for cortical cells increases steadily with contrast, while the spatial significance of their outputs is invariant. This is a serious matter, for it implies that the response characteristic of individual channels is nonlinear over the whole contrast range, and this conclusion makes the modelling of visual responses much more intractable, but I have so far been unable to come up with a viable alternative. One might opt, for example, for a threshold nonlinearity where, as contrast decreased, the number of active units would also decrease. However, since high spatial frequency channels are less sensitive than low ones, we would have to expect high frequency units to fall below threshold sooner, just as the higher harmonics of a square-wave grating become invisible at low contrast while the fundamental is still visible (Campbell & Robson 1968). In that case the distribution of responses should shift to lower frequency channels and patterns should look coarser at low contrasts, which is just the opposite of the truth.

Physiologically, the question of response tuning as a function of contrast has not been directly investigated, but in a sample of cat cortical cells Movshon *et al.* (1978) found that the few cells tuned to high spatial frequencies did exhibit an upward shift in their optimum frequency when the contrast was high. This result is consistent with the explanation offered above.

(b) A general rule

To add to the growing list of variables, it has also been found (Tynan & Sekuler 1974; Kulikowski 1975) that gratings look finer with brief presentations (e.g. 20 ms) than with longer ones (e.g. 200 ms). It therefore appears that from this whole set of results we can infer a very general rule: *when retinal spatial frequency is held constant, any other manipulation that takes the stimulus closer to threshold also increases its apparent spatial frequency.*

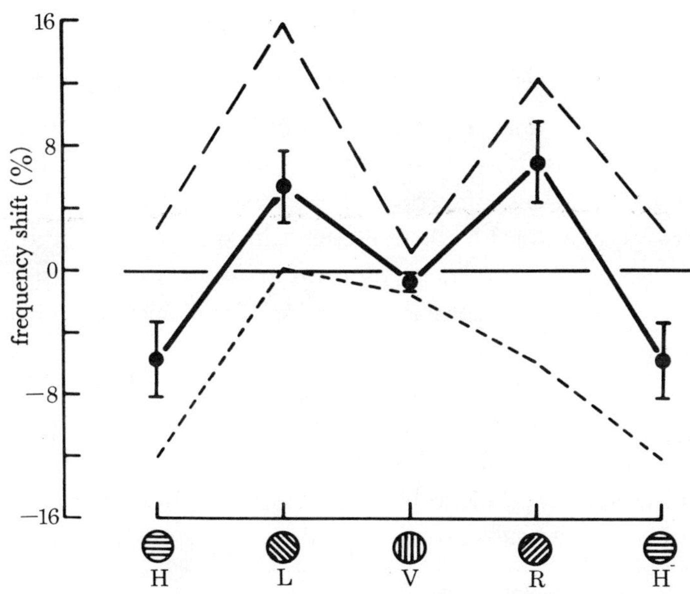

FIGURE 7. Spatial frequency matching as a function of test orientation. Test frequency, 16 cycles/deg; contrast, 12 %; foveal successive viewing of test and comparison gratings for 0.5 s each, with 0.5 s delay. Solid symbols and lines show means (± 1 s.e.) of six subjects. Broken lines illustrate two subjects; see text.

(c) Effects of grating orientation

In normal observers, sensitivity for high-frequency oblique gratings is lower than for horizontal (H) or vertical (V) ones (Campbell *et al.* 1966). From the rule given above, we can predict that obliques should also look finer than H or V. Figure 7 shows the results from an experimental test of this prediction.

Subjects adjusted the spatial frequency of a vertical grating to appear to match that of a test grating presented at any one of four orientations: H, V, left oblique or right oblique. Solid symbols show the mean results from six subjects. Oblique gratings did indeed look finer than V, but unexpectedly H was apparently coarser than V on average. The mean results, however, cannot be taken at face value, since we are dealing with a heterogeneous group of subjects. Data from individual subjects are illustrated by the two extreme cases (figure 7, broken lines). A subject with normal vision (upper curve) shows no H–V asymmetry, but a powerful oblique effect as predicted. At the other extreme, an optically corrected, astigmatic subject (the author) shows just the reverse. Fortunately this result supports the rule rather than contradicting it, for this subject is less sensitive to V than to H (Georgeson & Sullivan 1975, figure 9) and for him V looks finer than H as expected from the rule. A closer investigation of these relations is in progress.

One could imagine that the results described here on the effects of luminance, tilt, eccentricity and duration were all consequences of lowered apparent contrast, showing itself in different guises. This is, however, most unlikely because Georgeson & Sullivan (1975) found that, despite their lesser sensitivity, dim, oblique or eccentric gratings did not normally appear to have lower contrast. Instead 'contrast constancy' prevailed. The frequency shifts are therefore associated with changes in sensitivity rather than apparent contrast. In the case of brief presentations, however, apparent contrast may well play an important role, since it is known that apparent contrast decreases at short durations (Kitterle & Corwin 1979).

4. Conclusions

(a) *Mismatch between the tuning of channels and their perceptual signs*

In summary, my hypothesis is this: in conditions where the visual system as a whole suffers an attenuation of contrast sensitivity (which in fact occurs particularly at high spatial frequencies), the individual channels undergo a corresponding transformation (figure 6) which mimics that of the overall system, and leads to changes in apparent size and spatial frequency. The perceptual changes occur because each channel carries an invariant perceptual 'sign' or meaning that does not alter when the spatial selectivity of the channel shifts. If the hypothesis is correct, it becomes interesting to ask why the system is unable to compensate for these changes. Why does 'spatial frequency constancy' not exist in conditions where contrast constancy does? It is tempting to suppose that the process underlying the frequency shifts is closely related to that of contrast constancy, for in peripheral vision and at higher spatial frequencies compensation for loss of sensitivity needs to be more powerful, and it is in these conditions that the influence of contrast on perceived spatial frequency is greatest (figures 3 and 5).

(b) *Retinal coordinates: constructed or projected?*

The phenomena discussed in this paper are inconsistent with the 'neural image' concept implied by the convolution profiles of figure 1. For even if the channel tuning did vary in the way proposed (figure 6), the periodicity in the response profile would not alter (compare the bottom two traces in figure 1c). A strong conclusion would be that such a neural image does not exist at all. On the other hand, if it does exist, it is unlikely that spatial relations are represented metrically in it. If a coordinate map is used as an early visual representation, then it might be constructed from the locally encoded picture fragments rather than transmitted intact from the retina. It would be rather like putting together a jigsaw by finding out what is on each piece, and which pieces match up, rather than by knowing *a priori* where each piece should go. In addition, we know that the retinotopic mapping in the cortex does not hold locally, for within the Hubel & Wiesel (1974) hypercolumn there is a random scatter of r.f. locations over a limited region of retina. Of course, neurons could be jumbled anatomically while being well ordered functionally, but in view of the psychophysical evidence I prefer the conjecture that the retinotopic mapping presents at best a rough indication of location and that the detailed construction of visual space is carried out by quite different coding principles.

References (Georgeson)

Bisti, S., Clement, R., Maffei, L. & Mecacci, L. 1977 Spatial frequency and orientation tuning curves of visual neurones in the cat: effects of mean luminance. *Expl Brain Res.* **27**, 335–345.

Blakemore, C. & Sutton, P. 1969 Size adaptation: a new after-effect. *Science, N.Y.* **166**, 245–247.

Boring, E. G. 1942 *Sensation and perception in the history of experimental psychology.* New York: Appleton Century Crofts.

Campbell, F. W., Kulikowski, J. J. & Levinson, J. Z. 1966 The effect of orientation on the visual resolution of gratings. *J. Physiol., Lond.* **187**, 427–436.

Campbell, F. W. & Robson, J. G. 1968 Application of Fourier analysis to the visibility of gratings. *J. Physiol., Lond.* **197**, 551–566.

Georgeson, M. A. & Sullivan, G. D. 1975 Contrast constancy: deblurring in human vision by spatial frequency channels. *J. Physiol., Lond.* **252**, 627–656.

Heeley, D. W. 1979 A perceived spatial frequency shift at orientations orthogonal to adapting gratings. *Vision Res.* **19**, 1229–1236.

Hubel, D. H. & Wiesel, T. N. 1974 Sequence regularity and geometry of orientation columns in the monkey striate cortex. *J. comp. Neurol.* **158**, 267–294.

James, W. 1890 *The principles of psychology,* vol. 2, reprinted 1950. New York: Dover.

Kitterle, F. L. & Corwin, T. R. 1979 Enhancement of apparent contrast in flashed sinusoidal gratings. *Vision Res.* **19**, 33–39.

Kulikowski, J. J. 1975 Apparent fineness of briefly presented gratings: balance between movement and pattern channels. *Vision Res.* **15**, 673–680.

Macleod, I. D. G. & Rosenfeld, A. 1974 The visibility of gratings: spatial frequency channels or bar-detecting units? *Vision Res.* **14**, 909–915.

Marr, D. 1976 Early processing of visual information. *Phil. Trans. R. Soc. Lond.* B **275**, 483–519.

Movshon, J. A., Thompson, I. D. & Tolhurst, D. J. 1978 Spatial and temporal contrast sensitivity of neurones in areas 17 and 18 of the cat's visual cortex. *J. Physiol., Lond.* **283**, 101–120.

Newsome, L. R 1972 Visual angle and apparent size of objects in peripheral vision. *Percept. Psychophys.* **12**, 300–304.

Rentschler, I., Hilz, R. & Grimm, W. 1975 Processing of positional information in the human visual system. *Nature, Lond.* **253**, 444–445.

Tynan, P. & Sekuler, R. 1974 Perceived spatial frequency varies with stimulus duration. *J. opt. Soc. Am.* **64**, 1251–1255.

Virsu, V. 1974 Dark adaptation shifts apparent spatial frequency. *Vision Res.* **14**, 433–435.

Discussion

K. H. Ruddock (*Biophysics Section, Physics Department, Imperial College, London SW7 2BZ, U.K.*).

1. Both Dr Campbell and Dr Georgeson cite the 'frequency shift effect', observed with linear gratings, as evidence for spatial frequency analysis by the human visual system, but there are at least two published studies (de Valois 1977; Burton *et al.* 1977) that show that adaptation effects involving the light bars of the gratings are independent of the dark bar width, and vice versa. Such independence appears to be directly contrary to the concept of spatial frequency analysis by the visual system.

2. In his experiments Dr Georgeson has measured the apparent bar widths of linear, sine-wave gratings presented at different contrast and mean illumination levels. His discussion implied that the spatial characteristics of the gratings are defined entirely by the light distribution in the retinal images. Yet, even if scattered light effects can be neglected, any nonlinearity involved in signal transmission along the visual pathways will distort the sine-wave grating profile causing the apparent bar width to depend on grating contrast and mean illumination level (Maudarbocus & Ruddock 1973).

References

Burton, G. J., Naghshineh, S. & Ruddock, K. H. 1977 Processing by the human visual system of the light and dark contrast components of the retinal image. *Biol. Cybernet.* **27**, 189–197.

de Valois, K. K. 1977 Independence of black and white: phase specific adaptation. *Vision Res.* **17**, 209–215.

Maudarbocus, A. Y. & Ruddock, K. H. 1973 Non-linearity or visual signals in relation to shape-sensitive adaptation responses. *Vision Res.* **13**, 1713–1737.

M. A. GEORGESON.

1. As I emphasized in my talk, there are two distinct issues: (*a*) what are the response properties of units in the visual system, and (*b*) what perceptual message do they convey? With respect to (*a*), the work cited supports earlier conceptions of the multiple-channel model, with additional emphasis on the subpopulations of on- and off-centre neurons. I see no contradiction here. On the other hand, if Dr Ruddock is saying that the evidence supports the idea that local width, and *not* spatial periodicity, is the message conveyed by the system, then I agree that this is an important contribution to the literature, and I am glad that he has brought his paper to my attention. Previous work could be interpreted in either way. It should be remembered, though, that after adaptation to gratings, threshold elevation is selective for test spatial frequency but not for the width of single test bars (Sullivan *et al.* 1972). Again, this is not a contradiction, but is to be understood in terms of the low sensitivity of high frequency channels (or, if you insist, small r.fs!).

2. In my experiments, subjects adjusted the *spatial frequency* (s.f.) of a comparison grating. It is not obvious to me that apparent variations in the *duty cycle* of the test grating, however caused, would lead the subject to alter his s.f. setting, nor why he should choose to increase the frequency (to match, say, light bar width) rather than decrease it (to match, in this case, dark bar width). Subjects report, and my impression is, that overall differences in texture density are observed. Moreover at 20 cycles/deg, any variation in duty cycle caused by harmonic distortion must surely be negligible, since the harmonics that define it (40 cycles/deg or more) would be invisible, especially at the low contrasts used (not more than 32%). Yet at 20 cycles/deg the effect of contrast on apparent s.f. is very powerful (figure 3). Harmonic distortion therefore cannot be the explanation. Bar-width encoding remains viable, however, provided that shifts in all the local width signals are integrated to produce a perceptually finer texture.

Reference

Sullivan, G. D., Georgeson, M. A. & Oatley, K. 1972 *Vision Res.* **12**, 383–393.

Phil. Trans. R. Soc. Lond. B **290**, 23–37 (1980)

Printed in Great Britain

Perceptual signs of parallel pathways

By P. Lennie

Centre for Research in Perception and Cognition, Laboratory of Experimental Psychology,
University of Sussex, Brighton BN1 9QG, U.K.

Previous physiological work has shown that the X and Y cells found in the visual pathways of cats and monkeys have properties that might explain the perceptual distinction between 'sustained' and 'transient' mechanisms. However, when the sensitivities of X and Y cells are measured under conditions comparable with those used in psychophysical experiments, one finds that the properties thought to be relevant to the perceptual dichotomy do not in fact distinguish the two types of cell.

One of the most important psychophysical grounds for distinguishing 'sustained' from 'transient' mechanisms is that there appear to be two distinct thresholds for detecting grating patterns, depending upon whether the observer is asked to detect the spatial or the temporal properties of the stimulus. However, if thresholds are measured under conditions where the observer's criterion is tightly controlled, the two thresholds converge.

These experiments question the existence of qualitatively distinct 'sustained' and 'transient' mechanisms.

Introduction

One of the most influential recent ideas in visual psychophysics is that qualitatively different mechanisms underlie the detection of grating patterns of low and high spatial frequency, and that these mechanisms have different temporal properties: the mechanisms sensitive to low spatial frequencies have a fast and 'transient' response, while those sensitive to higher spatial frequencies have a slower, more 'sustained' response (Tolhurst 1973; Kulikowski & Tolhurst 1973). It has also been suggested that the 'transient' pathway might be specialized to convey information about movement, while the 'sustained' pathway conveys information about form (Tolhurst 1973, 1975).

The distinction between two classes of mechanism has drawn considerable support from recent phsyiological work, which shows that in the principal pathway from the retina to the cortex there exist populations of neurons that are physiologically quite distinct. Two of the cell types discerned in the cat, the X and the Y cells (Enroth-Cugell & Robson 1966; Cleland *et al.* 1971), which probably have counterparts in the macaque monkey (De Monasterio 1978), possess properties that have made them popular substrates of the 'sustained' and 'transient' mechanisms distinguished psychophysically. However, few of the physiological results are of a type that permit comparison with psychophysics.

In the first part of this paper I take for granted the psychophysical distinction, and examine the differences between X and Y cells that are thought to be relevant to it; I shall show that, when stimulated under conditions comparable with those used in psychophysical experiments, several properties thought to underlie their distinctive perceptual roles do not reliably distinguish the two types of cell. In the second part of the paper I examine some of the psychophysical evidence for distinct 'sustained' and 'transient' mechanisms. I shall describe the results of two experiments that I think weaken the psychophysical basis of the distinction.

Physiological substrates of 'sustained' and 'transient' mechanisms

Psychophysical experiments that bear upon the distinction between 'sustained' and 'transient' mechanisms have been reviewed by Breitmeyer & Ganz (1976), MacLeod (1978), Legge (1978) and Graham (1979). Here I shall deal only with those findings that have been thought to reflect a physiological distinction between X and Y cells. The relevant psychophysical observations fall broadly into two groups: (1) those that show a pronounced loss of sensitivity to gratings of low spatial frequency when their temporal frequency is low, and (2) those that suggest faster transmission of information by mechanisms sensitive to gratings of low spatial frequency.

These observations are consistent with the idea that the perception of high spatial frequencies depends upon X cells, which are thought to have slow responses and good sensitivity to low temporal frequencies, while the perception of low spatial frequencies, especially at higher temporal frequencies, depends upon Y cells, which are thought to have fast responses and poor sensitivity to low temporal frequencies. The following experiments examine these suggestions.

Methods

The general techniques were conventional. Adult cats were anaesthetized initially with an injection of Vetalar (ketamine hydrochloride, 20–25 mg kg^{-1}, intramuscular) and preparatory surgery was carried out under Saffan anaesthesia (alphaxalone and alphadolone acetate, intravenous). A loading dose of urethane (300 mg kg^{-1}) was given, and during the experiment further urethane (20 mg kg^{-1} h^{-1}) was given in a saline mixture containing dextrose and Flaxedil (gallamine triethiodide, 10 mg kg^{-1} h^{-1}) to immobilize the eyes. The cervical sympathetic trunks were cut and a small hole was made in the skull above the optic tract.

The pupils were dilated with atropine sulphate and the corneae were protected with transparent contact lenses. An artificial pupil (diameter 2 mm) was placed immediately in front of each eye, behind such supplementary lenses as were necessary to bring stimuli into focus on the retina. Action potentials, recorded by glass-coated tungsten microelectrodes placed stereotaxically in the optic tract, were counted by a computer.

Visual stimuli

Sinusoidal gratings patterns were generated by standard techniques (Campbell & Green 1965) on the screen of an oscilloscope that had a P31 phosphor. The computer generated a waveform to modulate the luminance of the screen, and also triggered each frame of the display. The phase of the modulating waveform, relative to the trigger pulse, could be varied as required, thus allowing the production of stationary grating patterns in any spatial phase, or of patterns that moved steadily across the screen. The contrast of the grating was controlled by multiplying the modulating voltage by a second signal from the computer, the product being fed to the Z-axis of the oscilloscope. In most experiments the screen subtended $16 \times 19°$ and, when no modulating signal was applied, was uniformly illuminated at 225 cd m^{-2}; in some early experiments the illumination was 45 cd m^{-2}.

Identification of X and Y cells

Two tests were used to establish the cell type unequivocally. In the first, grating patterns moved steadily across the receptive field. If the spatial frequency of the patterns was less than about

0.7 cycles/deg all cells gave modulated responses to the passage of bars across the receptive field, but if the spatial frequency was higher, the modulated responses of Y cells gave way to a steady discharge more rapid than that occurring in the presence of the uniformly illuminated screen (Enroth-Cugell & Robson 1966; Hochstein & Shapley 1976a). In the second test, stationary sinusoidal gratings of spatial frequency higher than that to which the cell was most sensitive were modulated by a temporal sinusoid to produce a standing wave. These stimuli were presented at different positions on the receptive field, and responses averaged for each position. One can find for X-cells a position of the pattern where temporal modulation elicits no response from the cell, but such a 'null' position cannot be found for Y cells (Hochstein & Shapley 1976a; Enroth-Cugell & Robson 1966). By the application of these tests all fibres studied in the optic tract were readily classified as X or Y type.

Sensitivity to temporal frequency

It is well established that the shape of the curve relating human contrast sensitivity to spatial frequency depends upon the temporal frequency; when patterns are moved or flickered rapidly, sensitivity to gratings of low spatial frequency improves. Sensitivity to gratings of intermediate and higher spatial frequencies is rarely improved by increasing temporal frequency (Robson 1966; Kelly 1977). This is consistent with the notion (Tolhurst 1973) that the mechanisms subserving the detection of low spatial frequencies are less sensitive to low temporal frequencies (i.e. they give more transient responses) than those sensitive to higher spatial frequencies. The 'transient' properties of such mechanisms relate only to their insensitivity to low temporal frequencies. A transient mechanism need not (although it has often been supposed to) have high sensitivity to high temporal frequencies.

X cells have smaller receptive fields than do Y cells and in general are more sensitive to high spatial frequencies (Enroth-Cugell & Robson 1966; Cleland et al. 1971). These properties suggest a possible connection between X cells and the 'sustained' mechanism and Y cells and the 'transient' one. However, to establish this link satisfactorily, we have to show that X cells are less sensitive than Y cells to low spatial frequencies (especially at higher temporal frequencies).

Figure 1 shows measurements of contrast sensitivity to moving gratings, made individually on nine X cells and eleven Y cells. Each curve shows the reciprocal of the contrast required for a discernible modulation of response plotted against the spatial frequency of the grating. Since within each of the two classes of cell there is no great scatter of curves on the abscissa (all receptive fields lay between 5° and 15° from the area centralis), it is convenient for our present purposes to consider the summary graph, which shows the sensitivities of X and Y cells averaged separately. It is clear that, for gratings moving at 2.6 Hz (close to the optimum rate for all units studied) the X cells are most sensitive to spatial frequencies of near 0.4 cycle/deg, while for Y cells the best spatial frequency is below 0.2 cycle/deg. Sensitivities of X and Y cells are strikingly different for spatial frequencies near 1 cycle/deg: the distributions do not overlap. At low spatial frequencies, however, Y cells are not significantly more sensitive than X cells, which causes one to ask whether the shapes of the curves depend upon temporal frequency, and whether Y cells were penalized by low temporal frequencies of stimulation.

I have made some measurements of spatial contrast sensitivity at different temporal frequencies, from which it appears that, except at the very highest temporal frequencies, the principal effect in both X and Y cells is to scale the contrast sensitivity equally for all spatial frequencies.

The question of whether Y cells are relatively less sensitive than X cells to stimulation at low temporal frequencies can therefore be answered by measuring contrast sensitivity for gratings of optimal spatial frequency at different temporal frequencies, and thus producing a graph relating contrast sensitivity to temporal frequency. Measurements of this kind made on seven X cells and eight Y cells are shown in figure 2. As in figure 1, the ordinate is the reciprocal of the contrast required for a threshold modulation of response. However, in this case the thresholds were calculated by computer because the experimenter could not guarantee a stable criterion for

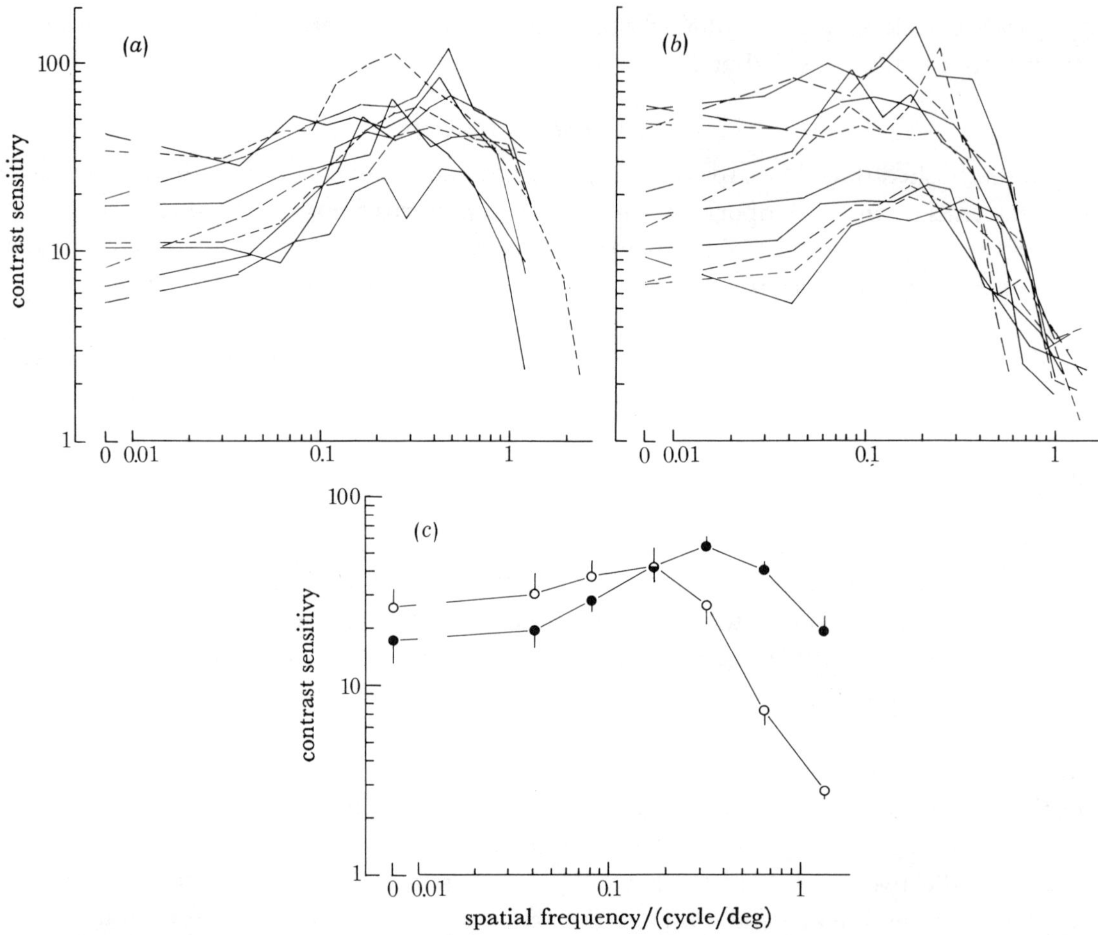

FIGURE 1. Spatial contrast sensitivities of X and Y cells, for gratings moving at 2.6 Hz. In all cases sensitivity was the reciprocal of the contrast required for the experimenter to hear a modulation of response. (*a*) Individual curves for X cells. (*b*) Curves for Y cells. (*c*) Curves averaged separately for X cells (●) and Y cells (○). Vertical bars mark 1 s.e. of the mean.

threshold at different temporal frequencies. The computer first analysed samples of the spontaneous discharge in the presence of the uniformly illuminated screen, to find the distribution of amplitudes of the Fourier components at the temporal frequencies used in the experiment. Then it set, for each frequency of interest, a criterion amplitude that had to be reached for a response to be detected reliably. Where this method of estimating threshold has been compared with the subjective method, it has given similar results.

The individual curves for X and Y cells (figure 2*a*, *b*), which are quite similar, are averaged separately in figure 2*c*. Plainly, the temporal contrast sensitivities of X and Y cells are indistinguishable at all but the highest temporal frequencies, where Y cells have a slight advantage.

The observations in figure 2 might be thought odd in view of the evidence (Cleland *et al.* 1971, 1973) that Y cells can be distinguished from X cells by their more transient responses,

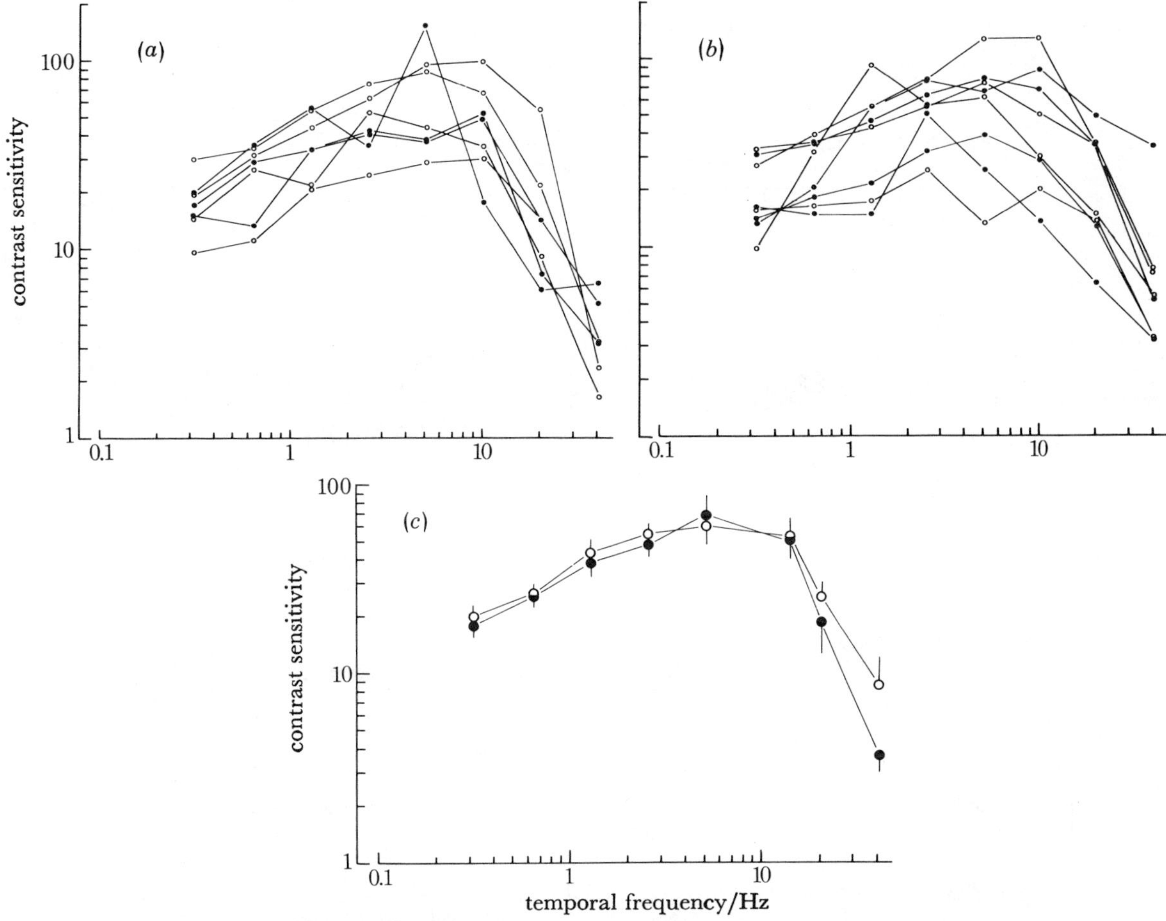

FIGURE 2. Temporal contrast sensitivities of X cells (*a*) and Y cells (*b*) for moving gratings of optimal spatial frequency. Open and closed symbols are used only for clarity. (*c*) Curves averaged separately for X cells (●) and Y cells (○).

which suggest poorer sensitivity to low temporal frequencies. Two factors probably account for the discrepancies. The observations that most clearly show Y cells to give more transient responses have generally used strong incremental (or decremental) spots of optimal size, and the time-scale of response has been of seconds. If one is interested in responses likely to be relevant to psychophysical thresholds, one should probably consider responses that are just strong enough to cause a reliable perturbation of the maintained discharge measured over a period of 1 s or less. Some such responses obtained from five X cells and five Y cells are shown in figure 3.

In each case the stimulus was an optimally positioned grating of optimal spatial frequency, which was switched on for one second then off again; its contrast just exceeded that required to elicit a threshold response on 50 % of stimulus presentations. The post-stimulus time histograms obtained from X cells (left) and Y cells (right) are quite different, but the difference lies principally in the rate of the underlying spontaneous discharge (very much higher in X cells) and not in the form of the response to the stimulus (the extra impulses above the spontaneous rate). The cell giving the most transient response is a Y cell and that giving the most sustained response is an X cell, but it would be hard to classify cells reliably by the 'transientness' of their responses to the threshold stimuli used here. Hochstein & Shapley (1976a) have also drawn attention to some difficulties associated with this index.

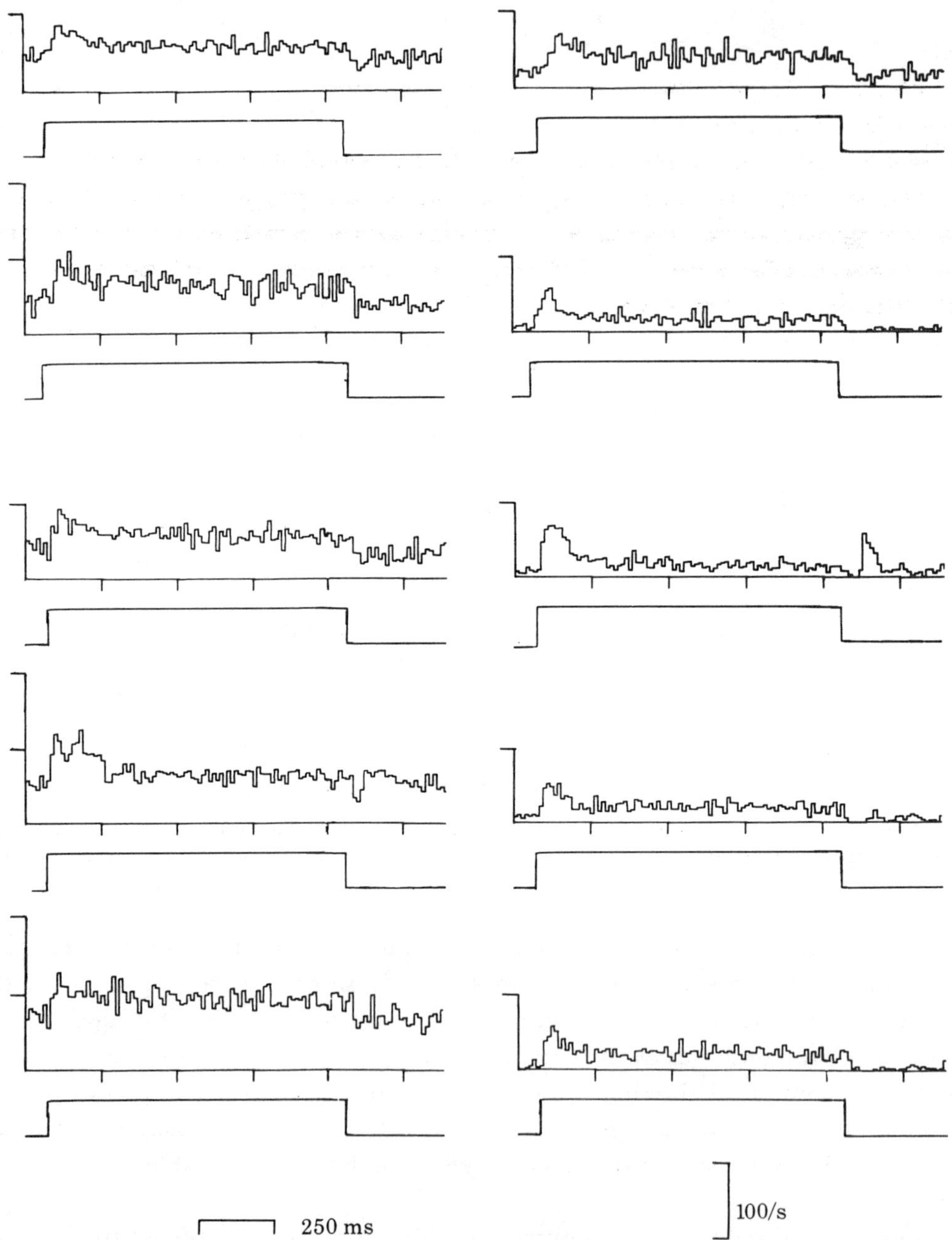

FIGURE 3. Averaged responses to 30 presentations for 1 s of gratings of optimal spatial frequency placed in even symmetry about the centre of the receptive field. Contrast was set to give a just suprathreshold response. Left, X cells, right, Y cells. Bin width, 10 ms.

The more transient responses of Y cells to strong stimuli are probably due to the action of the 'subunits' that exist within and beyond the classical receptive field (Hochstein & Shapley 1976b). These mechanisms generate rectified responses (i.e. they increase the discharge of a cell at both onset and offset of a stimulus), are relatively insensitive to low temporal frequencies and are probably densely distributed throughout the receptive field and beyond it. Although the manner in which subunits bring about more transient responses in Y cells is complex (Shapley & Victor 1978), they seem to be relatively much more effective when stimulated by gratings of high contrast.

Other factors explain why, despite the insensitivity of subunits to low temporal frequencies, the temporal contrast sensitivity curves of X and Y cells are so similar when measured by using continuously moving gratings (figure 2): a moving grating of spatial frequency optimal for the classical receptive field is not a particularly effective stimulus for subunits (its spatial frequency is too low). Moreover, it excites different subunits at different times, so the population of them contributes an unmodulated component to the discharges of Y cells.

It might be argued that, since subunits endow Y cells with the temporal properties that can distinguish them from X cells, the temporal properties of subunits are of greatest interest in drawing parallels with psychophysics. I think that this is wrong, because the spatial frequency for which a Y cell has the highest contrast sensitivity (and presumably therefore the greatest chance of contributing to vision) reflects the properties of the classical receptive field and is generally too low to be an effective stimulus for subunits.

These results suggest that unless signals from X and Y cells in the retina are subjected to different temporal filtering at higher stages in the visual pathway, they cannot provide the properties required of the presumed 'sustained' and 'transient' mechanisms, respectively.

Latency of response

The simple reaction time to the onset of a grating pattern is appreciably shorter when the gratings are of low spatial frequency than when the frequency is high, implying that mechanisms sensitive to low spatial frequencies transmit information faster (Breitmeyer 1975; Vassilev & Mitov 1976; Lupp *et al.* 1976). Other psychophysical results concerning backward masking (Breitmeyer & Ganz 1976; Rogowitz 1978) and saccadic suppression (Matin 1974) have also been interpreted in terms of the activity of a fast-responding mechanism sensitive to low spatial frequencies and a slower-responding mechanism sensitive to higher spatial frequencies. These ideas are consistent with the notion that X and Y cells respectively are the mechanisms sensitive to high and low spatial frequencies, for it is well established (Cleland *et al.* 1971) that the axons of Y cells conduct impulses faster than do those of X cells. Thus, other things being equal, one would expect impulses originating in Y ganglion cells to reach the lateral geniculate nucleus (l.g.n.) and cortex sooner.

However, the important functional latency is not conduction time, but the latency of a response to light. Since the bulk of the visual latency arises in the retina distal to the ganglion cells, differences between the conduction speeds of X and Y cells could be trivial. Ikeda & Wright (1972) found X cells to have the shorter visual latencies when stimulated by spots, but in their experiments X cells were probably more strongly stimulated.

J. B. Troy and I have made some measurements of the latencies of responses of X and Y cells to the abrupt onset of a grating pattern of optimal spatial frequency and spatial phase, and of contrast that produced small responses of peak amplitude about 50 impulses/s above the spontaneous discharge: a little stronger than would be required for threshold.

Latency was measured by the method shown in the inset to figure 4. One starts by counting, from some arbitrary time, the number of impulses discharged spontaneously in the presence of the uniformly illuminated screen; a cumulative count of impulses discharged is then plotted against time from the start of the counting period. The averaged counts are shown by filled circles and the slope of the straight line drawn through them gives the rate of the maintained

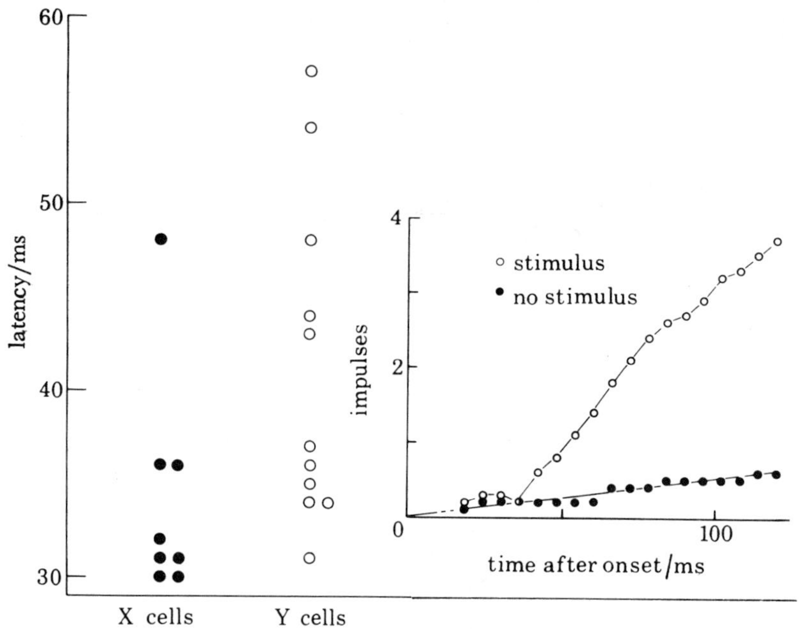

FIGURE 4. Latencies of just suprathreshold responses to the onset of gratings, measured by the method illustrated in the inset and described in the text. Counts were accumulated in 5 ms intervals. The latencies of X cells (average 34.2 ms) were significantly shorter than those of Y cells (average 41.2 ms).

discharge. If a stimulus is now presented and impulses are counted from the moment of its delivery, we find, as we should expect, that initially the stimulus has no effect upon the discharge and the cumulative counts follow the line for the spontaneous discharge. However, at some point there is an abrupt change of slope, indicating a change in discharge rate. The point of divergence of the two lines, usually sharply defined, marks the onset of response, and this we take as the latency. This measurement was made on eight X cells and eleven Y cells, with the result shown in figure 4. X cells have shorter latencies on average. Bearing in mind that these latencies were measured at a point in the optic tract just anterior to the l.g.n., by which time Y cells have a conduction advantage of perhaps 3 ms, it is unlikely that between the l.g.n. and cortex the faster conduction of impulses by Y cells could reverse the difference; neither are Y cells in the l.g.n. likely to be capable of exerting a prior inhibitory influence on X cells when weak visual stimuli are used (cf. Singer & Bedworth 1973).

It would be unwise to conclude from these results that the X system is functionally faster than the Y system, because the measurements take no account of the variability of response, which has a substantial effect on the latency for a reliable change in discharge. Moreover, the work of

Shapley & Victor (1978) suggests that, as stimulus contrast is raised, the latencies of responses of Y cells decrease faster than those of X cells. It seems most likely that the difference between the conduction velocities of X and Y cells has little significance for the speed of visual responses.

These observations suggest that, unless their responses become relatively very much faster with increasing contrast, Y cells cannot be the embodiment of the 'fast' mechanism hypothesized by Breitmeyer & Ganz (1976) to produce masking, and by Matin (1974) to produce saccadic suppression.

PSYCHOPHYSICAL EVIDENCE FOR 'SUSTAINED' AND 'TRANSIENT' MECHANISMS

The weakening of the apparently close relationship between physiological and psychophysical results prompts one to review the psychophysical evidence for the distinction between 'sustained' and 'transient' mechanisms. A good deal of it is based on observations that show a graded change in temporal properties with increasing spatial frequency. It is therefore worth asking if any of the psychophysical results could reflect the operation of a single class of mechanisms all having the same temporal properties.

One notion consistent with many of the observations is that mechanisms sensitive to high spatial frequencies have the same temporal properties as those that detect low spatial frequencies, but that small eye-movements, even those occurring during attempted steady fixation, introduce a temporal modulation of the retinal image sufficient to render quite visible the image of a grating that is stationary on the oscilloscope. Thus the apparently 'sustained' response arises from these fortuitous movements of the image (Arend 1976). This idea accounts qualitatively for the changes in shape of the spatial contrast sensitivity curve that accompany changes in temporal frequency (Robson 1966), for the effect of exposure duration on the shape of the spatial contrast sensitivity curve (Legge 1978) and for some effects of subthreshold summation (Tolhurst 1975). It is also rendered attractive by the physiological observation (see above) that changes in temporal frequency seem to affect contrast sensitivity of ganglion cells uniformly at all spatial frequencies. However, quantitative considerations are less encouraging: 'sustained' properties have been inferred for mechanisms subserving the detection of spatial frequencies as low as 1.5 cycles/deg (Legge 1978), where eye movements during fixation would be expected to have little effect upon sensitivity. The explanation in terms of eye movements is also weakened by the finding that, when the retinal image is stabilized (Kelly 1977; Tulunay-Keesey & Bennis 1979) sensitivity for intermediate and high spatial frequencies is only slightly reduced at low temporal frequencies.

A second possibility, which has not been explored experimentally, is that the progression to more transient properties with decreasing spatial frequency reflects a change in the retinal distribution of mechanisms that detect the gratings. Suppose that peripheral mechanisms are less sensitive to low temporal frequencies. In a typical experiment where grating displays are, say, 10° in diameter, regions more than a small distance from the fovea will contribute little to the detection of patterns of high spatial frequency, at any temporal frequency, but may contribute much more to the detection of low spatial frequencies when the temporal frequency is higher, i.e. there is greater probability summation across space when the temporal frequency is high.

A number of observations showing low temporal sensitivity in mechanisms sensitive to low spatial frequencies might be explained by one or other of the above ideas, but some others are more difficult. The most compelling argument for there being *qualitatively* different mechanisms that have different visual functions is based on the observation that there appear to be two distinct thresholds for perceiving grating patterns: when low spatial frequencies are presented, the temporal properties of the stimulus are easily seen at the threshold for detection, but one requires supra-threshold contrast to discern the spatial structure (van Nes *et al.* 1967; Keesey 1972; Tolhurst 1973; King-Smith & Kulikowski 1975). For higher spatial frequencies, on the other hand, the spatial structure of the stimulus seems to be readily discerned at the threshold for detection but supra-threshold contrast is required for perception of the temporal properties.

Perceptually distinct thresholds might arise because observers find it hard to maintain a stable criterion as spatial and temporal properties are varied. If an observer is forced to maintain a stable criterion (as in Nachmias's (1967) experiment where spatial contrast sensitivity was measured by a forced-choice technique that required the observer to identify the orientation of a grating), there is little fall in sensitivity for spatial frequencies below the optimum. It therefore seemed worthwhile to establish whether distinct thresholds are revealed in experiments where the observer's criterion is constrained.

Qualitatively distinct threshold percepts

Detection of the movement of threshold stimuli

This experiment was undertaken to establish the conditions under which the direction of movement of a grating could be discerned at the threshold for detection. I was particularly interested to know how the spatial frequency of the gratings affected performance.

The observer sat with his head held steady by a chin rest and temple support, and viewed binocularly an oscilloscope screen (mean luminance 27 cd m^{-2}) on which could appear side by side two gratings (each 4° wide by 4° high, viewed from 57 cm). These were separated by a narrow region of uniform illumination with a fixation spot in the middle. The threshold for detection of gratings was established in the first part of the experiment: on each trial a moving grating was presented in one or both halves of the screen, and the observer had to indicate, by pressing a key switch, whether one grating or two had appeared. A trial lasted 5 s, during which time gratings appeared at full contrast for 1.5 s with slow onset and offset (figure 5, inset). A single experimental session consisted of 560 trials, in which one or two gratings were presented equally frequently in random order (if a single grating was presented it appeared randomly on the left or right while the other side of the screen remained uniformly illuminated) at seven different levels of contrast. The results were plotted as a graph of the frequency with which one or two gratings were correctly detected, against the contrast of the stimulus. A probit regression line was fitted to these points, and threshold was taken as the contrast giving 80% correct detection.

In the second part of the experiment exactly the same procedure was followed, but this time two gratings were always presented. On a single trial they moved either in the same direction (both leftwards or both rightwards) or in opposite directions (one leftwards, one rightwards) and the observer had to decide whether they moved in the same or opposite directions.

The experiment therefore provides estimates of two thresholds, one for the detection of a grating and one for identifying its direction of movement. Figure 5 shows for one observer (the author) the ratio of threshold for identification to that for detection plotted against the rate of movement of the grating, for gratings of spatial frequency 0.5, 2.0 and 8.0 cycles/deg. A ratio greater than 1 means that discrimination requires more contrast than detection. Consider first the results for the highest spatial frequency (8.0 cycles/deg). When the grating was moved at 1 cycle/s the threshold for identifying its direction is nearly 1.4 times that for detection, which is in line with the previously reported observation. But notice that as gratings moved faster the difference disappeared (the horizontal bars on the graph mark limits beyond which the threshold ratio is significantly different from unity). Watson *et al.* (1980) have observed the same effects in similar experiments.

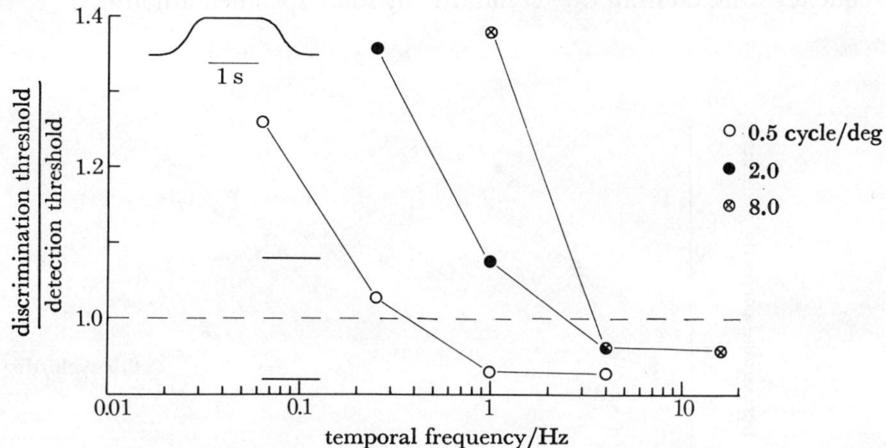

FIGURE 5. Relative thresholds for detecting a grating and discriminating its direction of motion, as a function of the rate of movement. Ratios greater than unity mean that direction of movement cannot be discerned at threshold for detection. Short horizontal lines bracket ratios not significantly different from unity. Inset shows the time course of a trial. Observer, P. L.

When gratings of 0.5 and 2.0 cycle/deg moved at 1 cycle/s, their direction of motion was identified correctly at the threshold for detection, but when these gratings moved more slowly the threshold for identifying direction of movement exceeded the threshold for detection, just as it did for the gratings of higher spatial frequency. Perhaps the simplest way to interpret these results is to suppose that the *velocity* of a grating determines whether or not its motion will be identified at the threshold for detection. Under the conditions of this experiment, motion was discriminated when the velocity was about $0.4° \text{ s}^{-1}$. It seems unnecessary to postulate qualitatively different mechanisms to account for the fact that gratings of high spatial frequency are not seen to move at the threshold for detection; this happens simply because their velocities are generally too low.

Detection of the form of threshold stimuli

The next experiment was designed to examine the observation that, at the threshold for detection, one apparently cannot with precision identify the spatial frequency of a low-frequency grating.

For this experiment the observer viewed an oscilloscope screen that subtended $10° \times 8°$ and had a space average luminance of 150 cd m^{-2}. In the first part of the experiment the threshold for detecting a grating was measured by a forced-choice procedure: on each trial (marked by a tone) either a grating was presented for 250 ms or the screen remained uniformly illuminated, and the observer had to decide which of these events had happened. In a session of 400 trials, gratings and blanks were presented equally often but in random order. When gratings were

presented they appeared with abrupt onset and offset. In any one experimental session gratings
were all of one contrast; different contrasts were used in different sessions, and a frequency-of-
seeing curve was constructed from the results of several sessions.

In the second part of the experiment the procedure was similar, but a grating appeared on
the screen on every trial. The observer's task now was to indicate whether the grating was of
'standard' spatial frequency of 'higher' spatial frequency, when all gratings were equally
detectable. In any one experiment the 'standard' frequency was 0.5 or 6.0 cycles/deg and the
'higher' frequency differed from the 'standard' by some specified amount. The 'standard' and

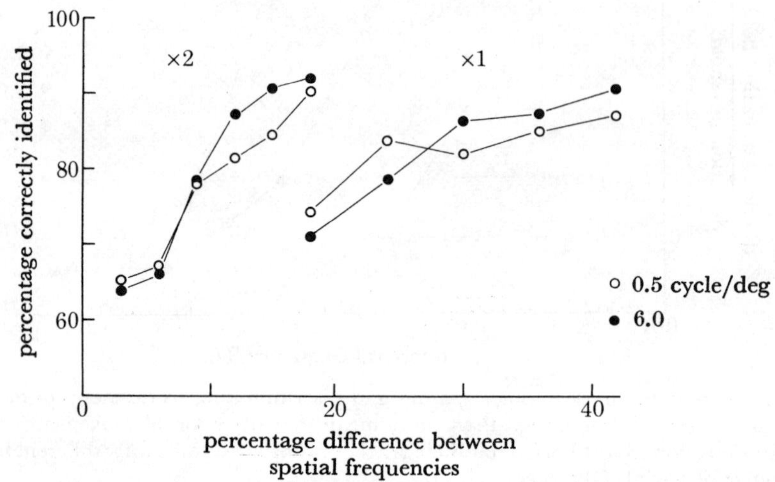

FIGURE 6. Identification of the spatial frequency of a grating at the threshold for detection (right-hand graphs)
and at twice the contrast required for detection (left-hand graphs), as a function of the percentage difference
between the two frequencies to be identified. ○, 'standard' frequency of 0.5 cycle/deg; ●, 'standard'
frequency of 6.0 cycles/deg. Observer, P. L.

'higher' frequency gratings appeared equally often, but in random order. This procedure was
repeated for a range of 'higher' frequency gratings. In figure 6 the results are plotted as graphs
showing the percentage of trials on which the different 'higher' frequency gratings could be
identified correctly, as a function of the degree to which their spatial frequencies differed from
that of the standard grating. The question of interest is whether the graphs made with a
standard frequency of 0.5 cycle/deg differ from those made with a standard frequency of
6.0 cycles/deg when all gratings are at the threshold for detection (in this case defined as the
contrast that gave 80% correct detection in the first part of the experiment). The pair of graphs
on the right-hand side of figure 6 show the percentage of trials on which gratings were correctly
identified, against the percentage difference between the 'standard' and the 'higher' frequencies.
Open circles show results for a 'standard' frequency of 0.5 cycle/deg, filled circles for a
'standard' frequency of 6 cycles/deg. It is clear that, for gratings that are equally detectable, the capacity to identify spatial frequency is no better when the 'standard' frequency is
6.0 cycles/deg than when it is 0.5 cycles/deg.

The capacity to identify spatial frequency improves as contrast is increased, but in step for
the gratings of 0.5 and 6.0 cycles/deg: the graphs on the left show the percentage of trials on
which gratings were correctly identified, as a function of the difference between spatial frequencies, when the contrast of all gratings was set to be twice that required for detection.

This experiment suggests that the mechanisms involved in detection of patterns of low and high spatial frequency are equally good at discriminating form. It therefore weakens the notion that the mechanisms are qualitatively different.

Conclusion

The physiological experiments described here all used stimuli that were just detected reliably. X and Y cells in the retina send more or less the same information about the temporal properties of threshold stimuli, and seem to transmit it effectively with the same speed, so unless the signals from X and Y cells are filtered differently at higher stages (for which Movshon *et al.* (1978) have provided some evidence) they seem weak candidates for the 'sustained' and 'transient' psychophysical mechanisms.

The results of the psychophysical experiments reported here suggest that the mechanisms subserving detection of spatial frequencies in the range 0.5–8 cycles/deg differ neither in their capacity to transmit information about movement, nor in their capacity to transmit information about form. Although these experiments do not impinge directly on the large body of evidence pointing to quantitative differences between the temporal properties of mechanisms subserving the detection of high and low spatial frequencies, they do weaken the evidence for the existence of *qualitatively* different mechanisms. But if one no longer requires that the underlying physiological mechanisms provide qualitatively different 'sustained' and 'transient' properties, the question remains open whether X and Y cells could subserve the detection of stimuli of low and high spatial frequency, respectively. It seems improbable that this could be the only visually significant function of a very clear-cut anatomical and physiological division of cell types. Perhaps one should look to other features that distinguish Y cells from X cells, such as their sensitivity to stimuli falling far from the classical receptive field (Fischer *et al.* 1975; Barlow *et al.* 1977; Derrington *et al.* 1979), or their different pattern of decussation (Levick 1977), for the key to their visual significance.

I am grateful to several colleagues who generously forsook the sun at Sarasota to comment upon the manuscript. This work was supported by a grant from the Medical Research Council.

References (Lennie)

Arend Jr, L. E. 1976 Temporal determinants of the form of the spatial contrast threshold MTF. *Vision Res.* **16**, 1035–1042.

Barlow, H. B., Derrington, A. M., Harris, L. R. & Lennie, P. 1977 The effects of remote retinal stimulation on the responses of cat retinal ganglion cells. *J. Physiol., Lond.* **269**, 177–194.

Breitmeyer, B. G. 1975 Simple reaction time as a measure of the temporal response properties of transient and sustained channels. *Vision Res.* **15**, 1411–1412.

Breitmeyer, B. G. & Ganz, L. 1976 Implications of sustained and transient channels for theories of visual pattern masking, saccadic suppression, and information processing. *Psychol. Rev.* **83**, 1–36.

Campbell, F. W. & Green, D. G. 1965 Optical and retinal factors affecting visual resolution. *J. Physiol., Lond.* **181**, 576–593.

Cleland, B. G., Dubin, M. W. & Levick, W. R. 1971 Sustained and transient neurones in the cat's retina and lateral geniculate nucleus. *J. Physiol., Lond.* **217**, 473–496.

Cleland, B. G., Levick, W. R. & Sanderson, K. J. 1973 Properties of sustained and transient ganglion cells in the cat retina. *J. Physiol., Lond.* **228**, 649–680.

De Monasterio, F. M. 1978 Properties of concentrically organized X and Y ganglion cells of macaque retina. *J. Neurophysiol.* **41**, 1394–1417.

Derrington, A. M., Lennie, P. & Wright, M. J. 1979 The mechanism of peripherally evoked responses in retinal ganglion cells. *J. Physiol., Lond.* **289**, 299–310.

Enroth-Cugell, C. & Robson, J. G. 1966 The contrast sensitivity of retinal ganglion cells of the cat. *J. Physiol., Lond.* **187**, 517–552.

Fischer, B., Krüger, J. & Droll, W. 1975 Quantitative aspects of the shift effect in cat retinal ganglion cells. *Brain Res.* **83**, 391–403.

Graham, N. 1979 Current psychophysics of spatial frequency channels. In *Perceptual organization* (ed. M. Kubovy & J. Pomerantz). Hillsdale, New Jersey: Erlbaum Associates.

Hochstein, S. & Shapley, R. M. 1976*a* Quantitative analysis of retinal ganglion cell classifications. *J. Physiol., Lond.* **262**, 237–264.

Hochstein, S. & Shapley, R. M. 1976*b* Linear and nonlinear spatial subunits in Y cat retinal ganglion cells. *J. Physiol., Lond.* **262**, 265–284.

Ikeda, H. & Wright, M. J. 1972 Receptive field organization of 'sustained' and 'transient' ganglion cells which subserve different functional roles. *J. Physiol., Lond.* **227**, 769–800.

Keesey, U. T. 1972 Flicker and pattern detection: a comparison of thresholds. *J. opt. Soc. Am.* **62**, 446–448.

Kelly, D. H. 1977 Visual contrast sensitivity. *Opt. Acta* **24**, 107–129.

King-Smith, P. E. & Kulikowski, J. J. 1975 Pattern and flicker detection analyzed by subthreshold summation. *J. Physiol., Lond.* **249**, 519–548.

Kulikowski, J. J. & Tolhurst, D. J. 1973 Psychophysical evidence for sustained and transient detectors in human vision. *J. Physiol., Lond.* **232**, 149–162.

Legge, G. E. 1978 Sustained and transient mechanisms in human vision: temporal and spatial properties. *Vision Res.* **18**, 69–81.

Levick, W. R. 1977 Participation of brisk-transient retinal ganglion cells in binocular vision – an hypothesis. *Proc. Aust. Physiol. Pharm. Soc.* **8**, 9–16.

Lupp, U., Hauske, G. & Wolf, W. 1976 Perceptual latencies to sinusoidal gratings. *Vision Res.* **16**, 969–972.

MacLeod, D. I. A. 1978 Visual sensitivity. *A. Rev. Psychol.* **29**, 613–645.

Matin, E. 1974 Saccadic suppression: a review and an analysis. *Psychol. Bull.* **81**, 899–917.

Movshon, J. A., Thompson, I. D. & Tolhurst, D. J. 1978 Spatial and temporal contrast sensitivity of neurones in areas 17 and 18 of the cat's visual cortex. *J. Physiol., Lond.* **283**, 101–120.

Nachmias, J. 1967 Effect of exposure duration on visual contrast sensitivity with square wave gratings. *J. opt. Soc. Am.* **57**, 421–427.

van Nes, F. L., Koenderink, J. J., Nas, H. & Bouman, M. A. 1967 Spatio-temporal modulation transfer in the human eye. *J. opt. Soc. Am.* **57**, 1082–1088.

Robson, J. G. 1966 Spatial and temporal contrast sensitivity functions of the visual system. *J. opt. Soc. Am.* **56**, 1141–1142.

Rogowitz, B. E. 1978 Backward masking with sinusoidal gratings: a look at spatial frequency and temporal response. *Invest. Ophthal. (suppl.)* **17**, 123.

Shapley, R. M. & Victor, J. D. 1978 The effect of contrast on the transfer properties of cat retinal ganglion cells. *J. Physiol., Lond.* **285**, 275–298.

Singer, W. & Bedworth, N. 1973 Inhibitory interaction between X and Y units in the cat lateral geniculate nucleus. *Brain Res.* **49**, 291–307.

Tolhurst, D. J. 1973 Separate channels for the analysis of the shape and the movement of a moving visual stimulus. *J. Physiol., Lond.* **231**, 385–402.

Tolhurst, D. J. 1975 Sustained and transient channels in human vision. *Vision Res.* **15**, 1143–1150.

Tulunay-Keesey, U. & Bennis, B. J. 1979 Effects of stimulus onset and image motion on contrast sensitivity. *Vision Res.* **19**, 767–774.

Vassilev, A. & Mitov, D. 1976 Perception time and spatial frequency. *Vision Res.* **16**, 89–92.

Watson, A. B., Thompson, P. G., Murphy, B. J. & Nachmias, J. 1980 Summation and discrimination of gratings moving in opposite directions, *Vision Res.* (In the press.)

Discussion

K. H. RUDDOCK (*Biophysics Section, Physics Department, Imperial College, London SW7 2BZ, U.K.*) In Dr Lennie's studies on the spatial properties of neural pathways selectively responsive to movement or to spatial patterns he used spatially periodic stimuli presented to a restricted retinal area. If moving, spatially non-periodic targets are employed, however, it is relatively easy to establish the activity of movement sensitive mechanisms with maximum response for spatial frequencies of around 5 cycles/deg (Barbur & Ruddock 1978). This supports Dr Lennie's thesis that movement sensitive (Y type) visual mechanisms are not characterized by low spatial frequency response. Has Dr Lennie considered employing spatially non-periodic stimuli in his own investigations?

Reference

Barbur, J. & Ruddock, K. H. 1978 The effects of background structure and target size on movement detection by the foveal and parafoveal retina, In *Proc. ICO-11 Conference*, Madrid, pp. 125–128.

P. LENNIE. Dr Ruddock imputes to me the suggestion that the Y system subserves the analysis of movement. I make no such claim; indeed my physiological results suggest that the Y system may be no better equipped to do this than the X system. My psychophysical results suggest that when a moving pattern is just detectable its movement can be discerned when a critical velocity is reached. I have no evidence to suggest that this critical velocity depends much upon the spatial frequency of the patterns.

Phil. Trans. R. Soc. Lond. B **290**, 39–55 (1980)

Printed in Great Britain

After-effects and the integration of patterns of neural activity within a channel

By B. Moulden

Department of Psychology, University of Reading, Earley Gate,
Whiteknights, Reading RG6 2AL, U.K.

Prolonged inspection of an adapting stimulus changes the appearance of a subsequent test stimulus. There are five distinct viewing conditions under which such 'after-effects' may be generated. These are MON–MON (inspect with one eye, test same eye), BIN–BIN (inspect with both eyes, test both eyes), BIN–MON (inspect with both eyes, test only one eye), MON–BIN (inspect with one eye, test with both) and TRANSFER (inspect with one eye, test with the other eye).

A model based upon the assumption of the linearly additive effects of adaptation generated in 'dominance classes' of cortical units that are driven either by one eye, or the other eye, or by either eye or both eyes together, is described. This model generates predictions concerning the expected relative magnitudes of after-effects generated under the five viewing modes described above, and experiments are described that confirm these predictions.

The model can be extended to generate predictions about other experimental conditions. A more complex version of the model is consistent with electrophysiologically derived estimates of the proportion of cortical units in each dominance class.

1. Introduction

(a) Background

The electrophysiological discoveries of the past two decades, and particularly the results of recordings from single units in the visual cortex of cat, monkey and other animals, have had the most profound impact upon our thinking about the mechanisms of human vision. The most important single finding was undoubtedly the discovery of stimulus-specific neurons. Such units respond selectively to stimuli which have a particular orientation, or which move in a particular direction, or which generate a particular degree of binocular disparity, and so on. This discovery led directly to the notion that early processing of visual information in man, too, might be carried out by 'channels' consisting of subsets of neurons specializing in the encoding of particular stimulus attributes, and it is in establishing, elucidating and extending this notion that the role of the psychophysicist has been pre-eminent.

In this work many paradigms have been used, such as subthreshold summation, masking and simultaneous interaction. But by far the commonest has been the adaptation–after-effect paradigm. Typically, an observer is exposed for several minutes to a high contrast stimulus, and this exposure affects the subsequent appearance of similar stimuli in some measurable way. It is assumed that if the adapting stimulus is generating activity in some restricted subset of neurons, then prolonged exposure should lead to a reduction in the sensitivity of those neurons. This should then be made manifest by the changed appearance of subsequently presented test stimuli whose encoding involves the participation of at least some of the adapted units.

Within this tradition, two distinct streams of research activity may be discerned. First, there is the search for consistency between psychophysical observations on man and the electro-physiological findings from animal studies. For instance, if adaptation to a particular stimulus attribute can be demonstrated, a channel for the encoding of that attribute is assumed to exist. As John Mollon neatly put it: 'If it adapts, it's there' (Mollon 1974).

Secondly, there are models that are intended to elucidate the relation between sensations and their neural correlates. One example of this approach is the attempt to discover whether the detection of movement depends simply upon the amount of activity generated in neurons tuned to a particular direction of movement, or upon the ratio of activity in neurons tuned to movements in opposite directions (see, for example, Sutherland 1961; Moulden & Mather 1978).

The research described here has its roots in both of these fields of activity, and correspondingly has two main aims. The first is to discover a simple rule which would describe how diverse patterns of activity within a channel might be integrated to yield a unitary percept: are those diverse patterns independent and linearly additive in their effects, or is some more complex algorithm required? The second aim is to try to draw rough quantitative parallels between phenomenology and inferred cortical structure: can visual phenomena be related in some quantifiable way to our assumptions about the functional organization of the human visual system?

The adaptation–after-effect paradigm has one peculiarity that is of special value. Unlike any other manipulation, the technique of adaptation provides a unique opportunity to make a unitary stimulus have more than one sensory consequence at one time, so we can examine the way in which two (or more) patterns of neural activity are integrated into a unified sensation. Non-unitary responses to unitary stimuli may be generated in at least two ways. In the first, the subject may be adapted to two or more stimuli simultaneously, so that a subsequent test stimulus is applied to a neural substrate in which two adapted states coexist. Each of these adaptive states on its own would produce a specific perceptual distortion, and by examining their joint effect one may draw powerful inferences concerning the linearity and additivity of the integration process. Experiments of this kind are currently being carried out in this laboratory, and the results will be described elsewhere. In the second technique, it is arranged that an inspection stimulus adapts only some of the neurons tuned to its particular characteristics, leaving others unaffected. In such a case, if a subsequent test stimulus produces activity in the whole of the appropriately tuned subset, of which some respond normally and some respond abnormally, the question arises: how are the 'normal' and the 'abnormal' signals integrated to give a single percept?

We investigated the after-effects of movement (m.a.e.) and of tilt (t.a.e.). After prolonged inspection of a stimulus moving steadily in one direction, a truly stationary test stimulus appears, for a short time, to be moving in the opposite direction; this is the m.a.e. Similarly, after prolonged inspection of a line or grating tilted, say, 10° clockwise from vertical, a truly vertical test line or grating appears, for a short time, to be tilted a few degrees anticlockwise; this is the t.a.e.

(b) Interocular transfer

Our starting point was an apparently minor phenomenon associated with the m.a.e., the t.a.e. and with other similar after-effects. This is the phenomenon known as interocular transfer (i.o.t.). If, instead of viewing the adapting and test stimuli with the same eye (or eyes), one adapts with only one eye open and then views the test stimulus only with the *other* eye, an after-effect is still seen, although its magnitude is reduced to about 50–60 % of the monoptic (expose one eye, test same eye) effect. Now the existence of this interocular transfer immediately raises three questions of some theoretical importance. What is the mechanism underlying i.o.t.? Why is i.o.t. smaller than the monoptic effect? Why is the magnitude of i.o.t. a *particular proportion* (about 50–60 %) of the monoptic effect?

This paper is mainly concerned with the third of these questions. The first two questions can be answered fairly easily, and the logic underlying the answer is central to the approach to be developed here.

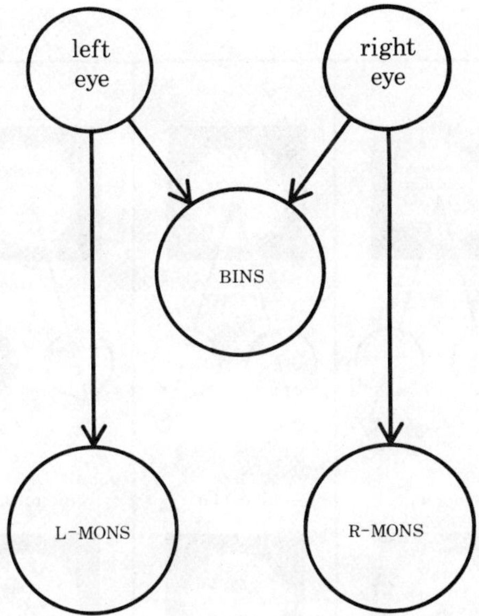

FIGURE 1. Scheme for the simplified three-unit model.

The key to the answers to the first two questions came from the electrophysiological discovery that in the cat and the monkey, cortical neurons could be classified into three broad groups. The neurons in one group could be driven only through the left eye (left monocular units, or L-MONS), those in the second group could be driven only through the right eye (right monocular units, or R-MONS), and those in the third group could be driven by either eye or by both eyes together (the binocular units, or BINS). These findings are schematized, albeit in a rather simplified manner, in the diagram in figure 1. Such a scheme can provide the basis of an explanation for i.o.t. Assume that the left eye only is adapted and the right eye only is tested. During the inspection phase the L-MONS and the BINS will become adapted; the R-MONS will not. During the test phase, the R-MONS and the BINS will be involved in signalling the test stimulus, and of these the BINS will be giving an 'abnormal' (adapted) signal while the R-MONS will give a 'normal' (unadapted) signal. As long as these two signals are integrated in some way, the resultant must be a signal that is neither 'normal' nor as 'abnormal' as if the R-MONS had also been adapted, as they would have been had the inspection phase involved the right eye and not the left. ..

Thus, our first two questions might be answered as follows: i.o.t. is mediated by adaptation of the BINS, and is smaller than the monoptic effect because only some of the units driven during the test phase are adapted.

(c) The three-class model

This model can in fact be extended, formalized and tested experimentally. The model can be extended by considering the monoptic and transfer conditions already described, and by adding three other possible viewing conditions. The five possible viewing modes are illustrated in figure 2. (It should be noted that for the four conditions that involve monocular viewing with the left or right eye in either the inspection or the test phase or both, there will be a symmetrical condition in which the other eye is used.) However, before predictions can be generated the notions employed in the explanation of i.o.t. must be formalized.

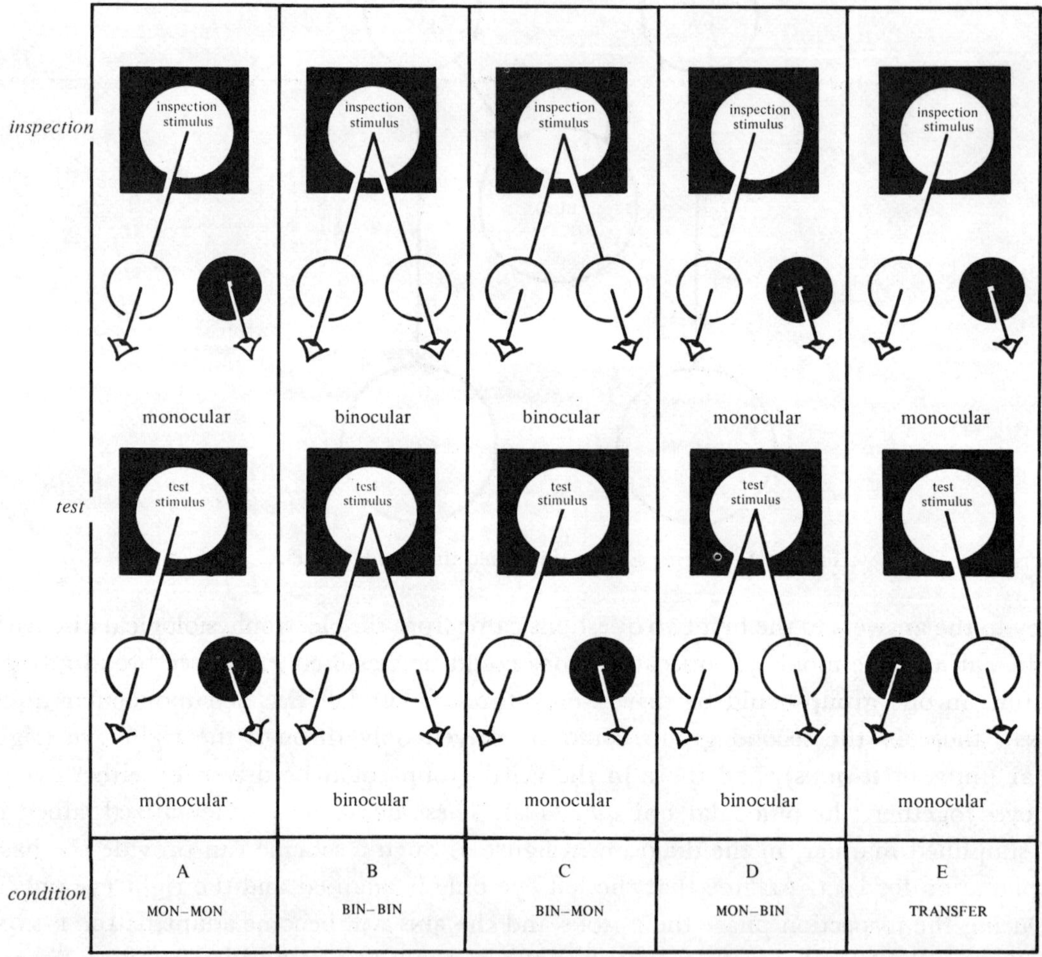

FIGURE 2. The five possible viewing modes involving inspection or test with either one eye, the other eye, or both eyes. For every case in which monocular viewing with the left eye was used for a condition, the symmetrical condition involving the right eye was also tested.

The formalization depends critically upon two key propositions, which are as follows:

(i) *The partitioning postulate*: the set of cortical units of which a channel is composed may be partitioned exhaustively into three mutually exclusive and independent subsets, namely the L-MONS, the R-MONS and the BINS.

(ii) *The ratio postulate*: the magnitude of an after-effect in a particular viewing mode depends upon the proportion of the units that are driven during the test phase that have previously been driven, and therefore adapted, during the inspection phase.

Two corollaries of the ratio postulate are that (1) units that are adapted during the inspection phase but that are not driven during the test phase do not contribute to the after-effect; and (2) units that are driven during the test phase but that have not been adapted during the inspection phase tend to reduce the after-effect.

The partitioning postulate is, of course, extremely naïve in electrophysiological terms. Electrophysiologists, following Hubel & Wiesel (1968), have generally classified cells into seven dominance classes. The units of class 1 are driven only by one eye, say the left; those of class 2 are driven by both eyes, but much more vigorously by the eye driving class 1; class 3 units are similar, but the dominance is less marked; class 4 contains units in which each eye is equipotential; and classes 5, 6 and 7 are symmetric with classes 3, 2 and 1, with the other eye dominating. Moreover, many binocular units are driven much more vigorously by both eyes together than by one eye alone (see, for example, Hubel & Wiesel 1968, p. 239). In fact, most of the objections that might be raised on these grounds are met by my five-unit model, involving three degrees of response vigour, which is described in §3a, and which generates precisely the same predictions as the simple three-unit model. In view of the greater tractability of the three-unit model it will continue to be used here for ease of exposition.

The ratio postulate is a plausible one, but is by no means inevitable. Lehmkuhle & Fox (1975), for example, have suggested that after-effect magnitude might depend solely upon the *total number* of units both adapted and tested. The essential assumption underlying the ratio postulate is that if unadapted cells respond during the test phase, then their veridical signals will tend to dilute the distorting effect of the adapted units.

TABLE 1. THE PREDICTION OF ORDER RELATIONS, THREE-CLASS MODEL: THE DERIVATION OF THE EXPRESSIONS USED TO PREDICT THE ORDER RELATIONS BETWEEN THE MAGNITUDES OF AFTER-EFFECTS GENERATED UNDER THE FIVE VIEWING MODES

condition	A (MON–MON)	B (BIN–BIN)	C (BIN–MON)	D (MON–BIN)	E (TRANSFER)
units tested	$M+B$	$2M+B$	$M+B$	$2M+B$	$M+B$
of units tested, those that have been adapted	$M+B$	$2M+B$	$M+B$	$M+B$	B
expression for relative A–E magnitude	$\dfrac{M+B}{M+B}$	$\dfrac{2M+B}{2M+B}$	$\dfrac{M+B}{M+B}$	$\dfrac{M+B}{2M+B}$	$\dfrac{B}{M+B}$
relative magnitude	$A = 1$	$B = 1$	$C = 1$	$D < 1$	$E < D$

Hence order relations: $A = B = C > D > E$.

Table 1 shows how the partitioning postulate and the ratio postulate can be combined to predict the order relations between the after-effects generated in the five viewing modes. For example, in the condition MON–BIN (adapt monocularly, test binocularly), the units driven during the test phase are the L-MONS, the R-MONS and the BINS; of these only the L-MONS and the BINS (or the R-MONS and the BINS, according to the sub-condition involved) will have been adapted during the inspection phase. The predicted relative magnitude of the after-effect is thus indicated by the expression $(M+B)/(2M+B)$, which is less than unity. Simple algebra will show that the expression $B/(M+B)$, the expression which relates to the TRANSFER condition (condition E in table 1) must be smaller than the expression $(M+B)/(2M+B)$. The predicted order relations between the after-effects in the five viewing modes are thus $A = B = C > D > E$.

This predicted relation was tested in two experiments, one with the m.a.e. and the other with the t.a.e.

2. EXPERIMENTAL TESTS

The stimulus was a disk with eight black and eight white sectors, the Michelson contrast C being 0.84; the disk subtended 9.5° at the eye and was surrounded by a radically striped stationary annulus 5° in width. The disk rotated at 25 rev./min in the inspection phase and was stationary in the test phase. Subjects viewed the rotating disk for 1 min and then recorded the duration of their m.a.e. by holding down a Morse key. By means of shutters it was arranged that viewing was either with the left eye, with the right eye, or with both eyes.

There were seven naïve subjects, each of whom attended for four 1 h sessions. During the first session, subjects were given their first experience of the m.a.e. and were given practice in establishing their criterion for its cessation. They were also given experience of the various viewing modes so that they could become accustomed to the operation of the shutters. No record was taken of m.a.e. durations during this session.

During each of the three remaining 1 h sessions, each viewing mode was presented three times, so that for each of the five conditions each of the seven subjects gave nine m.a.e. durations. Each block of five conditions was presented in a different random order, with a recovery period of at least 2 min between each condition. The mean duration for each condition was thus based upon 63 observations, and these means are summarized in figure 3.

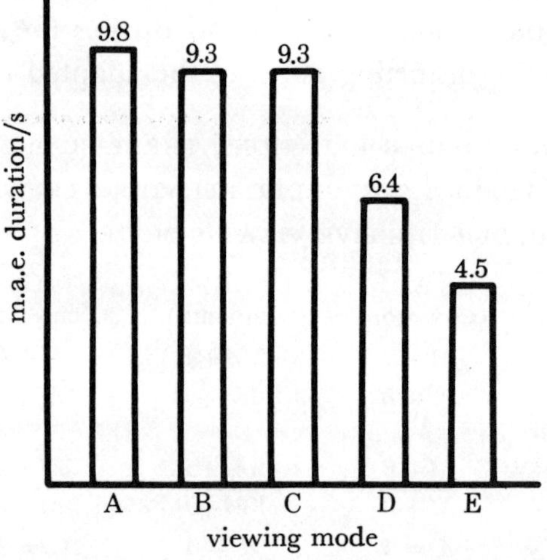

FIGURE 3. Mean m.a.e. durations in seconds for each viewing mode ($N = 7$, 63 observations per condition). A, MON–MON; B, BIN–BIN; C, BIN–MON; D, MON–BIN; E, TRANSFER. Standard errors: A, 2.38; B, 1.99; C, 2.13; D, 1.46; E, 1.60.

(b) The t.a.e. experiment

The inspection and test stimuli were back-projected square-wave gratings having a spatial frequency of 1.52 cycles/deg and a Michelson contrast of 0.9. There were three viewing fields each 8.0° in diameter; one field was to the right of the subject and was potentially visible only to the right eye via a half-silvered mirror; a similar field to the left of the subject was potentially visible only to the left eye via a second mirror. These were the inspection fields and contained gratings which, when viewed by the subject, were tilted 10° anticlockwise. These fields were illuminated only during the adaptation phase of the experiment. The third field was located straight ahead of the subject and was viewed through the half-silvered mirrors. This field was the test field and contained a grating whose orientation could be adjusted by the subject, and which was illuminated only during the test phase. By means of shutters it was arranged that during the inspection phase either the right eye only, or the left eye only, viewed its respective inspection field, or both eyes together viewed their respective, optically aligned, inspection fields. Similarly, in the test phase the test field could be made visible either to the right eye only, or to the left eye only, or to both eyes together. There were 15 subjects in all, each of whom was experienced in the use of this apparatus. Each subject attended for a total of about 2 h, and each yielded two data points for each condition (one based upon the use of the right eye and one based upon the use of the left eye in each condition involving monocular viewing; the BIN–BIN condition was also presented twice). These data were each based upon five settings, as described below, and were pooled to give a single measure for each of the five conditions. The mean t.a.e. for each condition was thus based upon 15 (subjects) × 2 (eyes) × 5 (settings) = 150 settings in all.

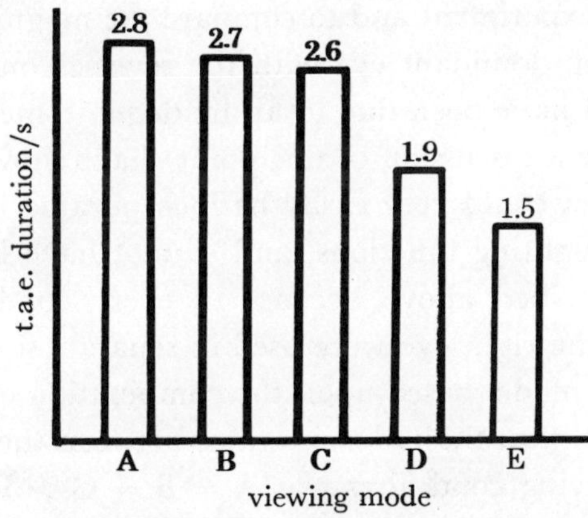

FIGURE 4. Mean t.a.e. magnitudes in degrees for each viewing mode ($N = 15$, 150 observations per condition). Symbols as for figure 3. Standard errors: A, 0.29; B, 0.28; C, 0.21; D, 0.20; E, 0.19.

The procedure in any one condition was as follows. Before adapting, and using the eye or eyes to be used in the later test phase, the subject set the movable grating to appear vertical; he made five such settings in succession, and the mean of these settings was taken as the baseline for that condition. He then viewed the tilted inspection stimulus with one eye or with both eyes, as appropriate, for 60 s. At the end of that time the test field was presented for 4 s, followed by the inspection field for 6 s and so on, with the shutters changing in synchrony with the illumination of the fields to give the appropriate viewing conditions in each phase. The alternating presentation of inspection and test fields was repeated until the subject had adjusted the test field to appear vertical. Five such adapted settings were made in succession; the difference between the mean of these settings and the mean of the baseline settings was taken as the measure of t.a.e. for that subject in that sub-condition.

The mean t.a.e. over all 15 subjects in each of the five conditions is shown in figure 4.

(c) Results

In the m.a.e. experiment (see figure 3), conditions A, B and C were not significantly different (Friedman's analysis of variance by ranks gave a χ_r^2 of 0.85; for $N = 7$, $k = 3$ a value of $\chi_r^2 = 6.00$ is required for significance at the 0.052 level). The smallest of these three (condition B) was compared with condition D; in all of the matched pairs for each subject the value for condition D was smaller than that for condition B. Similarly, each value for condition E was smaller than that for condition D. In the t.a.e. experiment (see figure 4), conditions A, B and C were again not significantly different (Friedman's test, $\chi_r^2 = 2.8$, $0.1 > p > 0.05$). On Wilcoxon's test, condition D was significantly ($0.005 > p$) smaller than condition B, the smallest of conditions A, B and C. Similarly, condition E was significantly ($0.025 > p > 0.01$) smaller than condition D.

A similar pattern of results was obtained from an experiment on the simultaneous tilt illusion, in which the inducing and test stimuli were presented simultaneously instead of successively. (In this experiment the condition equivalent to TRANSFER was a dichoptic condition in which one eye viewed the tilted inducing grating while the other eye viewed the test grating). The results, in degrees of induced tilt, were: condition A, 0.96°; B, 1.12°; C, 1.12°; D, 0.69°; E, 0.42°.

It is worth mentioning that an attempt was made to measure the eye dominance of the 15 subjects used in the t.a.e. experiment and to compare the magnitude of interocular transfer from the dominant to the non-dominant eye with the reverse condition. No consistent effect was found, but this may well have been due to an inadequate measure of dominance. Other workers (see Wade (1976) for a discussion of this point) have shown that there is an effect of eye dominance. Such an effect could very easily be incorporated into the model offered here by the simple addition of weighting functions, and cannot have been a source of systematic bias in the experiments described above because in every condition involving monocular inspection both the left and the right eye were used in separate sessions.

It will be recalled that the model based upon the combination of the partitioning and ratio postulate led to the prediction that the order relations between the magnitudes of after-effects generated under the five viewing conditions was A = B = C > D > E. This prediction has been confirmed. The notion that sensations depend upon the linearly additive effects of the activity of independent groups of detectors within a channel appears to be well founded.

(d) A further prediction

The simple algebraic expressions shown in table 1 allow a further quantitative prediction of the precise relative magnitudes of the MON–BIN (D) and TRANSFER (E) effects where 'relative magnitude' means the magnitude of the after-effect generated under conditions D and E expressed as a proportion of the after-effects generated under conditions A, B and C. If $D = (M+B)/(2M+B)$ and $E = B/(M+B)$, it can be shown by simple substitution that $D = 1/(2-E)$. In other words, the structure of the model requires that there should be a fixed and specifiable relation between the relative magnitude of the MON–BIN effect and that of TRANSFER. Table 2 shows the obtained and predicted magnitudes based upon the findings from the two experiments described earlier and upon an earlier m.a.e. experiment similar to that described above. Figure 5 shows the function $D = 1/(2-E)$ for all values of D, together with the individual subject data on which the means of table 2 are based. The straight line is the best linear fit for the data. The agreement is good, and this, together with the correct prediction of the order relations between the five viewing modes, lends considerable support to the model.

TABLE 2. PREDICTING MON–BIN FROM TRANSFER: THE RELATION BETWEEN THE MON–BIN (D) AFTER-EFFECT AND THE TRANSFER (E) AFTER-EFFECT, WHEN BOTH ARE EXPRESSED AS PROPORTIONS OF THE MON–MON, BIN–BIN AND MON–BIN EFFECTS, IS DESCRIBED BY THE EXPRESSION $D = 1/(2-E)$

	obtained value of E (TRANSFER)	if	predicted value of D (MON–BIN)	obtained value of D (MON–BIN)
m.a.e. experiment I	0.47		0.65	0.67
m.a.e. experiment II	0.43	$D = 1/(2-E)$	0.64	0.65
t.a.e. experiment	0.56		0.69	0.70

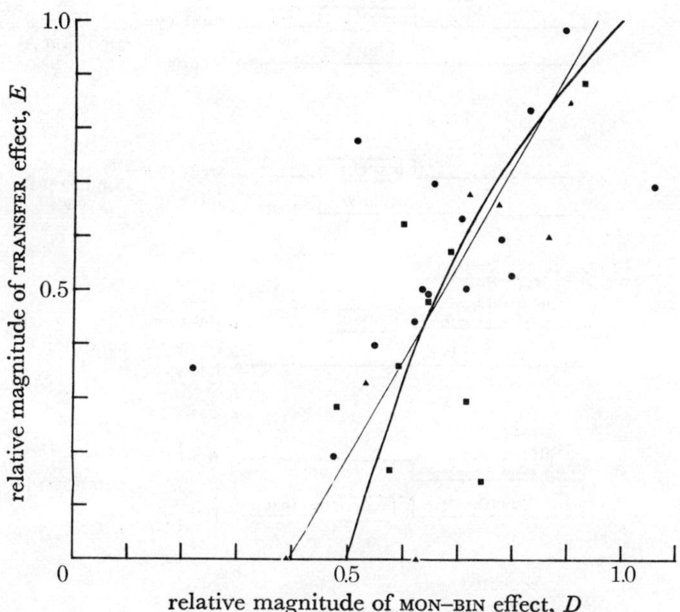

FIGURE 5. Function showing the predicted relation (curved line) between the relative magnitude of the MON–BIN condition (D) and that of the TRANSFER condition (E), according to the expression $D = 1/(2-E)$. Data points are individual subjects' measures from experiment 1 (m.a.e.), experiment 2 (t.a.e.) and a similar m.a.e. experiment not described here. The straight line is the line of best fit to the data determined by the method of least squares.

(e) A further experimental manipulation: the r.a. experiment

The use of a novel technique developed in our laboratory permits a further manipulation: this technique permits one to vary the magnitude of an after-effect generated in particular subsets of detectors in response to a constant adapting stimulus. Consider the effects of adapting, either alternately or simultaneously, to two identical stimuli moving in opposite directions. This will produce, of course, no *differential* state of adaptation in the detectors tuned to those directions of movement, and consequently no m.a.e. However, *both* sets of detectors will be adapted to some degree, and the differential adaptive effect of a subsequent unidirectional stimulus will be less than it would have been had that stimulus been applied to an unadapted system. In short, the effects of 30 s of adaptation should be less after a period of 'repeated alternations' (r.a.) than it would have been before it. Now if r.a. is applied to only some of the detectors involved in a particular viewing mode, it should be possible to predict the relative magnitudes of the after-effects so generated by considering the altered relative contributions of the sets of detectors involved.

The scheme of such an experiment is illustrated in figure 6. Conditions A and B are baseline MON–MON and TRANSFER conditions respectively. Condition C is a MON–MON condition preceded by r.a.; the predicted magnitude of the after-effect from this condition should be less than for condition A. Condition D is also a MON–MON condition, but one that is preceded by a period

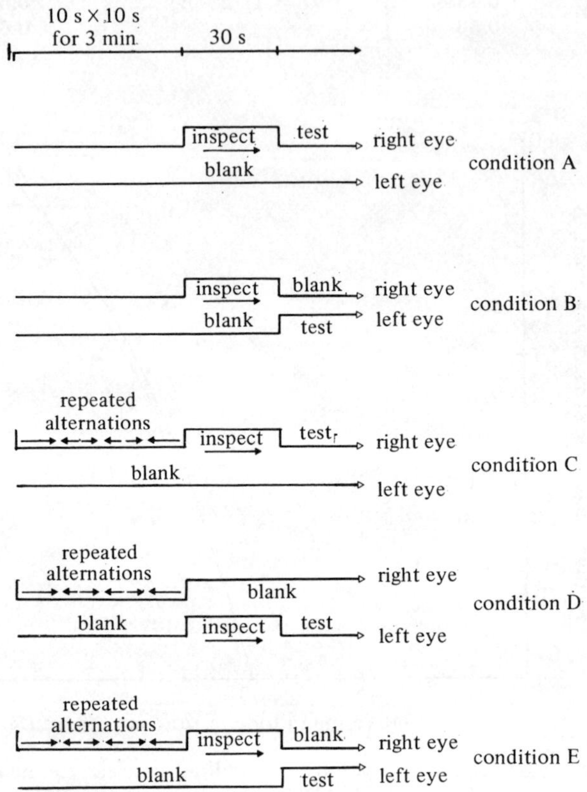

FIGURE 6. The procedure employed in each of the five conditions of experiment 3.

of r.a. applied to the eye *not* involved in the main adapt–test procedure. This procedure involves one set of MONS and the BINS; of these, the BINS will have been affected by r.a. and their contribution to the after-effect will be thereby reduced.

The after-effect from D should be less than that from A, but greater than that from C, in which *all* of the units contributing to the after-effect will have been affected by r.a. Condition E is a TRANSFER condition with the eye used in the inspection phase being exposed to r.a. beforehand. This should reduce the magnitude of the differential adaptation generated in the MONS and BINS that are driven during the inspection phase; of these, the BINS mediate the transferred effect, which should therefore be less than that in the baseline condition, condition D. The predicted size of the after-effect in the five conditions is thus $A > D > C$ and $A > B > E$.

The details of the experiment were precisely the same as those for the m.a.e. experiment described earlier, with the following exceptions. There were ten subjects, each of whom received a brief period of training to establish their criterion for the cessation of m.a.e. Whenever an r.a. condition was administered, the temporal sequence was as follows. For 3 min the subject viewed with only one eye (left or right according to the condition) a disk whose direction of rotation reversed every 10 s. At the end of this period, he viewed unidirectional rotation for 30 s again with the appropriate eye, and then viewed the stationary disk through the eye appropriate to the test phase, holding down a Morse key for as long as he could see an m.a.e. There was a 5 min recovery period after every condition involving repeated alterations, and a 2 min recovery period after other conditions. Each subject attended for two $1\frac{1}{4}$ h sessions, and during each session he experienced each of the five experimental runs twice, the ten conditions within a run being presented in a different random order for each subject. Each mean m.a.e. duration is thus based on 40 observations. The results are shown in table 3.

TABLE 3. RESULTS OF REPEATED-ALTERNATION EXPERIMENT

(Mean after-effect durations in seconds generated under the conditions represented in figure 6 and described in the text. $N = 10$.)

condition	A	B	C	D	E
mean m.a.e. duration/s	9.90	5.91	4.21	6.34	2.09
s.e.	1.19	0.83	0.67	0.82	0.43

The first set of predictions was that $A > D > C$; ideally, then, the rank order of these conditions should be 1, 2, 3 for each subject. Eight of the ten subjects showed this pattern of results. The probability of such a result occurring by chance is given by the binomial expansion for $N = 10$, $x = 8$, $p = \frac{1}{6}$, $q = \frac{5}{6}$. The associated p value is very much less than 0.001, and the first set of predictions is confirmed. The second set of predictions was that $A > B > E$; this was true for all ten subjects, and no statistical analysis is necessary. The experimental predictions are, therefore, all confirmed.

(f) Summary

So far, then, it has been possible to account for the existence of i.o.t., to account for the fact that it is smaller than the monoptic effect, to predict the rank order of the magnitudes of the after-effects in all five viewing modes, both with and without r.a., and to predict the precise relative magnitude of the MON–BIN and TRANSFER effects.

All of this, however, has been achieved within the framework of a three-class model, and it remains to be demonstrated that the predictions derived from this simple model may also be derived from a five-class model based upon more plausible assumptions, particularly with regard to the relative responsivity of binocular units to input either from one eye only or from both eyes together.

3. EXTENDING THE MODEL

(a) The five-class model

The units in the five classes of this extended model are assumed to have the following properties. Units in classes 1 and 5 are purely monocular. Units in class 3 may be driven equally by either eye but more strongly by both eyes together. Classes 2 and 4 contain units that are similar to those in class 3 except that one eye is more effective than the other. Assume for simplicity that a maximum of four different relative firing rates may be produced in a unit, depending upon the viewing conditions, and that the degree of adaptation generated in a class of units (and therefore the contribution of that class to the after-effect) is proportional to the relative firing rate. Let the maximum possible firing rate be unity, the minimum zero, and let two intermediate values be $1-x$ and $1-y$, where $y > x$. Let purely monocular units, those in classes 1 and 5, have only two possible levels of firing: zero or unity according to the input mode (ignoring other possible determinants of firing rate such as stimulus contrast). Let equipotential binocular units, those in class 3, have three possible relative firing rates: zero, $1-x$ (when driven by one eye only) and unity (when driven by both eyes together). Let unequal-dominance binocular units, those in classes 2 and 4, have four possible firing rates: zero, $1-y$ (when driven by the non-dominant eye), $1-x$ (when driven by the dominant eye) and unity (when driven by both eyes together). Let the degree of adaptation generated in each class of unit in a particular condition be directly proportional to the firing rate, so that after adaptation a unit will have either unit gain (if it has not been driven during the adaptation phase); a high gain, H, if it has been driven at the relative rate of $1-y$; a medium gain, M, if it has been driven at the relative rate of $1-x$; or a low gain, L, if it has been driven at its maximum (relative firing rate of unity).

TABLE 4. FIRING RATES AND SUBSEQUENT GAINS, FIVE-CLASS MODEL: THE RELATIVE FIRING RATES ASSUMED TO BE GENERATED IN EACH DOMINANCE CLASS BY EACH OF THE THREE INPUT MODES, TOGETHER WITH THE GAINS OF THE CLASSES AFTER ADAPTATION

dominance class ...	1	2	3	4	5	
L—MON						
firing rate	1	$1-x$	$1-x$	$1-y$	0	1
subsequent gain	L	M	M	H	1	2
R—MON						
firing rate	0	$1-y$	$1-x$	$1-x$	1	3
subsequent gain	1	H	M	M	L	4
BIN						
firing rate	1	1	1	1	1	5
subsequent gain	L	L	L	L	L	6

This argument is summarized in table 4, which shows the dominance classes (classes 1–5), the various potential firing rates (unity, 1-x, 1-y, zero) for each class in each possible viewing condition (right monocular, left moncular or binocular), and the various gains (unity, H, M of L) resulting from these firing rates. The relative firing rate in a unit after adaptation in a particular condition will be given by the product of its potential relative firing rate in that condition and the gain of the unit after adaptation. For example, in a left monocular adaptation phase, a class 4 unit will have been driven at a relative firing rate of $1-y$ (see line 1 of table 4); its gain will subsequently be H (line 2). If the unit is now driven in a right monocular test phase, which would normally drive the unit at a relative firing rate of $1-x$ (see line 3), the post-adaptation relative firing rate will be $H(1-x)$. In this way it is possible to describe the post-adaptation relative firing rates of the units driven in a particular test phase. If the magnitude of an after-effect in any condition is proportional to the ratio (in terms now of *relative firing rates*) of units driven in both adapt and test phase to units driven in test phase, then the relative magnitudes of the after-effects will be reflected by the ratios in table 5. The first three ratios are obviously unity, since of the units driven during the test phase, all are adapted during the inspection phase. D is clearly less than unity, and it can be demonstrated quite simply that E must be smaller than D. It is clear that the predictions from this five-class model are identical with those from the three-class model, but it is not open to the objections to the latter described in §1c.

TABLE 5. THE PREDICTION OF ORDER RELATIONS, FIVE-CLASS MODEL: THE EXPRESSIONS, DERIVED FROM THE ASSUMPTIONS REPRESENTED IN TABLE 4 AND DESCRIBED IN THE TEXT, THAT CAN BE USED TO PREDICT THE ORDER RELATIONS BETWEEN THE MAGNITUDES OF AFTER-EFFECTS GENERATED UNDER THE FIVE VIEWING MODES

adaptation condition	test condition			
L–MON	L–MON	$\dfrac{L+M(1-x)+M(1-x)+H(1-y)}{L+M(1-x)+M(1-x)+H(1-y)}$	$=1$	A
BIN	BIN	$\dfrac{L+L+L+L+L}{L+L+L+L+L}$	$=1$	B
BIN	L–MON	$\dfrac{L+L(1-x)+L(1-x)+L(1-y)}{L+L(1-x)+L(1-x)+L(1-y)}$	$=1$	C
L–MON	BIN	$\dfrac{L+M+M+H}{L+M+M+H+1}$	<1	D
L—MON	R–MON	$\dfrac{M(1-y)+M(1-x)+H(1-x)}{M(1-y)+M(1-x)+H(1-x)+1}$	$<D$	E

(b) The proportion of units in each class

Up to this point, the issue of the relative proportions of units in each dominance class has been ignored, because the prediction of order relations between the magnitudes of after-effects generated by the five viewing modes is quite independent of this factor, with two constraints. First, if a subject had no BINS, then the mechanism for the mediation of transfer would not exist; TRANSFER would be zero. (It is: subjects with a history of strabismus, who are stereoblind, and who by inference have failed to develop binocular units, do not show transfer; see, for example, Movshon *et al.* (1972) and the cautionary note by Hess (1978).) If equal numbers of monocular units were associated with each eye, the MON–BIN effect should be exactly 50 % of the MON–MON, BIN–BIN and BIN–MON effects. Secondly, if *all* of the units in a channel were binocularly driven, transfer would be 100 % and so would the MON–BIN effect.

Nevertheless, although the order relations are independent of the proportions of units in each class, it is obvious that the *precise relative magnitudes* of the TRANSFER and MON–BIN effects must be dependent upon this factor. This consideration raises the question of whether it might be possible to estimate those proportions given the exact relative magnitude of these effects. It is, but only at some cost in terms of the plausibility of the assumptions adopted. It is necessary to assume that class 3 units are driven equally strongly by either eye alone or by both eyes together, and that class 2 and class 4 units are driven as strongly by their dominant eye as both eyes together. Given these assumptions, the argument may be developed as follows.

It is assumed that the magnitude of the after-effect generated in a particular condition is a linearly additive function of the 'contribution' of each class of unit driven during the test phase. It is further assumed that the contribution of a class of unit depends first on the proportion of units in a particular class, and secondly upon the degree to which the units in that class have been adapted during the inspection phase, this in turn being directly proportional to the degree to which those units have been driven during the inspection phase.

In figure 7, the five classes of unit described above are represented along the abscissa, and the ordinate represents the proportion of units in each class; this proportion is of course unspecified, so that the overall shape of the distribution is entirely hypothetical. The width, again unspecified, of each column represents the maximum firing rate and hence the maximum potential degree of adaptation for each class of unit. The shaded areas represent the amount of firing in each class as a function of the three types of presentation mode, left monocular, binocular, or right monocular. The width of the shaded areas may take one of three values: zero, unity, and some unknown value k. This value k represents the degree to which units in classes 2 and 4 are driven by the non-dominant eye; consequently $1-k$ represents the degree (as a function of maximal firing rate) to which a unit in that class is *not* driven by input from the non-dominant eye.

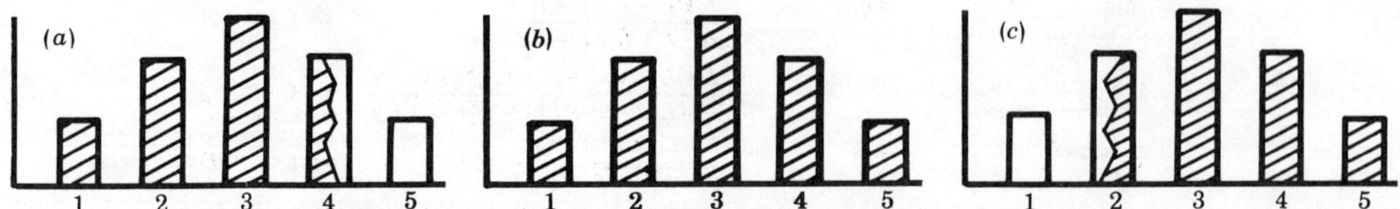

FIGURE 7. Illustrating the concept of the area $1 > k$. On the abscissa are the five classes of eye dominance described in the text; the ordinate represents the (purely imaginary) proportion of units in each class; the hatching represents the degree to which a class of units is driven (and therefore adapted) by a particular viewing mode. The unhatched area in classes 2 and 4 represents the quantity $1 > k$, being the degree to which a class of units is not driven by monocular exposure through its non-dominant eye. (*a*) L-MON presentation; (*b*) BIN presentation; (*c*) R-MON presentation.

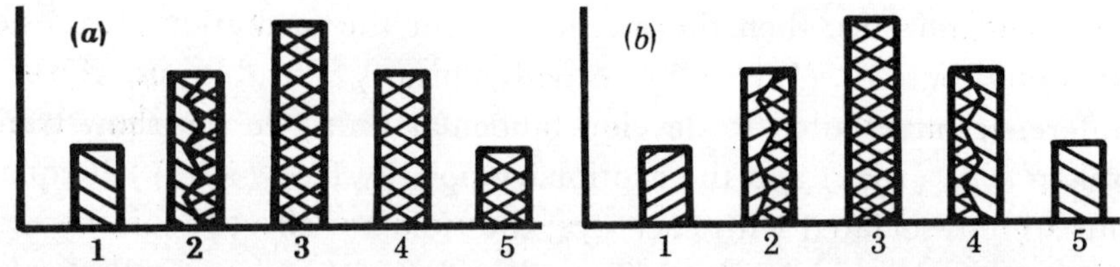

FIGURE 8. Conventions as for figure 7. The figure shows the degrees of overlap between the amounts of firing generated in the inspection phase and in the test phase in the various dominance classes. (*a*) The overlap in the condition R-MON–BIN; (*b*) the overlap in the condition TRANSFER.

The magnitude of an after-effect is a function of the extent to which the area representing the amount of adaptation generated during the inspection phase overlaps the area representing the amount of firing generated during the test phase. (This 'degree of overlap' is simply a spatial representation of the ratio postulate described in §1*c*.) The three possible extents of overlap are, first, *complete* (as in MON–MON, BIN–BIN and BIN–MON, when all of the tested cells have previously been adapted); secondly, *intermediate* (as in MON–BIN, where the whole of the area in class 1 and the area $(1-k)$ in class 2 is non-overlapping); and thirdly, *small* (as in TRANSFER, where the whole of the areas in classes 1 and 5, and the two areas $(1-k)$ in classes 2 and 4, are non-overlapping). The overlap in the MON–BIN and the TRANSFER cases are illustrated in figure 8. Let the sum of the area in class 1 (or 5) and the area $(1-k)$ in class 2 (or 4) be called W. Then the overlap in MON–MON, BIN–BIN and BIN–MON is unity; the overlap in MON–BIN is $1-W$; and the overlap in the case of TRANSFER is $1-2W$. If the sum of the areas taken over all classes is unity, than a quantity $V = 1 - 2W$ may be defined. A set of expressions representing the relative magnitude of the after-effect in each condition may now be derived; these expressions are in terms of areas V and W, and are given in table 6. These ratios are obviously isomorphic with the expressions derived from the three-class model (see table 1), and differ only in that the symbols

V and W, representing areas derived from the five-class model, replace the symbols M and B, representing class types in the three-class model.

V and W are in terms of proportional areas; the after-effects are expressed as proportions of the maximal after-effect, so the expressions may be treated as true equations. In the expression for the MON–BIN after-effect,

$$D = (V+W)/(V+2W); \quad V+2 = 1; \quad D = V+W; \tag{1}$$

similarly $E = V/(V+W)$; from (1),

$$E = V/D; \quad V = DE. \tag{2}$$

Therefore, from (1) and (2),

$$D = DE+W, \text{ or } W = D-DE. \tag{3}$$

Now let the proportion of units in class 1 (and class 5) be a; let the proportion of units in class 3 be b; then the proportion of units in class 2 (and class 4) must be $\frac{1}{2}(1-2a-b)$. In the L–MON–BIN paradigm, class 1 is driven at its maximum; its contribution to the after-effect is therefore simply equal to the proportion of units in that class, namely a. Similarly, the contributions of class 2 and class 3 are respectively $\frac{1}{2}(1-2a-b)$ and b. The contribution of class 4 is equal to

TABLE 6. THE PREDICTION OF ORDER RELATIONS IN TERMS OF THE QUANTITIES V AND W

(Note the isomorphism of this set of expressions with the set shown in table 1.)

BIN–BIN	MON–MON	BIN–MON	MON–BIN	TRANSFER
$\dfrac{V+2W}{V+2W}$	$\dfrac{V+W}{V+W}$	$\dfrac{V+W}{V+W}$	$\dfrac{V+W}{V+2W}$	$\dfrac{V}{V+W}$

that part of area W that is not accounted for by the proportion of units in class 5, which is a; class 4 therefore contributes $(W-a)$. But $W = D-DE$ (equation (3) above), so the contribution of class 4 is $(D-DE-a)$. All of these contributions are hypothesized to be linearly additive, so that the relative magnitude of the after-effect in the MON–BIN condition (D) may be expressed as

$$D = a+\tfrac{1}{2}(1-2a-b)+b+(D-DE-a).$$

Making this explicit for b, we obtain

$$b = 2DE+2a-1. \tag{4}$$

In other words, given only an estimate of the proportion of units in class 1 (that is, of a) and an estimate of E (the TRANSFER effect), it is possible first to calculate a value for D (since $D = 1/(2-E)$) and then a value for b, the proportion of units in class 3. Since the sum of the proportions in each class must be unity it is simple to derive an estimate for classes 2 and 4 by subtraction.

The data of Hubel & Wiesel (1968) provide a means of testing this model. They classified monkey cortical cells into seven dominance classes and their text-figure 14 shows how their sample of 177 units were distributed among these classes. These data, however, describe dominance classes in terms of whether the dominant eye was ipsilateral or contralateral to the hemisphere from .which the recordings were made, rather in terms of their being left-eye or right-eye dominant. Assume that all of these recordings were taken from the left hemisphere; then units described as contralaterally driven would be driven by the right eye, and units described as ipsilaterally driven would be driven by the left eye. Now assume that a similar distribution could be found in the right hemisphere: 'contralateral' would mean left-eye driven and 'ipsilateral' right-eye driven. To obtain an estimate of the proportions of cells, in both hemispheres taken together, that are driven by a particular eye, it would be necessary to take the two hypothetical identical distributions described above and to fold one on to the other. In this way the so-called ispilateral units from the left hemisphere (left eye driven) would be added to the so-called contralateral units from the right hemisphere (also left-eye driven), so that the classes are added as follows: $1+7$, $2+6$, $3+5$, $4+4$, $5+3$, $6+2$, $7+1$. If the distributions resulting from this 'foldover' transform are then collapsed so that the new classes 2 and 3, and 5 and 6 are combined, a five-class categorization results in which the characteristics of the units in each class matches those of the units in the five-class model described above.

TABLE 7. ESTIMATING THE PROPORTION OF UNITS IN EACH DOMINANCE CLASS

(The upper row shows the data from Hubel & Wiesel (1968), text-figure 14, transformed as described in the text. The lower row shows the distribution estimated from the model given the value of 17.3 % for a, the proportion of units in class 1 and class 5, and the value of 52.4 % for the relative magnitude of the TRANSFER (E) effect, based upon expression (4) in the text: $b = 2DE + 2a - 1$.)

dominance class...	1	2	3	4	5
distribution from Hubel & Wiesel	17.3%	30.2%	5%	30.2%	17.3%
estimated distribution	(17.3%)	29.9%	5.6%	29.9%	(17.3%)

The proportion of units in class 1 and in class 5 computed in this way is 0.173 (17.3%). From three m.a.e. experiments and one t.a.e. experiment (a total of 41 subjects and 289 observations) an average value for the TRANSFER effect (E) of 0.524 (52.4%) was obtained. (The data from these experiments are given in full in Moulden (1974).) The derived value for the MON–BIN effect (D), from the expression $D = 1/(2 - E)$, is 0.678 (67.8%). These values may be substituted in (4) to give $b = 2(0.678)(0.524) + 2(0.173) - 1 = 0.056$. The estimated proportion of units in class 3 is thus 5.6%, and by subtraction the proportions in class 2 and in class 4 are 29.9%. In table 7 these estimates are compared with the observed values from Hubel & Wiesel (1968).

The agreement is at first sight very impressive, but a number of qualifying factors must be borne in mind. The predicted distribution is actually derived from the prediction of only one value, that for the proportion of units in class 3 (5.6%). While the difference between this figure and the observed value of 5% is apparently small, the discrepancy of 0.6%, when expressed as a proportion of the predicted value, actually represents an error in prediction of 12%. Moreover, the statistical reliability of the Hubel & Wiesel estimates is indeterminate; the estimates derived above are based upon the implausible assumption that binocular units fire as strongly to one eye as to both together; and the obtained values depend critically upon the obtained value of transfer (here 52.4%), and a difference of a small percentage in this value makes a dramatic difference to the predictions. The agreement in this case should perhaps be taken as indicating only that the model outlined here is not inconsistent with electrophysiologically derived dominance distributions.

4. CONCLUSION

The model described here is based upon the assumptions that sets of cortical units making up a channel in the human visual system may be partitioned exhaustively into five mutually exclusive subsets of specified dominance, and that effects generated within these subsets are independent and linearly additive. An after-effect generated in a particular viewing mode thus depends upon the ratio between the number of tested units that have previously been adapted and the total number of units tested.

A few details remain to be settled. First, several workers (see, for example, Henry *et al.* 1969; Creutzfeldt *et al.* 1971; Noda *et al.* 1971) have described a very few binocular units for which stimulation via one eye was excitatory while stimulation via the other eye was inhibitory; it is difficult to assess the impact of this discovery upon the plausibility of the model described here. Secondly, Lehmkuhle & Fox (1976) have shown that interocular transfer is increased in magnitude if the non-adapted eye, rather than being occluded (as it was in the experiments described here), views a homogeneous bright field during the inspection phase. The present model can offer no explanation for this phenomenon. Finally, Wade & Wenderoth (1978), using a homogeneous field rather than occlusion for the unadapted eye during the inspection phase, failed to confirm that the condition MON–BIN results in a smaller tilt after-effect than either MON–MON, BIN–BIN or BIN–MON. The reason for this discrepancy is unclear.

Nevertheless, the broad features of the model appear to be well established, and it has two particular merits, namely simplicity and explicitness, which make it easy to test. One particularly intriguing possibility concerns the use of cyclopean stimuli, which would permit one to drive the binocular units without involving the monocular units. By using purely cyclopean stimuli in the inspection (or test) phases and monocular or binocular stimuli in the test (or inspection) phases, it would be possible to derive an independent estimate of the contribution of binocular units to an after-effect; this should agree with the estimates put forward in this paper.

My thanks are due to Professor N. S. Sutherland for his support and encouragement at every stage of the preparation of this paper.

REFERENCES (Moulden)

Creutzfeldt, O. D., Pöppel, E. & Singer, W. 1971 Quantitiver Ansatz zur Analyse der funktionallen Organisation des visuellen Cortex. In *1970 Kybernetik* (ed. O. J. Grüsser), pp. 81–96. Berlin: Springer.

Henry, G. H., Bishop, P. O. & Coombs, J. S. 1969 Inhibitory and subliminal excitatory receptive fields of simple cells in cat striate cortex. *Vision Res.* 9, 1289–1296.

Hess, R. 1978 Interocular transfer in individuals with strabismic amblyopia: a cautionary note. *Perception* 7, 201–205.

Hubel, D. H. & Wiesel, T. N. 1968 Receptive fields and functional architecture of monkey striate cortex. *J. Physiol., Lond.* 195, 215–244.

Lehmkuhle, S. W. & Fox, R. 1975 Binocular interaction of the motion after-effect: a simple model. Paper presented to A.R.V.O., Sarasota.

Lehmkuhle, S. W. & Fox, R. 1976 On measuring interocular transfer. *Vision Res.* 16, 428–430.

Mollon, J. 1974 After-effects and the brain. *New Scient.*, 21 Feb., pp. 479–482.

Moulden, B. 1974 Ph.D. thesis, University of Reading.

Moulden, B. & Mather, G. 1978 In defence of a ratio model for movement detection at threshold. *Q. Jl exp. Psychol.* 30, 505–520.

Movshon, J. A., Chambers, B. E. I. & Blakemore, C. 1972 Interocular transfer in normal humans and those who lack stereopsis. *Perception* 1, 483–490.

Noda, H., Creutzfeldt, O. D. & Freeman, R. B. 1971 Binocular interaction in the visual cortex of awake cats. *Expl Brain Res.* 12, 406–421.

Sutherland, N. S. 1961 Figural after-effects and apparent size. *Q. Jl exp. Psychol.* 231, 222–228.

Wade, N. J. 1976 On interocular transfer of the movement after-effect in individuals with and without normal binocular vision. *Perception* 5, 113–118.

Wade, N. J. & Wenderoth, P. 1978 The influence of colour and contour on the magnitude of the tilt after-effect. *Vision Res.* 18, 827–835.

Phil. Trans. R. Soc. Lond. B **290**, 57–69 (1980)
Printed in Great Britain

The persistences of vision

By M. Coltheart

Department of Psychology, Birkbeck College, Malet Street, London WC1E 7HX, U.K.

Human observers continue to experience a visual stimulus for some time after the offset of that stimulus.

The neural activity evoked by a visual stimulus continues for some time after its offset.

The information extracted from a visual stimulus continues to be registered in a visual form of memory ('iconic memory') for some time after its offset.

We may thus distinguish three distinct senses in which a visual stimulus may be said to persist after its physical offset: there is phenomenological persistence, neural persistence and informational persistence. Various assumptions have been made about the relation between these three forms of visual persistence. The most frequent assumption is that they correspond simply to three different methods for studying a single entity. Detailed consideration of what is known about the properties of these three forms of persistence suggests, however, that this assumption is not correct. It can reasonably be proposed that visible persistence is the phenomenological correlate of neural persistence occurring at various stages of the visual system: photoreceptors, ganglion cells and the stereopsis system. Iconic memory, on the other hand, does not correspond to visible persistence, nor to neural persistence in any stage of the visual system. Recent work, in fact, suggests that iconic memory is a property of some relatively late stage in the visual information-processing system, rather than being a peripheral sensory buffer store. This suggestion raises some fundamental theoretical issues concerning the psychology of visual perception, issues with which cognitive psychology has yet to come to grips.

Three persistences of vision

Visual scientists have for a century or more used the term *persistence of vision* to refer to a variety of visual phenomena having in common that they suggest that visual sensation is prolonged for some time after the physical offset of the visual stimulus. In this paper I wish first of all to show that there are three qualitatively different types of visual phenomenon that have been described as persistences of vision. This ambiguity in the usage of the term persistence of vision has not always been recognized.

When this ambiguity *has* been recognized, the assumption has been made that the ambiguity is not important because the three types of visual effect are merely three sides of the same coin: three different ways of looking at the same entity. I shall suggest that this is not so, and that if confusion is to be avoided one must distinguish between these three senses of the term 'visual persistence', and acknowledge that they may be mediated by different mechanisms.

I shall begin by explaining what I mean by the claim that there are three kinds of visual persistence. Two were known to Newton in the seventeenth century, as the quotation from the *Opticks* reveals:

And when a Coal of Fire moved nimbly in the circumference of a circle makes the whole circumference appear like a Circle of Fire; is it not because the Motions excited in the bottom of the Eye by the Rays of Light are of a lasting nature, and continue till the Coal of Fire in going round returns to its former place?

Here Newton proposed two things. The first is that the sensation produced by a visual stimulus continues to be experienced for some time after the physical offset of that stimulus. This observation belongs to the realm of phenomenology. Observations of this kind are often adduced in discussions of visual persistence. To refer to these effects I will use the term *visible* persistence.

Secondly, Newton hypothesized that the retinal activity produced by a visual stimulus continues to occur for some time after the physical offset of the stimulus. This is a hypothesis about neurophysiology, and the effect Newton speculated about will here be termed *neural* persistence.

Newton argued that visible persistence was explained by neural persistence in the retina. Clearly, however, this is only a hypothesis, and the relation between 'visible persistence' and 'neural persistence' must be elucidated by experiment. Furthermore, even if visible persistence is caused by neural persistence in the visual system, this persistence need not be entirely retinal; it need not be retinal at all.

The third form of persistence of vision was discovered by Sperling (1960). This discovery relied upon a methodological innovation, which I shall describe briefly. Suppose a visual display consisting of a 3×4 matrix of letters is presented to an observer for a brief period, say 50 ms. If the observer is asked to report as many of these letters as he can, he will average about 4.5 correct. This value is reasonably invariant across observers, laboratories, and indeed centuries, since experiments of this kind were carried out in the nineteenth century, with comparable results. Why is it that only about one-third of the letters in a brief 12-letter display can be reported? The answer to this question still eludes us; but certain obvious answers can be ruled out. Firstly, it might be that the visual recognition of items in a multi-item display is a serial process, and a display time of 50 ms permits only four of five individual acts of recognition. This can be ruled out, because if one shortens the display duration to 15 ms, or increases it to 500 ms, the number of items reported scarcely changes at all.

A second idea might be that the visual recognition of items is a parallel process, but one with limited capacity: it can deal with only four or five items at once, and after this some form of refractoriness intervenes. Thus only four or five of the items are stored in memory; the remaining seven or eight simply go unregistered.

Sperling's methodological innovation, *the partial-report technique,* provided evidence that ruled out this idea. When this technique is used, the subject is asked to report, not the entire display, but only some subset of the items. For example, on a particular trial he might be asked to report the items in the top row, or the red items, or the items containing a curved contour, or the highest-contrast items. Take the first of these as an example: one actually does the experiment by training an observer to associate a tone of high frequency with the top row, a medium frequency tone with the middle row and a low frequency tone with the low row.

Suppose, now, that the cue tone is presented to the subject immediately *after* the display has been switched off, and that the selection of high, medium and low tones is completely random. Under these conditions, the observer will be unable to predict during the physical presence of the display which of its three rows he will be asked to report. It will therefore be impossible for him to favour the items he is to report over other items in his visual processing during the physical duration of the display.

Now, if only four or five items from such a display can be registered in memory, and if these must be a random selection with respect to the row which will be cued, then it follows that the observer should be able to report 4.5/3 = 1.5 items from the row which is cued. This was not so with Sperling's observers: they averaged three out of a maximum possible of four. This must mean that, at the time at which the observer learns from the cue which row he is to report, he must have available in memory at least three items from each of the three display rows, that is, at least nine items are registered in memory. This is so in spite of the fact that when observers attempt to report all of the items from the display, they average only 4.5 items. The difference between the estimates of items in memory obtained with the partial report and the full report method is known as the *partial-report superiority*. When Sperling studied the effect of varying the delay between display offset and cue onset, he found that the size of the partial-report superiority declined as the cue delay increased; at delays of several hundred milliseconds or a few seconds (depending upon experimental conditions) no superiority is observed.

These results suggest the following interpretation. Immediately after the offset of the display, most of its items are held in a form of memory which is of high capacity but which is subject to rapid decay. Any item that is to be reported must be transferred to a second form of memory which is not subject to rapid decay, and hence which permits leisurely report. Only about four or five items can be transferred in this way, but the observer is capable of choosing which of the items in the transient high-capacity memory are to be transferred to the more durable memory. For example, he can choose to transfer the top row of items, or the red items, or the items containing a curved contour, or the high-contrast items.

The transient high-capacity memory responsible for the partial report superiority was subsequently named *iconic memory* by Neisser (1967) and his term will be adopted here. This memory is our third form of persistence of vision. It is not phenomenologically defined, as is visible persistence; it is not a neurophysiological entity, as is neural persistence; its essential characteristic is that it is *informational*: it preserves in rapidly decaying form the information that was present in a visual display.

There are thus three distinct senses in which a visual stimulus may be said to persist after its physical offset: the stimulus may continue to be experienced (visible persistence); the responses of stages of the visual system may go on occurring (neural persistence); and the visual information contained in the stimulus may continue to be available (iconic memory).

Consider now what relations may exist between these three visual phenomena. Newton believed, as we have seen, that visible persistence is the phenomenal manifestation of neural (specifically retinal) persistence. It is widely assumed that visible persistence is the phenomenal manifestation of iconic memory – that is, that iconic memory is visible. For example: 'the "short-term visual memory" of Sperling (1960) is a detailed texture memory but fades out in 0.1 sec like the afterglow of a cathode ray tube, and is merely an afterimage' (Julesz 1971, p. 103); and '(an) indicator of the visual persistence of a flash . . . yields data of the same high order of reliability and magnitude found by the far more laborious and indirect procedures of Sperling (1960)' (Haber & Standing 1970). Finally, iconic memory has been identified with neural persistence: 'the information about the icon is stored primarily inside the rod photo-receptors' (Sakitt 1975). A conflation of the views of Newton, Julesz, Haber and Sakitt results in the claim that visible persistence, neural persistence and iconic memory, are different manifestations of a single entity – the persistence of vision.

Despite the widespread nature of this claim, it has never been investigated or defended, except by Sakitt, whose work is discussed later. In particular, the identification of visible persistence with iconic memory is an assumption that has not been questioned, let alone defended.

One way of attempting to discover what the relations are between visible persistence, neural persistence and iconic memory is to determine what properties characterize each of these entities and to consider whether the three sets of properties coincide, as they must if visible persistence is neural persistence and neural persistence is iconic memory. I approach this by first surveying what is known about visible persistence.

VISIBLE PERSISTENCE

Methods for the study of visible persistence

Visible persistence has received much attention in the past 15 years, though its investigators have proceeded with a curious independence and a fine disregard for each other's findings. The basic phenomenon is that a visual stimulus goes on being visible for some time after its physical offset; and seven different experimental methods have been used in recent years to investigate this phenomenon.

(1) *Judgement of synchrony.* The physical offset of a visual test stimulus is followed after some delay by a brief probe stimulus. The observer adjusts this delay until the onset of the probe stimulus coincides exactly in time with the apparent disappearance of the visual test stimulus. The delay between test stimulus offset and probe stimulus onset is taken as a measure of the duration of visible persistence. This method has been used by Sperling (1967), Efron (1970 *a, b, c*), Haber & Standing (1970) and Bowen *et al.* (1974).

(2) *Onset-offset reaction times.* In one block of trials, the observer responds as rapidly as he can to the onset of a visual stimulus. In another block, he responds as rapidly as he can to the offset of the stimulus. On the assumption that offset responses are made to the termination of the visible persistence of the stimulus, substraction of onset reaction time from offset reaction time provides a measure of the duration of visible persistence. This method has been used by Rains (1961), Pease & Sticht (1965), Bartlett *et al.* (1968) and Briggs & Kinsbourne (1972).

(3) *Stroboscopic illumination of a moving stimulus.* If a moving object is stroboscopically illuminated, and if velocity and flash rate are suitably chosen, the nth illumination of the object will occur while the visible persistence generated by the $(n-1)$th illumination is still present. Thus two objects will be seen. Increases in velocity or flash rate will cause three, four or more objects to be seen. From the maximum interflash time at which two objects are seen one can calculate the maximum duration of visible persistence. This method has been used by Allport (1966, 1970), Mollon (1969), Efron & Lee (1971) and Dixon & Hammond (1972).

(4) *Viewing through a moving slit.* When you walk beside a paling fence and look at a cricket match through the interstices of the fence, an appropriate speed of walking will allow you to see the scene as a whole, even though at any one instance only half of it, divided up into a series of vertical slices, is available to your retina. A simplification is to look at a figure hidden behind an opaque card on which a vertical slit is cut. As the slit is moved to and fro across the figure, the whole figure can be seen, provided the eyes are stationary with respect to the figure. This occurs because visible persistences of adjacent figure segments are generated on adjacent retinal areas. The slowest slit traverse time at which the whole figure remains continuously visible is a measure of the duration of visible persistence. This method has been used by Anstis & Atkinson (1967), Haber & Nathanson (1968), Haber & Standing (1969) and Stanley & Molloy (1975).

(5) *Phenomenal continuity.* When a visual stimulus is repeatedly switched on and off, it appears to be present continuously if the off-time is short enough, since the visible persistence of the

stimulus bridges this temporal gap. The maximum off-time at which the stimulus is phenomenally continuously present is a measure of the duration of visual persistence. This method has been used by Haber & Standing (1969), Meyer *et al.* (1975) and Meyer (1977).

(6) *Temporal integration of form parts.* This is Newton's coal-whirling technique. If a visual form is broken up into parts, and the different parts displayed at different times, the whole form will be seen, provided that the part displayed first is still visibly persisting at the time of presentation of the part displayed last. The maximum temporal interval between first and last parts at which the form is seen as a whole is a measure of the duration of visible persistence. This method has been used not only by Newton but also by Eriksen & Collins (1967, 1968), Pollack (1973), Hogben & di Lollo (1974), di Lollo (1977), di Lollo & Wilson (1978) and di Lollo (1980).

(7) *Stereoscopic persistence.* This method has been described in an important but neglected paper by Engel (1970). It has been known for many years that, if the two members of a stereoscopic stimulus-pair are briefly displayed to their respective eyes at different times, stereopsis can be experienced if the interstimulus interval is brief enough. This indicates that information from the leading stimulus must be available to the stereopsis mechanisms for some time after the offset of that stimulus. Engel's contribution was to investigate the persistence of the stereoscopic sensation itself. Given that two asynchronous stimuli, one to each eye, have generated a stereoscopic sensation, how long can one wait before re-presenting the two stimuli, without causing a discontinuity in the experience of stereopsis? Visible persistence of stereoscopic depth measured in this way can last as long as 300 ms after the offset of the lagging monocular stimulus.

Properties of visible persistence

Studies with the use of these seven methods show that a visual stimulus continues to be visible for some hundreds of milliseconds after its physical offset. More importantly, these studies provide information about the relation between the duration of such visible persistence and two parameters of the stimulus: its duration and its intensity. In both cases, the relation is counter-intuitive. The greater the duration of the stimulus, the *shorter* is the time for which it continues to be visible after its offset (Efron 1970*a*, *c*; Haber & Standing 1970; Bowen *et al.* 1974; Briggs & Kinsbourne 1972; di Lollo 1977). The greater the luminance or contrast of the stimulus, the *shorter* is the time for which it continues to be visible after its offset (Bowen *et al.* 1974; Pease & Sticht 1965; Bartlett *et al.* 1968; Allport 1970; Efron & Lee 1971; Dixon & Hammond 1972; Haber & Standing 1969; Pollack 1973). I shall refer to these two results as the *inverse duration effect* and *the inverse intensity effect*. They provide a signature for visible persistence. Any phenomenon that is said to be reducible to visible persistence must itself display both of these effects; if it does not, then it cannot be identified with visible persistence. In addition, any hypothesis that seeks to explain visible persistence must be able to explain why there are inverse effects of duration and intensity.

Having described the methods used to study visible persistence, and the two properties of visible persistence revealed by experiments with the use of these methods, I turn now to the second persistence: neural persistence. My comments will be brief, since my acquaintance with visual neurophysiology is a superficial one. Nevertheless, I attempt to consider whether neural persistence occurs, and, if it does, at what locus or loci in the visual system it occurs. A discussion of this kind provides a basis for evaluating Newton's hypothesis that visible persistence is due to the lasting nature of the Motions excited in the bottom of the Eye by Light.

Neural persistence

The first locus that I shall consider is the late receptor potential (r.p.) of rods and cones. Recordings in the macaque monkey by Whitten & Brown (1973 *a*, *b*, *c*) as well as in other species (rat, cat, mudpuppy) by Steinberg (1969), Penn & Hagins (1972) and Fain & Dowling (1973) have shown that both the rods and the cones continue to transmit signals for some time after stimulus offset. The cone signal, however, decays away rapidly, whereas the rod signal has a relatively long constant of decay (see, for example, Whitten & Brown 1973 *a*, figs. 7, 9 and 14 *a*). Therefore neural persistence exists at the photoreceptor level, especially in the rods. Consequently, one might make Newton's hypothesis more specific by identifying 'Motions excited in the bottom of the Eye' with 'receptor potentials', and proposing that visible persistence is due to the prolongation of the receptor potential.

Any hypothesis about the neural basis of visible persistence must be capable of explaining the inverse intensity and duration effects. This appears to present problems for a hypothesis based on the receptor potential, since Whitten & Brown (1973 *a*) found that as stimulus intensity increased, both the rod r.p. and the cone r.p. increased in duration: in other words, there was a *direct* relation, not an inverse one, between stimulus intensity and duration of neural persistence. However, it may be possible to deal with this problem. It has been suggested by Whitten & Brown (1973 *b*), Makous & Boothe (1974) and Stabell & Stabell (1976) that cones inhibit rods. In mesopic conditions, rod r.ps last longer than cone r.ps. As one increases intensity within the mesopic range, cones will respond more and more strongly, and hence exert greater and greater inhibition on rods. The net effect of this could be that the rod r.p. becomes shorter and shorter as intensity increases in the mesopic range, if the inhibitory effect of cones outweighs the direct effect of increasing intensity on the duration of the rod r.p. and since in the mesopic range the rod r.p. lasts longer than the cone r.p., the maximum duration of the r.p. could show an inverse intensity effect.

This argument cannot apply to scotopic or photopic vision; it therefore makes the strong prediction that the inverse intensity effect will only be obtained with intensities in the mesopic range, a prediction that would be simple to investigate. It seems probable that the studies of visible persistence demonstrating the inverse intensity effect have used intensities generally within the mesopic range; if there are any that have not, they would provide data relevant to the r.p. hypothesis.

Thus something (albeit speculative) can be said about the way in which the r.p. hypothesis can explain the inverse intensity effect. But what of the inverse duration effect? One might argue that the cone inhibitory effect accumulates while the stimulus is present. This could be investigated in experiments like those of Whitten & Brown if stimulus duration were varied systematically, something that they did not try. An alternative possibility is that, if the intensity effect operates at the r.p. stage, perhaps the duration effect operates the next stage – the ganglion cell?

When one records from retinal ganglion cells, at least two types of cell can be distinguished: transient cells and sustained cells. Sustained cells respond during the presence of the stimulus; after stimulus offset, their activity begins to diminish, and decays away relatively more slowly to the pre-stimulus level. This form of neural persistence might produce visible persistence.

It has been proposed by, for example, Breitmeyer & Ganz (1975) that transient cells inhibit sustained cells. If so, transient cells could act to curtail visible persistence. This might explain why visible persistence duration is shorter for low-frequency grating stimuli than for high-frequency grating stimuli (Meyer & Maguire 1977): transient cells are known to be selectively sensitive to low spatial frequencies.

Evoked-potential results reported by Servière *et al.* (1977*a*, *b*) might be taken as evidence that, when stimulus duration is varied, the latency of the transient off-response decreases linearly as stimulus duration increases, up to a stimulus duration of about 60 ms. At longer durations, off-response latency was independent of stimulus duration. If this off-response curtails visible persistence, then the relation between visible persistence duration and stimulus duration will be an inverse one up to some critical value, after which visible persistence duration will be independent of stimulus duration; this is the result obtained by Efron (1970*a*, *c*).

Thus the hypothesis that neural persistence of the sustained class of retinal ganglion cells is one basis for visible persistence may provide an explanation of the inverse duration effect. The hypothesis that persistence of the receptor potential is also a neural basis for visible persistence may provide an explanation of the inverse intensity effect. Even two neural loci are not enough, however, because the stereoscopic visible persistence studied by Engel (1970) must have a cortical locus.

These suggestions, the neurophysiological speculations of a cognitive psychologist, can be evaluated directly, simply by detailed comparisons between appropriate psychophysical data (obtained in experiments on visible persistence) and neurophysiological data (obtained in experiments studying neural persistence), and it is to be hoped that such data will become available. In the meantime, one can take the view that Newton may have been correct in proposing that visible persistence is due to neural persistence, although he would have to admit now that the neural persistence is not only in the 'bottom of the Eye' (receptors and ganglion cells) but also in the cortex (stereopsis system).

ICONIC MEMORY

Having made some suggestions as to the relation beween visible persistence and neural persistence, we are left with two questions. The first is, what is the relation between iconic memory and visible persistence? The second is, what is the relation between iconic memory and neural persistence?

Iconic memory and visible persistence

There is a fairly direct way of assessing the assumption (Julesz & Chiarucci 1973; Haber & Standing 1970) that iconic memory *is* visible persistence. If this assumption is correct, the duration of iconic memory will be greater for short or weak stimuli than for long or intense stimuli.

It has been demonstrated by Keele & Chase (1967), Eriksen & Rohrbaugh (1970), Scharf & Lefton (1970) and Adelson & Jonides (1978) that the duration of iconic memory does *not* diminish when stimulus intensity is increased. It has been demonstrated by Sperling (1960) and di Lollo (1978) that the duration of iconic memory does *not* diminish when stimulus duration is increased. Thus the inverse intensity and duration effects characteristic of visible persistence are not properties of iconic memory. In my view this represents a conclusive demonstration that iconic memory and visible persistence are completely different phenomena.

Further work relevant to this question which has been done is the investigation of iconic memory with direction of movement as the stimulus feature used in partial report. Russell

(1977), Treisman *et al.* (1975) and Demkiw & Michaels (1976) showed that when a display of moving stimuli was presented and followed by a cue requesting report of the direction of movement of the cued stimuli, typical iconic memory results were obtained. There was a partial report superiority which diminished as cue delay increased. Russell (1977) notes that his subjects did not report seeing a persisting impression of movement; yet their iconic memories included information about movement. A more rigorous argument could be developed if one carried out an experiment in which, by using one of the methods described earlier, the duration of visible persistence of movement was actually measured.

The third and final point to be made here concerns comparisons between the durations of visible persistence and of iconic memory. It is sometimes argued that these durations have been found to be roughly equal in magnitude, and this is offered as evidence that the two phenomena are really one. Such claims overlook an important factor in partial-report experiments: cue-decoding time. The subject must decode the partial-report cue to determine which subset of the items in iconic memory are requested for report. The decoding process cannot be instantaneous; it must take time. In fact, the time required to decode a partial report cue was measured by Averbach & Coriell (1961), and in their experiment this time was about 270 ms. This means that a cue presented simultaneously with display offset is not applied to the contents of iconic memory until 270 ms later, and during this time iconic memory will have decayed considerably. Hence estimates of the lifetime of iconic memory as derived from partial report experiments will be underestimates; they must be corrected by adding cue-decoding time, which can be as much as 270 ms. When this is done, then there is no longer much coincidence between the duration of iconic memory (as measured by partial report experiments) and the duration of visible persistence (as measured by any of the seven methods described earlier). Visible persistence durations are much shorter than iconic memory durations. This is clearest in data provided by Averbach & Sperling (1961), indicating an iconic memory lasting for some seconds; in all studies of visible persistence, its duration is considerably less than a second.

The relation of iconic memory to visible persistence needs further investigation, but, in view of the three points made here, it seems most unlikely that the claim of identity between iconic memory and visible persistence will be salvaged by further work.

Iconic memory and neural persistence

Considerations of the relation between iconic memory and neural persistence have been brought into sharp focus by the work of Sakitt (1975, 1976 *a, b*). Her view is that iconic memory and visible persistence are the same thing and that their neural basis is persistence of activity in rods and cones, the important factor being the neural persistence of rods, since cone persistence is much briefer than rod persistence. Here I shall consider her view that iconic memory depends upon photoreceptor persistence, especially rod persistence. It seems to me that there are a number of difficulties for this view.

The first point is that iconic memory includes information about direction of rotary or linear movement (Russell 1977; Treisman *et al.* 1975; Demkiw & Michaels 1976). How could the persisting activity of photoreceptors encode this kind of dynamic information?

Secondly, it seems unlikely that a brief visual stimulus could evoke in the rod system a burst of activity that persists for a second or more. None of the recordings of photoreceptor persistence in non-human species suggest that its duration can approach the duration of iconic memory as measured in partial report experiments.

Thirdly, experiments by Eriksen & Hoffman (1973) and Eriksen & Eriksen (1974) are difficult to interpret if one argues that the iconic memory for a visual display consists of a complex pattern of persistences in photoreceptors, and selection from iconic memory consists of selection of a part of this pattern for further analysis, the remainder of the sensory data receiving no further analysis. Eriksen and his colleagues used a row of three letters as a visual display. The subject's task was to classify the central letter; for example, to move a lever one way if it was an H or an M, and a different way if it was an A or U. The latency of this movement was influenced by the nature of the flanking non-target letters; latency was reduced if they belonged to the same category as the target letter, and increased if they belonged to the opposite category. Therefore on some occasions at least the non-target letters must have been categorized too. This shows that, even when there is no uncertainty at all as to which information in iconic memory is to be selected for further analysis and which is irrelevant, nevertheless the irrelevant information is also given further analysis to a profound level. The most natural interpretation of this is that all of the information in iconic memory has been given full analysis, and that iconic memory is not an early sensory stage in the information-processing sequence, but a late stage that *follows*, not precedes, stimulus identification. This is discussed further below.

Decisive work relevant to the assertion that iconic memory is photoreceptor (primarily rod) persistence remains to be carried out, however. There are at least two clear avenues to be pursued here. The first concerns iconic memory for colour. If cone persistence is very brief, then colour information should be available only very briefly in iconic memory. Therefore, if one can show that colour information persists in iconic memory for a relatively long time, this would be evidence against a photoreceptor locus for iconic memory. Several studies of this issue have recently been published (Banks & Barber 1977; Adelson 1978), but it is not yet established whether colour information does persist for relatively long durations in iconic memory.

A second important topic here is stereoscopic iconic memory. The general idea is that, if an iconic memory is generated by stereoscopic stimulation, it must be a cortical and hence not a retinal iconic memory. It would not be sufficient, however, to show that partial-report superiority occurs when a display is presented as a stereo pair. Persistence of the individual monocular stimuli at the photoreceptor level would be sufficient to account for a partial-report superiority in this stereoscopic situation. What is required is to adopt the methods of Engel (1970): these methods allow independent measurement of monocular persistence and stereoscopic persistence. If such an experiment showed that the duration of a stereoscopically generated iconic memory is too long to be accounted for in terms of persistence in monocular channels feeding the stereopsis system, then definitive evidence would have been obtained for the existence of an iconic memory whose neural locus is cortical, and hence evidence obtained against the view that iconic memory is photoreceptor persistence.

The nature of iconic memory

In contemporary models of the psychology of perception, iconic memory is regarded as a peripheral buffer store which holds unprocessed visual information, allowing the processing mechanisms sufficient time to perform operations upon visual input in conditions where the display duration itself is too short to allow the completion of these operations. The partial report superiority is interpreted as an indication that the perceiver can perform these operations selectively, on certain items in iconic memory rather than on others.

It has been pointed out by van der Heijden (1978) that this view of the nature of iconic memory is at variance with another body of literature on the psychology of perception, namely, work showing that visual identification is non-selective and automatic. For example, the work of Eriksen described above indicates circumstances in which a subject cannot direct his processing operations to a certain item and away from other items, even when to do so would improve his performance. Van der Heijden (1978) showed that a subject's rapid naming of a colour patch presented to one side of a fixation point was affected by the nature of a printed word presented to the other side of the fixation point, even though the subject was not required to process the word in any way. These two examples suggest that subjects cannot use a spatial criterion to select certain unprocessed visual inputs for further processing and to prevent further processing of unwanted visual inputs. Instead, it appears that given adequate visual registration *all* inputs are processed, and selection follows this processing.

An attempt at demonstrating this directly is reported by Allport (1978). His tachistoscopic display consisted of four words. One was always the name of an animal. Subjects were asked to report as many words from a display as they could, but to give special priority to animal names. Suppose that the stage at which the information extracted from a visual display decays rapidly is before the stage at which items are identified. If this is so, requiring subjects to favour items belonging to a particular semantic category will be ineffective: the favouring of items operates at the rapidly decaying stage, whereas the semantic category of an item is not known until a subsequent stage. On this reasoning, which relies on the usual view of iconic memory as an early sensory buffer store, the subjects in Allport's experiment should be no better at reporting animal names than any other words from the display. However, report of animal names *was* superior. This suggests that there is significant rapid decay of information at some stage *after* the meanings of briefly displayed words have been established. If this rapid decay, responsible for partial report superiority, is the signature of iconic memory, then iconic memory is not a peripheral buffer store, but a much later stage in the system.

In my view, this conceptualization of the nature of iconic memory will gain ground rapidly in the future; experiments like those of Eriksen, van der Heijden and Allport will provide a body of evidence indicating that iconic memory is not an entirely pre-categorical or pre-identificatory system. At the same time, it must be admitted that this approach to the nature of iconic memory raises extremely difficult theoretical problems, which will be very briefly sketched here.

The meanings of words are represented in some form of permanent long-term memory; this will here be termed the *internal lexicon* (see Coltheart 1978; Coltheart *et al.* 1978). An individual word is represented in this lexicon as a *lexical entry*. To understand a printed word one must gain access to its lexical entry. Clearly this process, lexical access, must proceed regardless of the particular visual form of the printed word: the lexical entry for 'tree' must be accessible from TREE, tree, handwritten forms of the word, and so on. It would be chaotic to have different lexical entries for different visual representations of the same word. However, if the same entry is accessed by a variety of visual forms, the lexical access process itself provides no information about the particular visual form of the word whose lexical entry is accessed. How then, when presented with (STEEL mouse), do we know that 'STEEL' was in capitals and 'mouse' in lower case? This difficulty can be described in terms of the distinction drawn by Tulving (1972) between semantic memory and episodic memory. Semantic memory is memory for facts about the world (such as the meaning of the word 'tree'). Episodic memory is memory for events that have happened to us (such as seeing a pair of words a few lines above, one in capitals and one in lower case). The difficulty to which I am drawing attention here is the coordination of semantic memory with episodic memory. Semantic memory tells us that one of (STEEL mouse) is a metal and the other an animal. Episodic memory tells us that what we saw was a word in capitals and one in lower case. What tells us that the metal was printed in capitals and the animal in lower case?

Presumably, in some way impossible to envisage at present, episodic information becomes temporarily attached to a lexical entry. If this temporary episodic information is subject to rapid decay when it has been obtained hurriedly from a brief display, then perhaps iconic memory consists of the attachment of episodic information to a lexical entry.

CONCLUSIONS

I began by distinguishing three senses in which one might say that vision persists. There is visible persistence: visual stimuli continue to be visible for some time after their physical offset. There is neural persistence: at various stages in the visual system, neural activity evoked by a stimulus continues to occur for some time after stimulus offset. There is informational persistence ('iconic memory'): the sensory information contained in a visual display remains available to an observer for some time after stimulus offset. The relation between these three persistences of vision has not been established. It has sometimes been claimed that all three are manifestations of a single process looked at from three different perspectives.

I have proposed that visible persistence is in fact the phenomenological correlate of neural persistence (in fact, of neural persistences, since persistences at the level of the receptor potential, the ganglion cell, and the stereopsis system may all generate forms of visible persistence). Iconic memory is another matter. There are reasons for rejecting an identification of iconic memory with visible persistence. There are also reasons for rejecting an identification of iconic memory with neural persistence, at least at the retinal level. The nature of iconic memory thus remains obscure. A possibility is that iconic memory, rather than representing an early stage in the information-processing sequence (a peripheral sensory buffer store), arises at a very late stage, after stimulus identification. To develop this possibility into a theory, it will be necessary to explain how episodic and semantic information about a stimulus may be coordinated. This is at present beyond the capabilities of cognitive psychology; it is the fundamental question for the psychology of perception.

REFERENCES (Coltheart)

Adelson, E. H. 1978 Iconic storage: the role of rods. *Science, N.Y.* **11**, 544–546.
Adelson, E. H. & Jonides, J. 1978 The psychophysics of iconic storage. Presented at Psychonomic Society meeting.
Allport, D. A. 1966 Studies in the psychological unit of duration. Ph.D. thesis, University of Cambridge.
Allport, D. A. 1970 Temporal summation and phenomenal simultaneity: experiments with the radius display. *Q. Jl exp. Psychol.* **22**, 686–701.
Allport, D. A. 1978 On knowing the meaning of words we are unable to report: the effects of visual masking. In *Attention and Performance*, vol. 6 (ed. E. Dornic), pp. 505–534. Hillsdale: Erlbaum Press.
Anstis, S. M. & Atkinson, J. 1967 Distortions in moving figures viewed through a stationary slit. *Am. J. Psychol.* **80**, 572–585.
Averbach, E. & Coriell, A. S. 1961 Short-term memory in vision. *Bell Syst. tech. J.* **40**, 309–328.
Averbach, E. & Sperling, G. 1961 Short term storage of information in vision. In *Information theory* (ed. C. Cherry). London: Butterworth.
Banks, W. P. & Barber, G. 1977 Color information in iconic memory. *Psychol. Rev.* **84**, 536–546.
Bartlett, N. R., Sticht, T. G. & Pease, V. P. 1968 Effects of wavelength and retinal locus on the reaction time to onset and offset stimulation. *J. exp. Psychol.* **78**, 699–701.

Bowen, R. W., Pola, J. & Matin, L. 1974 Visual persistence: effects of flash luminance, duration and energy. *Vision Res.* **14**, 295–303.

Breitmeyer, B. & Ganz, L. 1975 Temporal studies with flashed gratings: inferences about human transient and sustained channels. *Vision Res.* **17**, 861–865.

Briggs, G. G. & Kinsbourne, M. 1972 Visual persistence as measured by reaction time. *Q. Jl exp. Psychol.* **24**, 318–325.

Coltheart, M. 1978 The internal lexicon and its access during reading. In *Conceptual analysis and method in psychology* (ed. J. P. Sutcliffe), pp. 71–81. Sydney: University Press.

Coltheart, M., Jonasson, J. T., Davelaar, E. & Besner, D. 1978 Access to the internal lexicon. In *Attention and performance*, vol. 6 (ed. S. Dornic), pp. 535–556. Hillsdale: Erlbaum.

Demkiw, P. & Michaels, C. 1976 Motion information in iconic memory. *Acta psychol.* **40**, 257–264.

di Lollo, V. 1977 Temporal characteristics of iconic memory. *Nature, Lond.* **267**, 241–243.

di Lollo, V. 1978 On the spatio-temporal interactions of brief visual displays. In *Studies in perception* (ed. R. H. Day & G. V. Stanley), pp. 39–55. Perth: University of Western Australia Press.

di Lollo, V. 1980 Temporal integration in visual memory. *J. exp. Psychol.: General* (In the press.)

di Lollo, V. & Wilson, A. E. 1978 Iconic persistence and perceptual moment as determinants of temporal integration in vision. *Vision Res.* **18**, 1607–1610.

Dixon, N. F. & Hammond, J. 1972 The attention of visual persistence. *Br. J. Psychol.* **63**, 243–254.

Efron, R. 1970a The relationship between the duration of a stimulus and the duration of a perception, *Neuropsychologia* **8**, 37–55.

Efron, R. 1970b The minimum duration of a perception. *Neuropsychologia* **8**, 57–63.

Efron, R. 1970c Effects of stimulus duration on perceptual onset and offset latencies. *Percept. Psychophys.* **8**, 231–234.

Efron, R., & Lee, D. N. 1971 The visual persistence of a moving stroboscopically illuminated object. *Am. J. Psychol.* **84**, 365–375.

Engel, G. R. 1970 An investigation of visual responses to brief stereoscopic stimulu. *Q. Jl exp. Psychol.* **22**, 148–160.

Eriksen, C. W. & Collins, J. F. 1967 Some temporal characteristics of visual pattern perception. *J. dev. Psychol.* **74**, 476–484.

Eriksen, C. W. & Collins, J. F. 1968 Sensory trace versus the organization of form. *Jl exp. Psychol.* **77**, 376–382.

Eriksen, C. W. & Hoffman, J. E. 1973 The extent of processing of noise elements during selective encoding from visual displays. *Percept. Psychophys.* **14**, 217–224.

Eriksen, C. W. & Rohrbaugh, J. 1970 Visual masking in multielement displays. *Jl exp. Psychol.* **83**, 147–154.

Eriksen, B. A. & Eriksen, C. W. 1974 Effects of noise letters upon the identification of a target letter in a nonsearch task. *Percept. Psychophys.* **16**, 143–149.

Fain, G. L. & Dowling, J. E. 1973 Intracellular recordings from single rods and cones in the mud-puppy retina. *Science N.Y.* **180**, 1178–1181.

Haber, R. N. & Nathanson, L. S. 1968 Post-retinal storage? Some further observations on Parks' camel as seen through the eye of a needle. *Percept. Psychophys.* **3**, 349–355.

Haber, R. N. & Standing, L. 1969 Direct measures of short-term visual storage. *Q. Jl exp. Psychol.* **21**, 43–54.

Haber, R. N. & Standing, L. 1970 Direct estimates of the apparent duration of a flash. *Can. J. Psychol.* **14**, 216–229.

Hogben, J. H. & di Lollo, V. 1974 Perceptual integration and perceptual segregation of brief visual stimuli. *Vision Res.* **4**, 1059–1069.

Julesz, B. 1971 *Foundations of cyclopean perception.* Chicago University Press.

Julesz, B. & Chiarucci, E. 1973 Short-term memory for stroboscopic movement perception. *Perception* **2**, 249–260.

Keele, S. W. & Chase, W. G. 1967 Short-term visual storage. *Percept. Psychophys.* **3**, 383–386.

Makous, W. & Boothe, R. 1974 Cones block signals from rods. *Vision Res.* **14**, 285–294.

Meyer, G. E. 1977 The effects of color-specific adaptation on the perceived duration of gratings. *Vision Res.* **17**, 51–56.

Meyer, G. E., Lawson, R. L. & Cohen, W. 1975 The effects of orientation-specific adaptation on the duration of short-term visual storage. *Vision Res.* **15**, 569–572.

Meyer, G. E. & Maguire, W. M. 1977 Spatial frequency and the mediation of short-term visual storage. *Science, N.Y.* **198**, 524–525.

Mollon, J. 1969 Two approaches to the perceptual moment hypotheses. Paper read to the Experimental Psychology Society.

Neisser, U. 1967 *Cognitive psychology.* New York: Appleton-Century-Crofts.

Pease, V. P. & Sticht, T. G. 1965 Reaction time as a function of onset and offset stimulation of the fovea and periphery. *Percept. Mot. Skills* **20**, 549–554.

Penn, R. D. & Hagins, W. A. 1972 Kinetics of the photocurrent of retinal rods. *Biophys. J.* **12**, 1073–1094.

Pollack, I. 1973 Interaction effects in successive visual displays: an extension of the Eriksen-Collins paradigm. *Percept. Psychophys.* **13**, 367–373.

Rains, J. D. 1961 Reaction time to onset and cessation of a visual stimulus. *Psychol. Rec.* **11**, 265–268.

Russell, R. J. H. 1977 Temporal coding in iconic memory. D.Phil. thesis, University of Oxford.

Sakitt, B. 1975 Locus of short-term visual storage. *Science, N.Y.* **190**, 1318–1319.

Sakitt, B. 1976*a* Iconic memory. *Psychol. Rev.* **83**, 257–276.

Sakitt, B. 1976*b* Psychophysical correlates of photoreceptor activity. *Vision Res.* **16**, 129–140.

Scharf, B. & Lefton, L. A. 1970 Backward and forward masking as a function of stimulus and task parameters. *Jl exp. Psychol.* **84**, 331–388.

Servière, J., Miceli, D. & Califret, Y. 1977*a* A psychophysical study of the visual perception of 'instantaneous' and 'durable'. *Vision Res.* **17**, 57–63.

Servière, J., Miceli, D. & Galifret, Y. 1977*b* Electrophysiological correlates of the visual perception of 'instantaneous' and 'durable'. *Vision Res.* **17**, 65–69.

Sperling, G. 1960 The information available in brief presentations. *Psychol. Monogr.* **74**, 1–29.

Sperling, G. 1967 Successive approximations to a model for short-term memory. *Acta psychol.* **27**, 285–292.

Stabell, U. & Stabell, B. 1976 Absence of rod activity from peripheral vision. *Vision Res.* **16**, 1433–1437.

Stanley, G. & Molloy, M. 1975 Retinal painting and visual information storage. *Acta psychol.* **39**, 283–288.

Steinberg, R. H. 1969 The rod after-effect in S-potentials from the cat retina. *Vision Res.* **9**, 1345–1355.

Treisman, A. M., Russell, R. & Green, J. 1975 Brief visual storage and shape and movement. In *Attention and performance V* (ed. P. M. A. Rabbitt & S. Dornic), pp. 699–721. London: Academic Press.

Tulving, E. 1972 Episodic and semantic memory. In *Organization of memory* (ed. E. Tulving & W. Donaldson), pp. 381–403. New York: Academic Press.

van der Heijden, A. H. C. 1978 Short-term visual information forgetting. Ph.D. thesis, University of Leiden.

Whitten, D. N. & Brown, K. T. 1973*a* The time courses of late receptor potentials from monkey cones and rods. *Vision Res.* **13**, 107–135.

Whitten, D. N. & Brown, K. T. 1973*b* Photopic suppression of monkey's rod receptor potential, apparently by a cone-initiated lateral inhibition. *Vision Res.* **13**, 1629–1658.

Whitten, D. N. & Brown, K. T. 1973*c* Slowed decay of the monkey's cone receptor potential by intense stimuli, and protection from this effect by light adaptation. *Vision Res.* **13**, 1659–1667.

Phil. Trans. R. Soc. Lond. B **290**, 71–82 (1980)
Printed in Great Britain

The absolute efficiency of perceptual decisions

By H. B. Barlow, F.R.S.

Kenneth Craik Laboratory, Department of Physiology, Cambridge CB2 3EG, U.K.

Our perceptions of the world around us are stable and reliable. Is this because the mechanisms that yield them are crude and insensitive, and thus immune to false responses? Or is it because a statistical censor that blocks unreliable messages intervenes between the signals from our sense organs and our knowledge of them? This question can be answered by measuring the efficiency with which statistical information is utilized in perception. It is shown that mirror symmetry can be detected in displays of otherwise random dots with an efficiency of up to 50 %; thus the statistical mechanisms are not crude and insensitive, and this aspect of sensory physiology and psychology may deserve more attention.

One would like to investigate higher peceptual mechanisms with types of psychophysical experiment that are as rigorous as those that have been used for investigating colour vision, absolute thresholds or acuity, but a glance at papers and textbooks is enough to show that this is not usually done. I want to suggest in this paper that it can be done. For simple tasks the physical or photochemical limits are known, and quantitative measurements are largely guided by this knowledge. If we knew what limited perception, this might prove a similar guide; hence the first question to discuss is the nature of the limits to the perception of more abstract properties of visual images than those involved in sensitivity, resolution or colour matching.

What limits perception?

The reasons for an instrumental system's failing to respond can be divided into two classes. In the first, the input causes no change at all in the output; the gain is insufficient or the pointer is jammed against its stop by too strong a return spring. In the second, a change is present at the output, but it cannot be measured, or even reliably detected, because it is small in comparison with the changes in the output that occur without any deliberately imposed change at the input of the type the system is supposed to measure. It is often assumed that perceptual failures belong to the first category because, when asked to make a difficult judgement, one is usually unaware of spurious perceptions that hinder the judgement. For instance, when deciding which of two hemifields is the brighter one does not, in a good photometer, see them as flickering in intensity, or non-homogeneous, so that at one moment and in one place one hemifield is brighter, at another moment and another place the other is brighter. The same often seems to be true of more complex perceptions. In judging collinearity of a vernier, or in recognizing the photograph of an acquaintance, one is not aware of a background of unstable misalignments or false facial resemblances from which the true impressions emerge; on the contrary, the true impression emerges in a secure way like a pointer rising from zero to a definitive reading. But I think that this common impression conceals the essential problem of perception, which is how reliable knowledge of the world around us is extracted from a mass of noisy and potentially misleading sensory messages. What I am suggesting is that the statistical step of extracting knowledge is often solved *before* we consciously perceive anything at all, and that is why our perceptions are usually reliable.

Let me give three prior reasons for believing that avoidance of spurious impressions is a major problem of perception, whether or not one is consciously aware of it. The first is simply that many psychophysicists would not agree with the description I gave in the previous paragraph of the way that weak perceptions arise. They would hold that spurious perceptions *do* occur, and that subjects can, if pressed, set their criterion for a particular perception at such a level that it will occur at almost any desired frequency in the total absence of the input signal. This is certainly my own subjective experience at the absolute threshold of vision (Barlow 1956), and Sakitt (1972) has demonstrated clearly that subjects can be persuaded to respond to very few quantal absorptions, at the expense of the increase in the proportion of false responses that signal detection theory leads one to expect (see Swets 1964). Thus a closer investigation of the way that weak perceptions arise tends to support the view that perception failures belong to the second class and do not result simply from inadequate gain or high thresholds.

The second prior reason for emphasizing the importance of noise in perception is a general argument: sensory nerve fibres must under ordinary conditions be responding with complex patterns of activity at immensely variable rates, and it is hard to conceive of any mechanism testing the patterns of activity for the presence of a perceptual property that would be immune to spurious responses and entirely avoid false alarms, unless of course it was very insensitive. The problem is how to reach a conclusion from a mass of fragmentary information: our senses give us *knowledge* of the world around us, and one recalls Fisher's remark that new knowledge can *only* be created by statistical testing. It is certainly true that the best way of analysing the sensory messages would be to apply a battery of statistical tests to them, and some proposals along these lines will be made later.

One may also remark that psychologists are well aware of the importance of statistical tests when it comes to submitting a paper for publication in a reliable journal; it would be strange if they denied the importance of statistical tests of incoming messages when a sensory system is submitting them to higher levels of the nervous system.

A third reason for preferring the view that perception is often noise-limited is illustrated in figure 1. As the quality of the type deteriorates, it becomes more and more difficult to identify the middle letter: is this because the necessary information has sunk below the threshold of a needlessly insensitive perceptual mechanism, or is it because noise has been introduced? In figure 2 the same letters are shown at greater magnification, but in spite of this, perception fails at about the same point. Magnification fails to help, presumably because the noise is magnified with the signal. In this case we know that we fail to see the letters because the noise level has risen too high, but it does not seem subjectively very different from many other cases where perception fails, so it is natural to suspect that noise is important there too.

These three reasons for believing that sensory messages are statistically tested before we become aware of them make the idea plausible, but we need quantitative tests to become more fully convinced. The real question is whether the postulated statistics are done well, for it would be possible to regard any crude criterion for eliminating weak sensory messages as some kind of statistical method. Suppose, for instance, that one asks one's research assistant to fit a line to a set of points, and he simply joins the two extreme values; is that to be regarded as a statistical

1	sat	set	sit	sot
2	sat	set	sit	sot
3	sat	set	sit	sot
4	sot	sat	sit	sot
5	sat	set	sit	sot
6	sat	set	sit	sot

FIGURE 1. The quality of the print makes it difficult to distinguish the letters in lines 5 and 6.

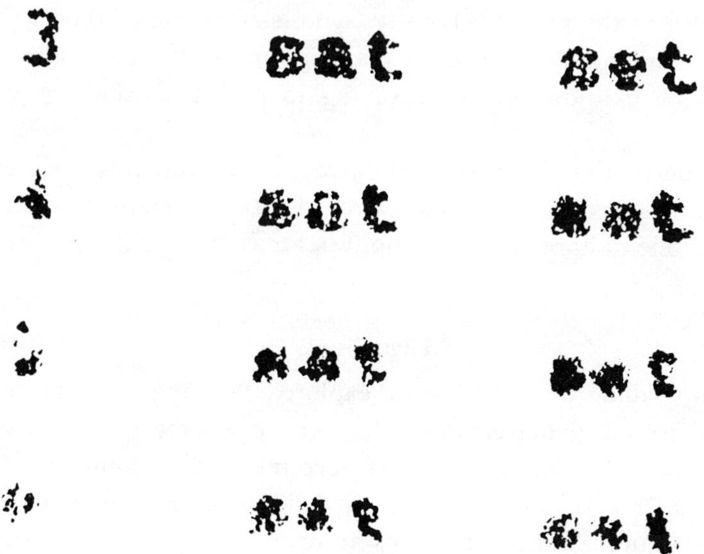

FIGURE 2. Magnification does not cure the problem of figure 1 because the noise is enlarged with the signal. Many perceptual limits are presumably set by noise, not by inadequate magnification or contrast.

method? Maybe, but it certainly is not a good one, and what is implied by the hypothesis is that *good* statistics are used in sensory systems to eliminate spurious, ureliable perceptions. To test this, we must measure how well the statistics are performed. This was the motive for the experiments that I shall now describe. The question is an important one, for the statistical limitations of induction may be as important a guide to understanding higher perceptual processes as the physical limits of image formation and light absorption are to the earlier steps of vision.

Choice of task

If you look at the three pairs of pictures in figure 3 you will agree, I think, that those on the left have a property in common with each other that enables them to be distinguished at once from those on the right. This property of bilateral symmetry is one that we can perceive very readily and directly, without conscious introspection to check whether a dot or small configuration on the left has its mate on the right. In this respect it is like simpler perceptions such as that of the colour of texture of a surface, or the collinearity of a row of dots, but it is a type of perception that seems to lead towards more complex tasks such as that of identifying a letter, or recognizing a face. For many of the simpler tasks, we have plausible ideas about the underlying phsyiology, but for symmetry I, at least, started out with no ideas at all about mechanism. But the detection of symmetry is a definite perceptual ability, and the characteristics of human performance at this task ought to give hints about the physiology, as has been the case with measurements of human sensitivity, acuity and colour vision.

Symmetry is also interesting because its detection is necessarily an associative process. If I cover up the right halves of each pattern in figure 3, there is nothing to tell which is symmetric; this can only be detected by comparing left and right halves, and this comparison may operate over the whole breadth of the pattern. Finally, symmetry is one of those 'Gestalt' processes which psychologists often employed 20 or 30 years ago to taunt and mystify innocent physiologists, and it would be extraordinarily gratifying to find a satisfactory explanation of its detection.

To summarize, the perception of symmetry in arrays of random dots as shown in figure 3 is a global, Gestalt, associative, process that is complicated enough to pose an interesting challenge, but simple enough for one to hope that psychophysics may throw light on the mechanism and what limits it.

Methods

The first experiments, done with B. Reeves, explored the range of conditions under which symmetry could be detected in patterns of dots, but we wanted quantitative answers so we usually did the experiments as follows (a fuller account is to be found in Barlow & Reeves 1979). The subject sat at a keyboard facing an oscilloscope screen, with a computer programmed to generate examples of dot patterns according to one of two paradigms. The two paradigms might be those illustrated in figure 3, that is either 100 dots were positioned entirely at randon as on the right, or 50 dots were placed at random and 50 as pairs to the first 50 mirrored about the midline vertical. Initially the subject could obtain samples generated according to either paradigm at will, and from these he learned the perceptual characteristics of each population. When he had seen enough known samples, the computer generated 100 selected at random from the two populations, and the subject's task was to classify them. The correctness of each trial was signalled so that his knowledge of the two populations was continually refreshed. From the results, the proportion correct for each class was calculated and expressed as d'; this is the measure of detectability used in signal detection theory, and is best regarded for present purposes as an estimate of the signal:noise ratio of whatever quantity in the nervous system is used for making the distinction between symmetric and asymmetric patterns. In terms of this quantity it is the separation of the means of the two populations divided by their standard deviation (see Swets (1964) for further details).

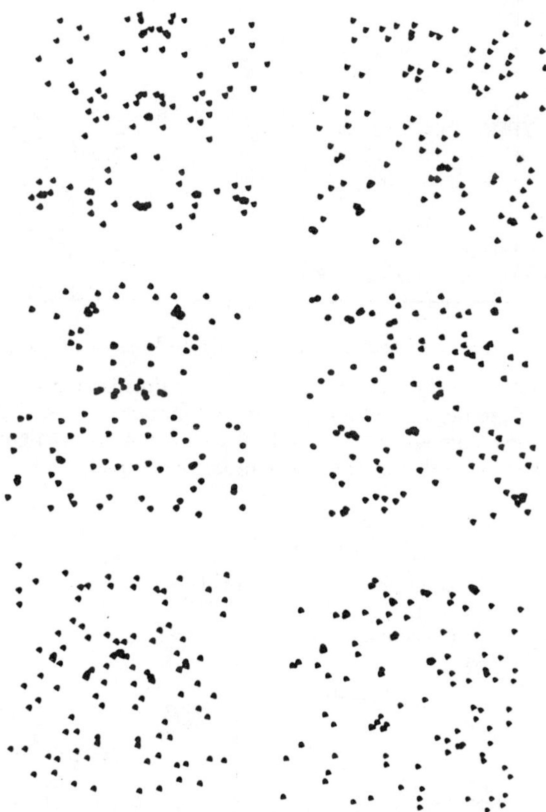

FIGURE 3. Examples of random patterns with mirror symmetry (left) and without mirror symmetry (right).

If the two populations shown in figure 3 had actually been used, a good subject would have made no errors; this corresponds to an infinite d', so the task must be made more difficult to ensure that the results lie within the range where the measure works properly. We have done this by arranging for only a proportion P of the dots to be in pairs, the remainder $(1 \times P)$ being placed at random over the whole pattern. With $P = 0.5$ or 0.8, enough errors are made for the d' to work satisfactorily.

RESULTS

Our first results showed that symmetry could be detected in brief exposures when the axis was not vertical (figure 4) and when it was displaced from the midline (figure 5), though both of these made the task harder. Clearly these results have important implications with regard to mechanism, for the task of detecting symmetry about the vertical midline of the visual field would have needed a much simpler and more stereotyped operation than what we now know is required. We also obtained evidence that the impression of symmetry could be graded over a considerable range and that the dots giving rise to it could lie some distance from the axis, not necessarily adjacent to it, thus confirming that it could not be performed by operations restricted to limited regions of the visual field.

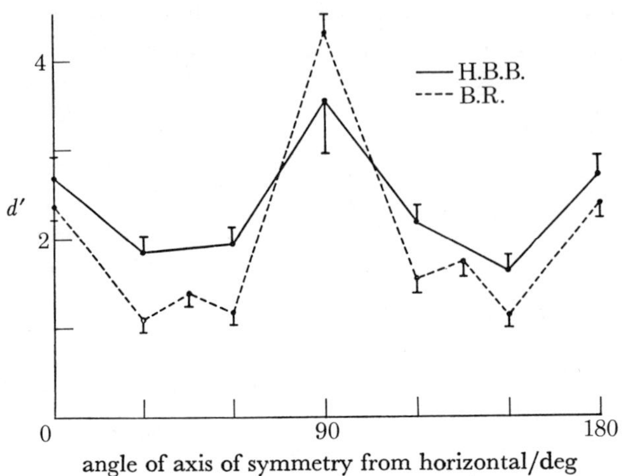

angle of axis of symmetry from horizontal/deg

FIGURE 4. Effect of the orientation of the axis of symmetry: 100 dots in a circular field (4.2°) with a proportion 0.8 in symmetric pairs were to be discriminated from 100 randomly placed dots after an optional number of familiarizing trials. Exposure time was 100 ms and the axis was constant in each run of 100 trials. Discriminability is best with the axis vertical, but the task can be performed at other orientations. (From Barlow & Reeves (1979).)

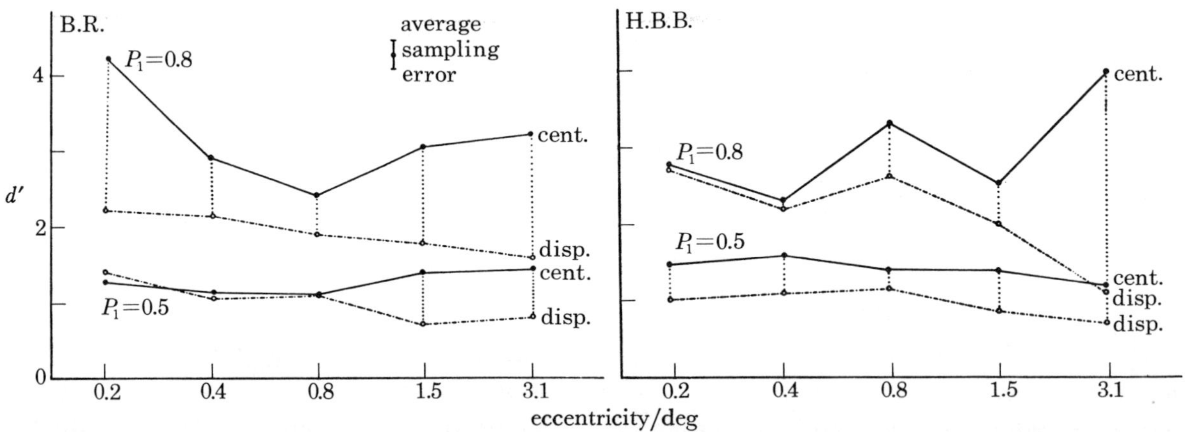

eccentricity/deg

FIGURE 5. Effect of displacement of the axis of symmetry. The two subjects fixated a mark; shortly after its disappearance the figure appeared for 100 ms either centrally (marked cent.) or displaced at random either to the left or right (marked disp.) by the movement shown on the abscissa. In all but two cases performance was worse on the displaced patterns, but the task can still be done even with displacement up to 3°. (From Barlow & Reeves (1979).)

These experiments showed that the mechanism was versatile, but told us little about its nature. We therefore started to think of possible ways of distinguishing symmetric patterns like those on the left of figure 3 from asymmetric ones. We paid particular attention to the factors that would set a limit to its detection, for if we understood this we should be able to assess how good human performance was in absolute terms, and thus obtain evidence on the issue whether the statistical testing of sensory messages is important.

For these computer-generated patterns we are in the strong position of knowing exactly the rules that generated them, and because of this we can also specify how best to detect them. Suppose, for example, that a list of the coordinates of the dots of a pattern in figure 3 is available. If the pattern is symmetric, the very first dot in the list will have a symmetric mate, and whether this is so can readily be found by searching through the coordinates of all other dots. Now a positive result of the search is not infallible evidence that the pattern belongs to the left-hand, symmetric, group, because a dot might, by coincidence, have been placed in the symmetric position even if all dots had been placed at random. The actual chance of this happening depends on the accuracy with which dots are positioned. In our system the accuracy both vertically and horizontally is normally 0.1% because we use 10 bit digital–analogue converters, and it will be seen that there is only a small chance that one of the 99 candidate-pair dots will be positioned in any of the 10^6 dot positions that would entitle it to be considered a pair to another dot.

The situation changes radically if the accuracy of placing the paired dots is less. For instance if the accuracy was only 10% in each direction, there would be only 100 distinct positions for a dot and there are very likely to be many dots positioned as pairs, even when every one is placed independently and at random. In this situation I do not think that one can do better than to count up the total number of qualifying pairs and use this count to decide whether a particular pattern is from the symmetric or non-symmetric population. It is clear, however, that when the accuracy of placing pairs is very poor the number of spurious pairs in totally random patterns will rise, and the variability in this number may obscure the difference between samples from symmetric and random populations. Corresponding to this limit to the discrimination of symmetric from random patterns from the coordinates of their dots, we may expect that the appearance of symmetry will vanish as the accuracy of placing the mirror dots is diminished. The question is, do the perceptual mechanisms do a good job in combating this possible factor limiting the detection of symmetry?

Figure 6 shows how reducing the accuracy of placing the symmetric dot impairs performance. The tolerance given on the abscissa scale indicates the range of positions within which the dot was placed, and it applied both vertically and horizontally. Thus for an angular tolerance range of 16′, the paired dot was placed at a random position in a square frame of side 16′ centred on the exactly symmetric position. It will be seen that performance drops off when the tolerance range is 8–16′, which is a surprisingly large figure compared with two point acuity of 1′ and the positional accuracy of 6″ or less attainable in a vernier task. Evidently symmetry detection does not depend upon a high-precision mechanism, but rather upon a low-resolution system.

The continuous line in figure 6 shows the performance predicted from counting the number of pairs that qualify as symmetrically placed for each tolerance range. For low tolerance ranges this can be calculated from simple geometric considerations, but the simple calculation is inaccurate at large tolerance ranges because the borders of the patterns spread out and the average dot density tapers off. This ideal curve was thus obtained by a computer simulation in which the coordinates were searched in the manner outlined previously. The ideal d′ is simply the difference between the mean numbers of qualifying pairs in the symmetric and unsymmetric patterns, divided by the standard deviation of the mean number.

For tolerance ranges above about 12′, the curve fits the points quite well, but note that the ordinate scale for the ideal curve is at the right, and the values are twice those on the left. Thus for moderate and large tolerances, the human subjects' d'_E is half the ideal d'_I. That corresponds to an efficiency of $\frac{1}{4}$ or 25%, because the ratio d'_E/d'_I must be squared if one wishes to express efficiency in the way that Fisher (1925) suggested. The figure then means that on average 25% of the information in a particular pattern is utilized in forming the decision as to which population it was derived from. I think that this is quite a high figure when one considers the nature of the task, and we started speculating on the type of mechanism that would achieve it.

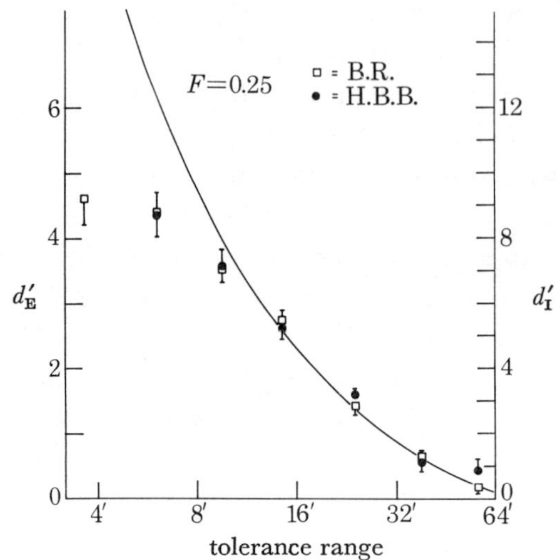

FIGURE 6. The accuracy of pairing was varied by placing the mirror pair to a dot at a random position in a square area centred on the true position and of side as given on abscissa. Ordinate shows d'_E for discriminating samples of the inaccurately paired population from a random population, with precautions taken to avoid other cues as to the origin of the sample. The continuous line shows the d'_I values obtained by counting the total number of pairs that would qualify as symmetric under the tolerance range being used, and basing the discrimination on this number in a computer simulation of the experiment. The scale for d'_E is at the right, and is twice the left-hand scale. For tolerances greater than about 12′, the points fit the curve. This means that the subjects used 25% of the statistical information in the patterns. (From Barlow & Reeves (1979).)

In the ideal method, every possible pair of dots was inspected to see if it qualified as a symmetric pair with the tolerance range in use. With 100 dots there are 4950 pairs, and it is hard to imagine a neural mechanism capable of conducting this search in the brief time required to detect symmetry, especially as the required pairing is determined by the position of the dots, not by positions in the visual field. Taking a hint from the fact that the system tolerates a good deal of inaccuracy in the placing of symmetric pairs, our first attempt to formulate a simpler model postulated comparisons of the numbers of dots falling in fixed areas of the visual field. Figure 7 shows the scheme. The 2° square within which the dots fall is divided up into sixteen $\frac{1}{2}° \times \frac{1}{2}°$ squares, and the numbers in mirror-paired areas are compared as indicated. A computer simulation of this model was run, and the results are shown in figure 8. The agreement was almost embarrassingly good, and (with K. Mullen) we started to do some other tests of the model.

If performance depended only on the numbers of dots in the squares shown in figure 7, it should drop to zero if the symmetric patterns were constrained to have equal numbers in each of the subsquares. There would still be evidence of symmetry in the detailed pattern within the subsquares, for this could be mirrored or not in the corresponding subsquare, but according to the model only the number in a subsquare is used and these were constrained to be all equal. The result was disappointing. Performance was only slightly impaired compared with the usual paradigm for producing patterns, so removing the only evidence used by the model had little influence on human performance.

Next we tried generating patterns in the usual way, but perturbing the arrangement of the dots within each subsquare by a re-randomizing process, leaving the number in each subsquare unchanged. The model says that performance is uninfluenced by the detailed arrange-

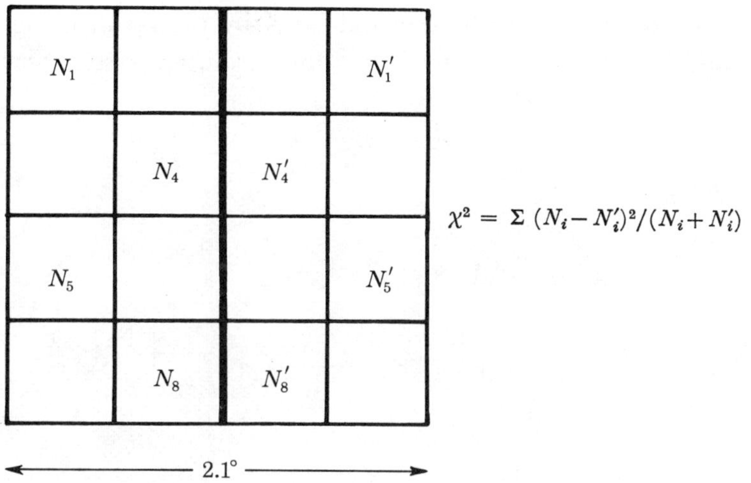

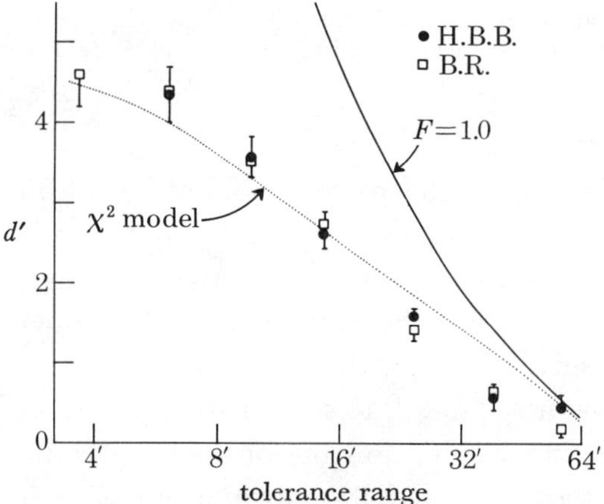

$$\chi^2 = \Sigma \ (N_i - N_i')^2/(N_i + N_i')$$

FIGURE 7. Model based on the idea that the human symmetry system counts the numbers of dots in large, fixed, areas rather than searching through all pairs, and bases discrimination on a χ^2 test performed on these numbers. It tests the hypothesis 'the numbers of dots are randomly divided between symmetric areas', and low values of χ^2 indicate symmetry.

FIGURE 8. The performance of the model of figure 7 obtained by computer simulation is compared with the data points of figure 6. The model appears to fit well, and thus could account for human performance, were it not for other results described in the text.

ment of the dots in these squares and should be equally good if their positions were re-randomized. This, however, had a devastating effect on performance, efficiency dropping to only 1 or 2%. We then thought that we might be able to avoid the additional noise caused by re-randomization by replacing all the dots in the square by a single square at the centre whose brightness or size was proportional to the number in the square. This was better, but the best efficiency was still no higher than 10%. We therefore decided to test the essential features of our model separately.

It is clear that many of the features are not only inessential but wrong. For instance, the model says that the areas that are compared between one side and the other across the mirror axis are square and do not overlap. The essential feature is that they are large, and at fixed positions in the visual field, not aligned on points of the image such as dot positions, because it is the large size and fixed position that greatly reduces the number of comparisons that must be made to assess whether symmetry is present. We were led to postulate this by the high tolerance or low accuracy of the symmetry mechanism indicated by the result of figure 6, and we therefore decided to test directly the idea that only a low-resolution system was required.

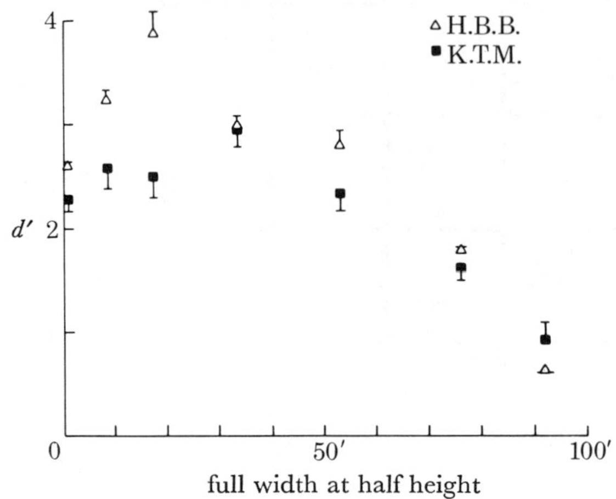

FIGURE 9. Patterns generated with a tolerance range of 15′ both vertically and horizontally were viewed through a diffuser placed in front of the oscilloscope screen. Ability to discriminate symmetric from random patterns was was only impaired seriously when the diffuser was at such a distance that the line spread function (abscissa) had a full width greater than 40′ at half height. This confirms that a low resolution system is involved in symmetry detection. However, it was not predicted that performance with moderate blurring would actually be better than with less blurring or none at all.

If that was the case, then blurring the dot patterns should have little effect on performance, for this would only cut out the high spatial frequencies that our model said were not used anyway. We set out to do this by placing a diffusing screen between the dot patterns and the viewer. By changing its distance from the screen the amount of high frequency reduction would be varied, and figure 9 shows the effect of doing this.

The abscissa gives the full width of the line spread function at half its peak height for a particular distance of the diffusing screen, and the ordinate gives the experimental value of d' obtained. As expected on almost any model, performance is impaired for large amounts of blurring, and as predicted by our model it is not impaired until the blur reaches $\frac{1}{4}-\frac{1}{2}°$. What was unexpected was that blurring actually improved performance up to a certain point: subjects do better at detecting symmetry when high spatial frequencies are eliminated. What this means with regard to the mechanism is not yet clear; one interpretation would be that the inaccurate positioning of mirror pairs introduces details on one side that are not mirrored on the other, and eliminating this detailed evidence for asymmetry by blurring makes it easier to detect symmetry in the coarse positioning of the dots. More thought will be needed to repair our battered model, and more experiments will be required to test the possibilities, but there is one implication with regard to the main purpose of these experiments.

Blurring the picture by interposing the screen removes information contained in high spatial frequencies and cannot make the task of detecting symmetry objectively easier. That is to say, it cannot improve the best attainable value of d'_{I}. So filtering out the high spatial frequencies must actually improve the efficiency of detecting symmetry.

Figure 10 shows a series of measurements with variable tolerance for placing the dots (cf. figure 6) with the diffusing screen at a distance that gave a line spread function of 25′ full width at half height; this corresponds to 50% attenuation at 0.76 cycle/deg in the modulation transfer function. The continuous curve gives ideal performance at an efficiency of 50%, and is a

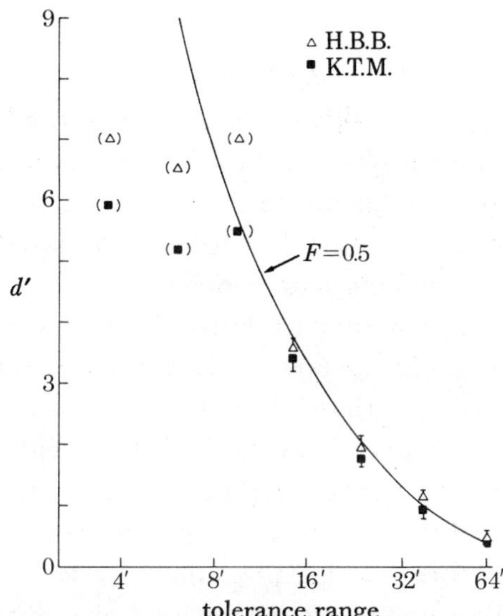

FIGURE 10. Performance with various tolerance ranges for symmetry production (cf. figure 6) when a diffusing screen is placed to produce a line spread of 25′ full width at half height. The continuous line represents utilization of 50% of the statistical information as to symmetry (see text). (Bracketed points are unreliable since subjects scored 100% correct on some of the trials.)

reasonable fit to the determinations made with tolerances down to about 10′. That is as high a figure as we have found for the performance of *any* psychophysical task, even ones in which much simpler judgements are made (Barlow 1978). There is not even any evidence that a simple threshold determinations, in which the subject does no more than decide whether a stimulus was presented or not, can be done any better, as I have argued elsewhere (Barlow 1977).

Detecting symmetry may not be a difficult task compared with recognition of a letter or a face, but it certainly has greater complexity than simply detecting the presence or absence of a specific type of signal; the difference, to my way of thinking, is similar to that between a χ^2 test for the adequacy of a hypothesis and the simplest of all statistical tests, that of deciding whether a sample belongs to a population of known parameters. The fact that the test of a more complex perceptual hypothesis, 'This pattern is symmetric', can be done with an efficiency of 50% shows that the limits to perception are often close to the statistical limits of induction. I think that the possibility that there is a statistical censor screening the messages from one's sense organs must make one take a new look at the anatomical structures and physiological mechanisms of sensory pathways, and perhaps also at the general psychological problems of perception.

I wish to thank B. Reeves, P. Mowforth and K. Mullen for their great help in these experiments.

REFERENCES (Barlow)

Barlow, H. B. 1956 Retinal noise and absolute threshold. *J. opt. Soc. Am.* **46**, 634–639.

Barlow, H. B. 1977 Retinal and central factors in human vision limited by noise. In *Vertebrate photoreception* (ed. H. B. Barlow & P. Fatt), ch. 19, pp. 337–358. London: Academic Press.

Barlow, H. B. 1978 The efficiency of detecting changes of density in random dot patterns. *Vision Res.* **18**, 637–650.

Barlow, H. B. & Reeves, B. C. 1979 The versatility and absolute efficiency of detecting mirror symmetry in random dot displays. *Vision Res.* **19**, 783–793.

Fisher, R. A. 1925 *Statistical methods for research workers.* Edinburgh: Oliver & Boyd.

Sakitt, B. 1972 Counting every quantum. *J. Physiol., Lond.* **223**, 131–150.

Swets, J. A. 1964 *Signal detection and recognition by human observers.* New York: Wiley.

Discussion

S. LAL (*Department of Physiology, Chelsea College, Manresa Road, London SW3 6LX, U.K.*). I should like to ask two questions. First, what kinds of statistical decision tests are being used by neural systems in detecting variations of image dot intensity, mirror symmetry, etc.? Secondly, what proportion of the false responses made can be ascribed to biased hypothesizing as compared with stimulus ambiguity or distorted measurement?

Neural systems cannot be simple-minded relative frequency theorists. For there would be obvious disadvantages for a species in calculating the long-term relative frequency odds that an object approaching was a lamb rather than a lion. In other words, decisions could not be made (or rather would be unlikely to be made) on the basis of repeated trials.

As to the problems of false responses, they could be due to biased hypothesizing by the neural detection–decision elements rather than to stimulus uncertainty or distorted measurement. Presumably one could test for these rival explanations by setting up detection tasks that involved the resolution of stimulus ambiguity or that used biased measurements.

H. B. BARLOW, F.R.S. Presumably the visual mechanism incorporates assumptions about the type of the distributions that it is called upon to handle, and it is only the parameters of the assumed distributions that it estimates from the nature of the messages received. I do not know what these assumptions are, and it is difficult to see how one might find out, for the kind of measurements that one can readily make yield estimates of barely sufficient accuracy even when aimed at means and variances. Much work would be involved in estimating skewness or kurtosis, but it is certainly worth while bearing in mind the possibility that a mismatch between the distribution assumed, and that which actually occurs, might be responsible for certain visual illusions or errors. Perhaps there are perceptual analogies to the errors of judgement that people frequently make when asked to guess the expectation of two or more members of a small group having the same birthday.

With regard to false responses, I am not sure that the distinction that is suggested is helpful, either in theory or practice. The psychophysical method that I use is very simple from the point of view of statistical decision theory, for all I ask the subject to do is select one of two 'hypotheses' on the basis of 'results'. The results are the pattern he has just seen, and the hypotheses are that this came from one or the other of two populations which I assume he knows all about. The method requires that the subject makes errors of both kinds – he must wrongly assign samples to both populations – and it works best when they are about equally frequent and around 10%. These restrictions are good from the point of view that they sharpen the probe with which I am testing the system, but the answer to the question raised would, I think, show up rather indirectly, as inefficiencies of performance under certain test conditions.

Phil. Trans. R. Soc. Lond. B **290**, 83–94 (1980)
Printed in Great Britain

Spatial nonlinearities in the instantaneous perception of textures with identical power spectra

By B. Julesz

Bell Telephone Laboratories, 600 Mountain Avenue, Murray Hill, New Jersey 07974, U.S.A.

In 1962, Julesz observed that texture pairs with identical second-order statistics but different third- and higher-order statistics were usually not discriminable without scrutiny. Since second-order (dipole) statistics determine the autocorrelation functions and hence the power spectra, this observation also meant that in preattentive perception of texture the phase (position) spectra were ignored. In the last two decades many new classes of texture pairs with identical power spectra have been invented that were not effortlessly discriminable; however, recently (Caelli & Julesz 1978; Caelli *et al.* 1978; Julesz *et al.* 1978) several counterexamples were found. In these texture pairs with identical power spectra some local structures of 'quasi-collinearity', 'corner', 'closure' and 'granularity' yielded strong discrimination. These features can be regarded as the fundamental building blocks of form, that is, the essential nonlinearities of the preattentive perceptual system. Here, it will be shown that these counterexamples are not independent of each other, but can be described by two elementary units: *bars* (line segments) and their *terminators*. Furthermore, the preattentive texture perception system can count the number of terminators but ignores their positions.

1. A quasi-linear conjecture of texture perception

The primary purpose of visual perception is to extract information from the visual environment. This requires irreversible, nonlinear decisions such as the separation of the visual world into figure and ground. As long as a visual subsystem is shown to be linear, no loss of information occurs (i.e. no decision is made), and this subsystem is merely a transmission cable that connects remote processing stages with each other. The only noteworthy property of such a linear cable or fibre bundle is its spatial–temporal spectral characteristics, often shaped to achieve optimal signal transmission in noise.

In 1962, I became interested in the question of whether texture pairs, presented side by side, could be effortlessly discriminated when their second-order statistics were identical, but their third- and higher-order statistics differed (Julesz 1962). In the language of random geometry the nth-order statistics is equivalent to the n-gon statistics. This is the probability that the n vertices of randomly thrown n-gons will land on a certain colour combination of the texture. For instance, the statistics that both endpoints of randomly thrown 2-gons (dipoles) would fall on black (or some other specific colour combination) is the second-order or dipole statistics; similarly, the statistics of the three vertices of a triangle falling on a specific colour combination is the third-order or trigon statistics. (A more detailed explanation is given by Julesz (1978).) A texture pair with identical second-order statistics (also called iso-dipole textures), but different third- and higher-order statistics are shown in figure 1. Here one texture consists of identical micropatterns (R's) thrown at random, while the second texture, embedded in one quadrant of the first texture, is composed of micropatterns that are the mirror-images of the micropatterns in the first texture. It has been shown (Julesz *et al.* 1973) that texture pairs composed of mirror-image dual micropatterns are iso-dipole, regardless of the micropattern chosen. As demonstrated in figure 1, such an iso-dipole texture pair cannot be discriminated without scrutiny, in spite of the fact that their third-and higher-order statistics differ. One way to avoid scrutiny by scanning eye-movements, or changes in focal attention, is to present the array for a brief flash (under 200 ms) and such that the boundaries between the texture pair are outside 1° from the centre of fixation.

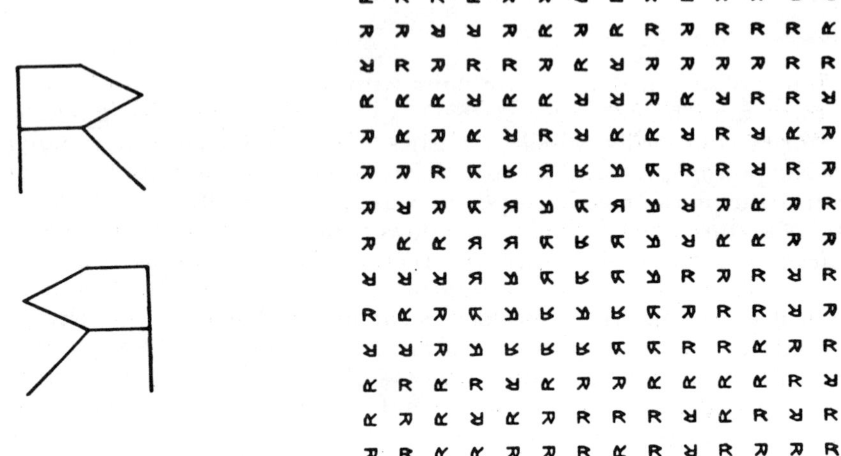

FIGURE 1. Non-discriminable iso-power-spectrum texture pair generated by the mirror-image dual method of Julesz *et al.* (1973).

Indeed, from 1962 to 1978 many other kinds of iso-dipole textures were generated that could not be effortlessly discriminated (Julesz 1962, 1971, 1975; Julesz *et al.* 1973; Caelli *et al.* 1978; Schatz 1978; Pratt *et al.* 1978). So, my observation that iso-dipole textures are usually not discriminable without scrutiny (Julesz 1962) gained the status of a conjecture.

Such a conjecture is not just a mathematical game. After all, the second-order statistics determine the autocorrelation function (what is more, for black and white textures the dipole statistics is identical to the autocorrelation function). In turn, the Fourier transform of the autocorrelation function is the power spectrum. Therefore, *iso-dipole textures* are also *iso-power-spectra textures*. In the light of this realization the conjecture is equivalent to the statement that 'in preattentive (effortless) perception of textures the phase (spatial position) spectra are ignored'. Thus texture perception is very different from figure perception for which the slightest distortion of phase spectra can render the figure unrecognizable. In a sense, visual texture perception resembles auditory perception, in which the phase information is usually ignored too.

Another iso-power-spectrum texture pair that cannot be effortlessly discriminated is shown in figure 2. The dual micropatterns that are the elements of the two textures, respectively, are depicted in the inset of figure 2, and were constructed according to a method devised by Caelli *et al.* (1978), and explained in figure 3. The inability of the preattentive texture system to perceive the spatial position spectrum is well demonstrated by the non-discriminable texture pair in figure 2. Indeed, one micropattern consists of two rectangles, each containing an X, while in the dual micropattern one rectangle is empty and the other contains two X's. While the dual micropatterns by themselves are perceived as different figures, the corresponding textures cannot be discriminated.

What could we learn about preattentive texture perception if the Julesz conjecture were corroborated? Obviously, it would mean that the preattentive perceptual system operates quasi-linearly, in the sense that only the simplest nonlinear decision is made. This is equivalent to taking the spatial Fourier transform of the input image, and performing one of the simplest nonlinear decisions, the throwing away of the phase spectrum.

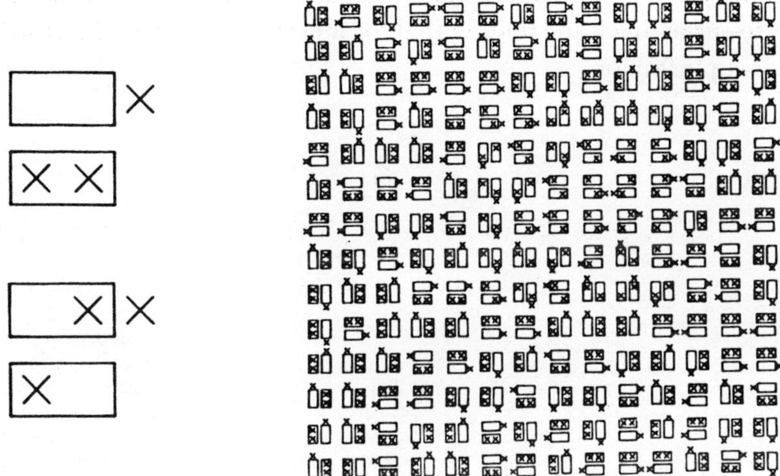

FIGURE 2. Non-discriminable iso-power-spectrum texture pair, demonstrating the insensitivity of texture perception to phase (position) information.

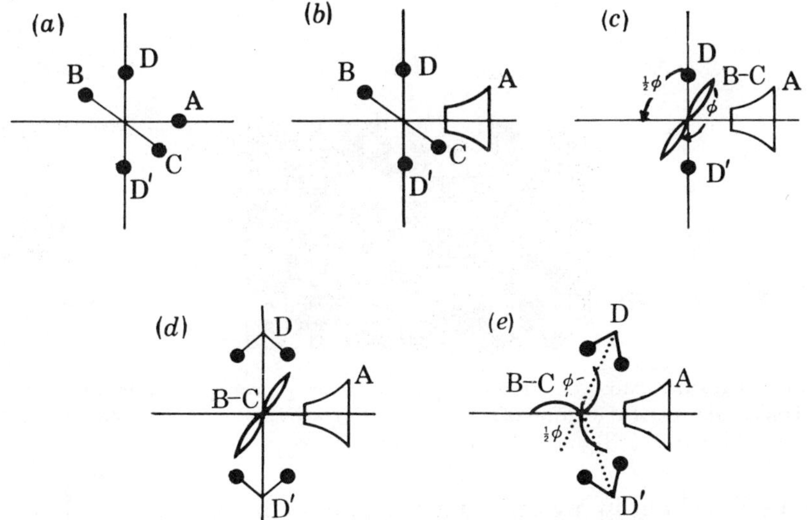

FIGURE 3. Methods for generation of iso-power-spectra textures (e.g. figures 2 and 5). General method for generating iso-dipole micropatterns, seen as a generalization of the four-disk method by four steps. Step (b) involves the generalization of disk A to any bilaterally symmetric shape. Step (c) converts the disks B and C into any 180° rotation invariant shape. Step (d) converts the disks D and D′ into two shapes where each shape is invariant under reflexions on the Y-axis and D′ is the x-axis reflection of D. The final step (e) demonstrates how B–C can be rotation invariant for 180°/n rotations, while D and D′ are symmetric with respect to axes determined by 360°/n rotations. (From Caelli *et al.* (1978).)

2. Counterexamples to the quasi-linear texture conjecture

As we have seen, the quasi-linear texture conjecture is equivalent to assuming that the system makes one of the simplest nonlinear decisions, the ignoring of the phase information. There are many physical systems, from quantum physics to Fourier crystallography, in which the only measureable quantity is the wave power spectrum, and this does not contain any phase information. What is so surprising is the finding that for most textures tried, the visual system appears to behave in this simple fashion.

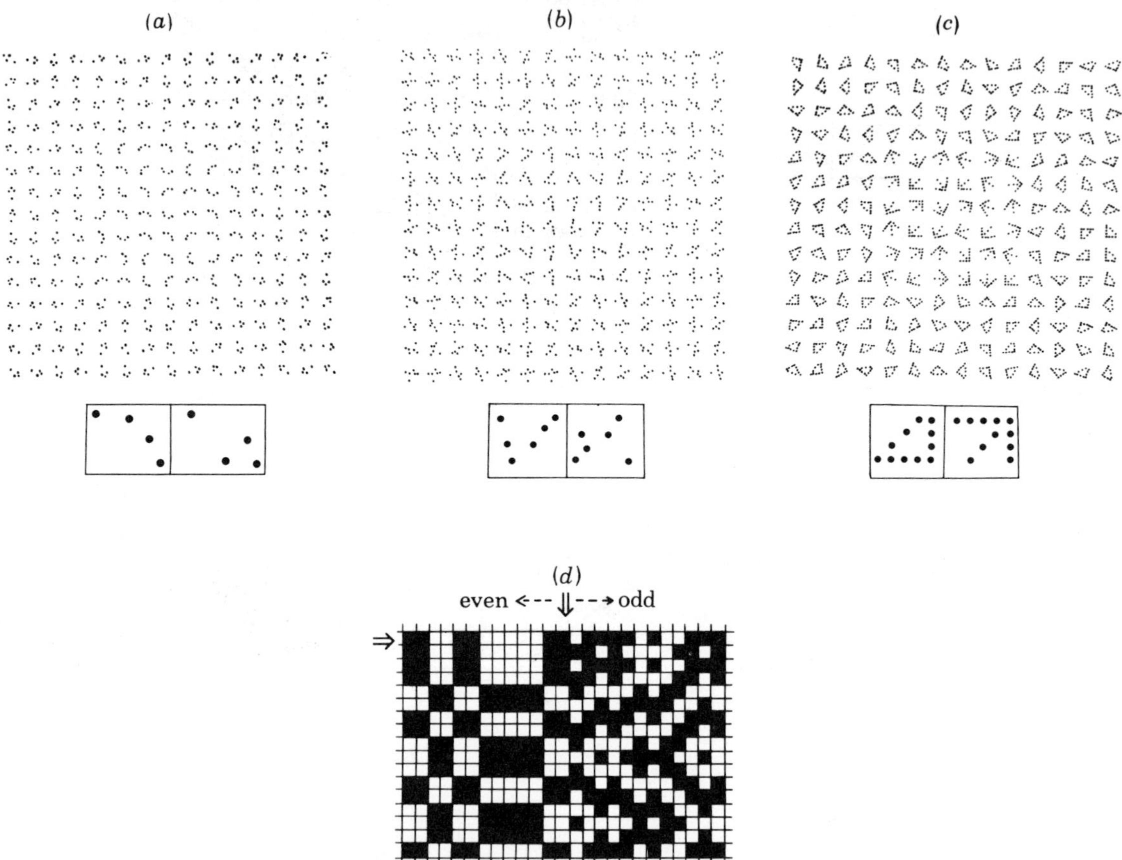

Figure 4. Discriminable texture pairs; counterexamples to the iso-power-spectra texture conjecture. Discrimination is based on nonlinear local features of: (a) quasi-collinearity, (b) corner, (c) closure, and (d) granularity (blobs). (From Caelli *et al.* (1978) and Julesz *et al.* (1978).)

Obviously, as I pointed out in my earliest articles on texture perception (Julesz 1962, 1965), it is most unlikely that any simple stochastic parameters, such as low-order statistics, could describe the many conspicuous *local* features to which a gamut of cortical analysers are selectively tuned, as revealed by single microelectrode recordings. How could one take seriously a 'Turing imitation game', in which the imitator uses n-gons as 'receptive fields' and measures the statistics of their *vertices*, while the real receptive fields in the monkey cortex measure complex properties that exist *inside* the receptive fields. Unfortunately, no mathematician knows how to extend stochastic geometry to more complex statistics than the vertices of n-gons. (An important first step was made by Victor & Brodie (1978) who invented texture pairs with iso-Buffon-needle statistics, where the *intersection* of an infinitely long line with the black texture elements is controlled.) Therefore, it is really remarkable that a second-order Turing imitation game (i.e. dipole statistics) mimics human texture perception to the extent that it does.

Recently, several new texture generation methods have been invented that have yielded strongly discriminable iso-power-spectra texture pairs. Discrimination is based on some local

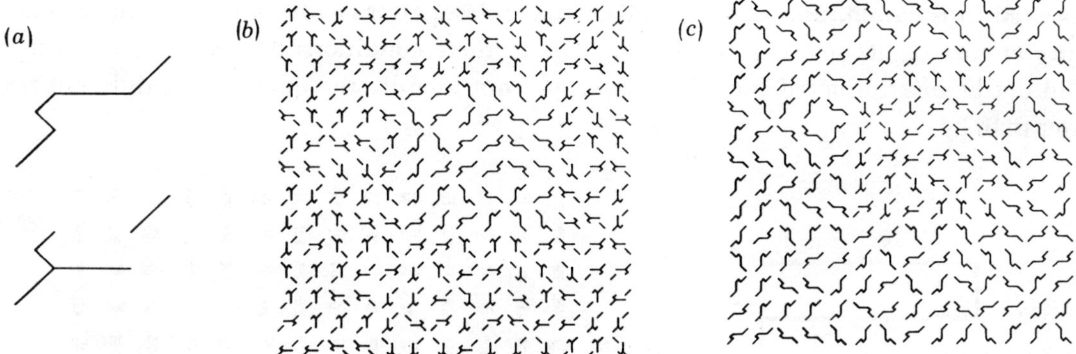

FIGURE 5. Discriminable iso-power-spectra textures based on connectivity.

conspicuous features such as quasi-collinearity, corner, closure and 'blobs' (granularity) (Caelli & Julesz 1978; Caelli *et al.* 1978; Julesz *et al.* 1978). These counterexamples to the Julesz conjecture are shown in figure 4*a*, *b*, *c* and *d*. The first three are based on the method described in figure 3, while figure 4*d* is not only an iso-dipole counterexample, but is an iso-trigon counterexample, based on a new method devised by Julesz *et al.* (1978). Another method with the use of iso-Buffon-needle textures – that are always iso-dipole textures as well – was invented by Victor & Brodie (1978). This juxtaposes disk textures with ellipsoid textures, and yields stong discrimination. This counterexample is similar to the different local blobs of figure 4*d*.

In figure 5 a new counterexample to the iso-power-spectra texture conjecture is published for the first time. This was constructed by using the method of figure 3*d* and discrimination is based on *connectivity*. Interestingly, discrimination is somewhat different when the unconnected micropatterns form the inside texture, and the connected ones the outside texture, than vice versa. In one case, it is easier to discriminate between the two textures, while in the other it is easier to perceive the location of the boundaries between them.

3. 'PERCEPTUAL QUARKS': BARS AND THEIR TERMINATORS

It was demonstrated in figures 4 and 5 how the counterexample to the iso-power-spectra texture conjecture yielded some of the essential local nonlinearities of the preattentive visual system. The 'blobs' in figure 4*d* are of particular interest, since they are in essence the features to which the simple '*bar detectors*' of Hubel & Wiesel (1962, 1968) are tuned. It is also interesting to note that, contrary to common belief, the 'granularity' of textures (e.g. in figure 4*d*) cannot always be described by the power spectrum, not even by the third-order statistics, but is a fourth-order, or perhaps even a fifth-order property (Julesz *et al.* 1978).

The quasi-collinear counterexample in figure 4*a* is a *line segment*, which in turn is a special case of a thin *bar*. So, figure 4*a, d* depicts those conspicuous local features that can be extracted by the elongated receptive fields of simple cortical units found in cat and monkey.

The question arises whether the counterexamples of corner, closure, and connectivity require the postulation of new feature extractor classes, or can be explained by existing ones.

To test independence of the counterexamples, a texture pair consisting of connected (open) and unconnected (closed) micropatterns (see figure 6) was tested by using a 200 ms flash. The micropatterns in the farthest corners of the array were made large enough to be resolved when presented in isolation, and care was taken that micropatterns within a 1° radius around the centre of gaze could not be used as clues. Under these conditions the texture pair in figure 6 could not be discriminated (i.e. observers could not identify the quadrant of different texture better than by chance).

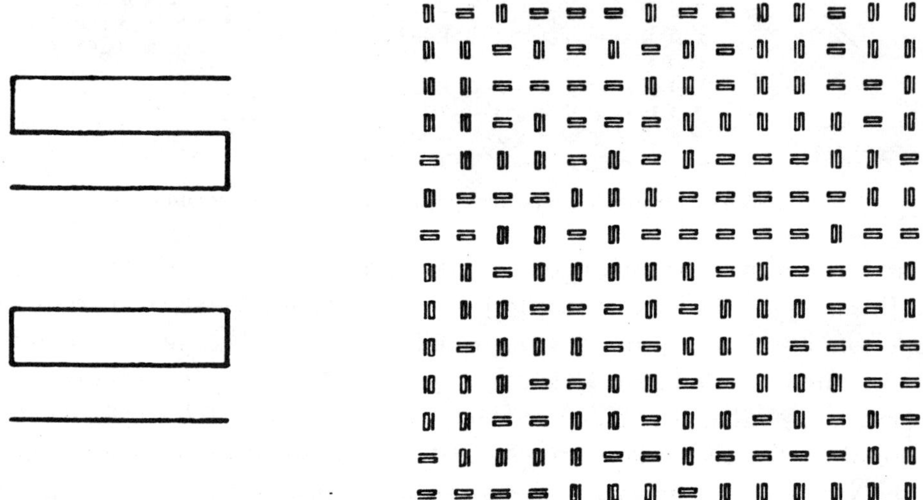

FIGURE 6. Demonstration that textures composed of connected (open) and unconnected (closed) micropatterns, respectively, cannot be effortlessly discriminated, if the number of their *terminators* agrees.

Since the micropattern duals in figure 6 are not iso-dipole, they were chosen to be elongated, to make their dipole statistics more similar. A second texture pair, shown in figure 7, however, permits discrimination. (Instead of a 25% correct guess, which is the chance performance for figure 6, observers of the texture pair in figure 7 guessed the quadrant 72% correctly.)

In figure 6 the dual micropatterns have the same number of line segment terminators (two); however, in figure 7 one micropattern has two terminators, while its partner has three. These experiments clearly show that the preattentive texture system cannot evaluate the exact position of the terminators, only their numbers. In figure perception the 'S'-shaped micropattern is very different from its '10'-shaped partner in figure 6, yet since they both have two terminators, the texture system can only count their numbers, not their exact positions. Discrimination in figure 7 reflects the difference in the terminator number of the micropattern duals. The very strong discrimination (97% correct guesses under tachistoscopic testing) in figure 5 illustrates that even for iso-dipole textures, a large difference in the terminator number of micropattern partners is a decisive parameter.

In a way, the original conjecture – that in texture perception, the phase is ignored – seems to be correct for terminators of bars (line segments). As the texture pair of figure 3 illustrates, even the spatial position of bars (line segments) is not well preserved. However, in many cases, adjacent line segments and blobs trigger wide bar detectors, and thus encode their relative positions to each other.

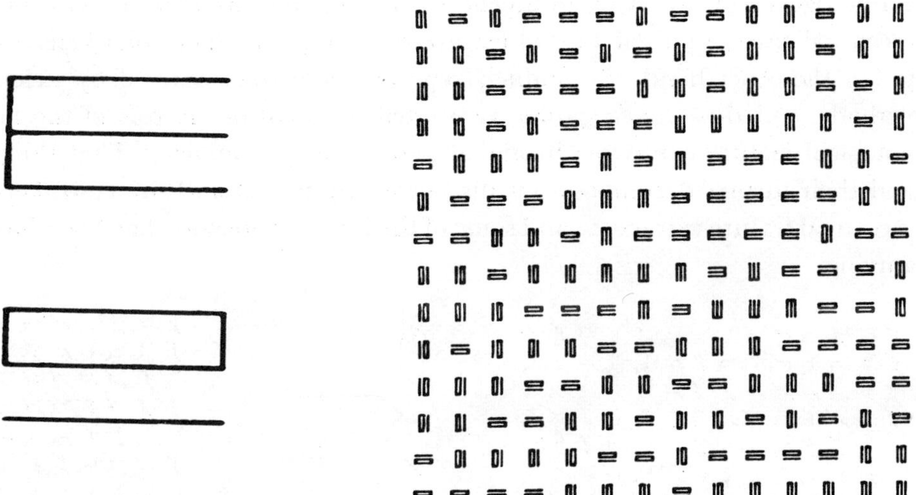

FIGURE 7. Discriminable texture pair, based on the difference of the number of terminators of the micropatterns.

Note that bar (edge, line segment) detectors tuned to specific width, orientation and aspect ratio, and detectors for their terminators are adequate to explain the counterexamples of corner, connectivity and closure. The 'corners' in figure 4*b* differ from their iso-dipole duals, that for the former the quasi-linear dots end in the crossing point (no terminators), while for the latter these dots protrude after the crossing point (two terminators). Similarly, for the closed and open micropattern partners in figure 4*c* and the connected and unconnected ones in figure 5 the difference between the numbers of terminators is three, which explains their strong discriminability.

So, in essence, we can describe the conspicuous local features in iso-power-spectra textures as the combination of bars (line segments) and their terminators. These two 'perceptual quarks', of bars (blobs) and their terminators, are probably the simple and the complex units of the neurophysiologists. Indeed, the simple units extract elongated blobs of specific orientations, widths and aspect ratios, while the complex (hypercomplex) units extract the terminators (corners, ends, gaps) of these blobs. If these bars make up micropatterns such that the bars have the same number, have similar width, orientation and length, and the number of terminators in the micropattern configuration is the same, then the resulting textures are not discriminable.

4. TOWARDS A THEORY OF TEXTURE PERCEPTION

It seems that the perception of line textures is based on some statistics of line segments (with the same orientation and extent) and their terminators, but the exact position of these line segments and terminators is not utilized. Indeed, Julesz *et al.* (1973) stated: 'It might be that the texture discrimination process takes only the first-order statistics of various simple feature extractors that might be segregated according to diameter (and for those with elongated receptive fields, according to width and orientation).' However, they did not know at the time the importance of terminators. It was Marr (1976) that first emphasized the importance of terminators, besides line segments, in the early processing of visual information. His 'primal sketch' model is very reminiscent of the ideas developed here. Nevertheless, there is a crucial difference between Marr's approach and mine. Marr developed his model within the framework of artificial intelligence (a.i.), trying to invent algorithms that are able to perform some well defined perceptual tasks, inspired by the feature extractors of single micro-electrode neurophysiology. On the other hand, the findings reported here were derived by strictly psychophysical methods, and these investigators were often sceptical of the role of the highly local neurophysiological feature extractors in global perceptual phenomena. That the perceptual elements and their further decompositions discovered by myself and my coworkers resemble some of the cortical feature extractors, and some of the feature detectors that Marr has invented, is most gratifying.

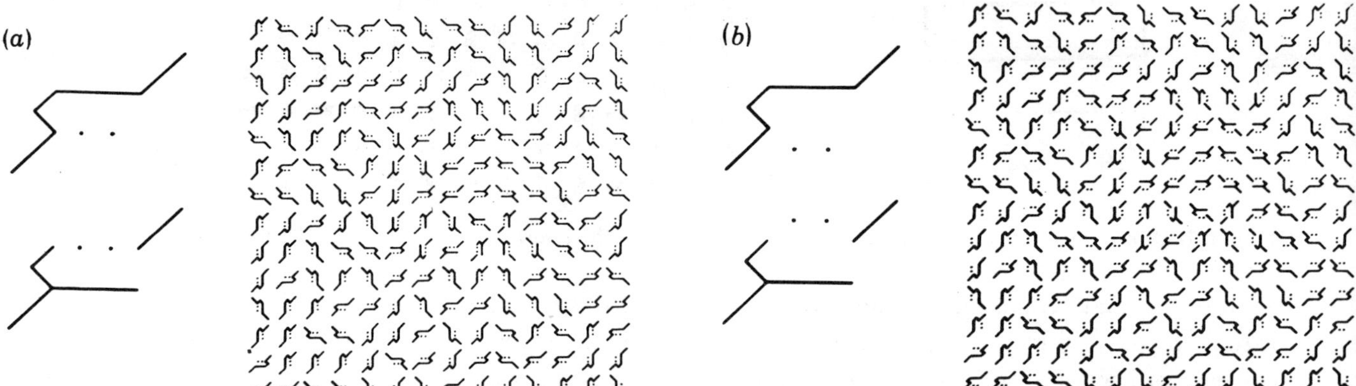

FIGURE 8. Demonstration of illusory (virtual) line segments acting as: (a) connectors (e.g. as real lines); and (b) non-connectors (e.g. remaining virtual lines), based on texture discrimination.

Nevertheless, it is most unlikely that the present enterprise of single microelectrode neurophysiology could have revealed the fact that the texture perception system ignores the position of terminators. Similarly, it is unlikely that an a.i. approach could have predicted the discrimination strength as a function of terminator difference. Also, the difference between real and virtual (illusory) line segments cannot be easily guessed, but requires careful psychophysical studies. For instance, we show in the next example how virutal line segments delivered by dots interact with real line segments, by using connectivity as the criterion. Let us take two dots and place them in 'strategic positions' in figure 5, as shown in figure 8a. These iso-power-spectra textures are now rendered not discriminable. It appears that when the two dots are collinear with the two corner points of the line segments, they act as connectors, that is as real line segments. However, if the two dots are placed elsewhere, as shown in figure 8b, the texture pair is strongly discriminable, which means that the virtual lines defined by the dots are not acting as connectors.

Up to now, we have studied conditions under which textures with iso-power spectra can or cannot be discriminated. On the other hand, as pointed out by Julesz (1962), texture pairs with *different* power spectra often cannot be discriminated. This means that preattentive vision does not utilize the entire second-order statistics, but only a subset of it. Recently, Caelli & Julesz (1979) studied the discriminability of non-iso-dipole textures, composed of pairs of dots (dipoles) as a function of the number (n) of such pairs. When one texture contained dot pairs (dipoles) of a single length and of all possible orientations from 0 to 180°, while the orientation range of the other texture was restricted to a θ interval, as shown in figure 9, a theoretical psychometric function could be derived for discrimination, such that $\ln \theta - \ln (\pi - \theta) \approx \ln n$. As figure 10 shows, data for two observers, and for two dipole lengths, accurately fall on the predicted

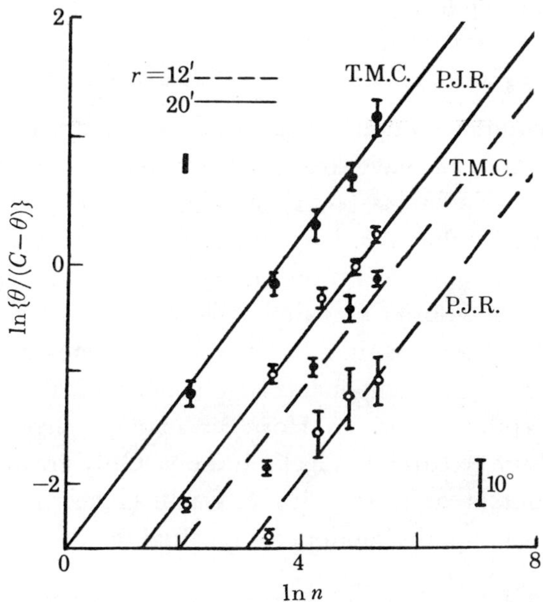

FIGURE 9. Two textures having uniform micropattern dipole orientation distributions. The left texture varies between 70° and 110°, the right between 0° and 180°. (From Caelli & Julesz (1979).)

FIGURE 10. Orientation (θ) discrimination on thresholds as a function of number of dipole elements. Lines correspond to theoretical predictions (n, number of micro-patterns; $C = 180°$ range; θ, threshold range for discrimination (degrees); bars represent standard deviations in degrees; r, length of dipole elements in arc minutes). (From Caelli & Julesz (1979).)

straight lines. This is one of the few known cases of globality in vision for which an increase in the number of texture elements leads to an improved texture discrimination.

However, as is demonstrated in figure 11, if one half field is composed of point pairs of constant length, while the second half field contains greatly varying dipole lengths (with the same mean length as the first half field), no effortless discrimination is experienced. So the texture system is sensitive to dipole orientation changes, but not to changes in dipole length. This finding shows that only a subset of the dipole statistics is utilized. Further psychophysical experiments of this kind are needed to determine the sensitivity of the texture system to the various blob parameter changes as a function of the number of texture elements.

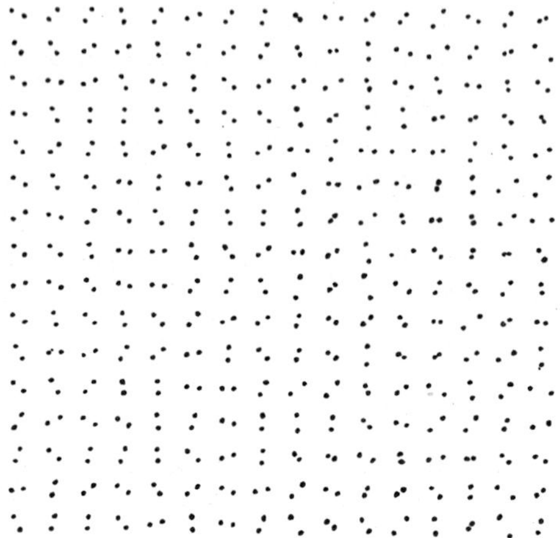

FIGURE 11. Demonstration that only a subset of the dipole statistics has perceptual significance. Left and right textures differ in dipole length variances (left is zero), and no discrimination occurs.

5. TEXTURES AND SPATIAL FREQUENCY CHANNELS

Let us note that the counterexamples to the 1962 conjecture of Julesz, particularly the discriminable textures in figure 4 d, have strong implications for research with sinusoidal gratings. For instance, Graham & Nachmias (1971) showed, by using the multiple-channel idea of Campbell & Robson (1968), that the detection of the sum of two gratings with 3:1 or higher spatial frequency ratio does not depend on phase. This finding appears to be equivalent to the Julesz conjecture in the Fourier domain; however, it fails for components that fall within a 'critical band' (i.e. that have less than 3:1 spatial frequency ratios).

Thus, these phase-dependent components within the critical bands can account for texture discrimination in some counterexamples. However, in others involving the terminators of bars, the use of gratings in vision research has its limitations. Only gratings that are confined to small subregions have terminators, and, as Julesz & Caelli (1979) have shown, the Fourier phase spectra of figure 4 c appear equally random for the dual textures with and without terminators.

6. TEXTURE PERCEPTION: THE SECOND VISUAL SYSTEM

In the light of these studies carried out over 17 years by myself and my coworkers, it appears that preattentive texture perception is an early warning system which triggers the attentive perceptual system. If there is some discontinuity in the power spectra of adjacent areas, or there is some conspicuous local change in the orientation, width and aspect ratio of blobs that constitute the texture, or in the number of the terminators of adjacent blobs, the figure perception system is switched on. So the preattentive system can be regarded as the 'ground' perception system, while the attentive system with scrutiny is the 'figure' system. Of course, scrunity requires foveal attention, which in turn is based on scanning eye-movements. On the other hand, to avoid scrutiny, preattentive texture perception is carried out by the peripheral visual system. However, in the periphery, stationary patterns are not well resolved, and they have to move, or be suddenly switched on, to be seen. So texture (or ground) perception can be thought of as the Y-system of transitory patterns pooled in parallel that bring serially into foveal attention the figure system carried out by the stationary, high-resolution X-system, as first discovered by Enroth-Cugell & Robson (1966).

Thus texture perception can be thought of as the second visual system according to most dichotomous subdivisions of the visual system. While the study of this second system is interesting for its own sake, it is my contention that it is the local nonlinear features of this system that are the building blocks of form perception.

7. Conclusion

We have seen how the search for counterexamples to the quasi-linear conjecture led to local conspicuous features of quasi-collinearity, corner, closure, connectivity and blobs which, in turn, could be reduced to bars and their terminators. These psychophysically defined entities ('perceptual quarks') are similar to those that excite the simple and complex feature extractors found in the monkey cortex (Hubel & Wiesel 1968). The importance of bars and their terminators was recognized by Marr (1976) in the framework of a.i. However, he did not distinguish between real and virtual lines (bars), and only after careful psychophysical studies will we know the conditions under which a virtual line segment acts as a real one.

Since the counterexamples of strong discrimination were obtained for textures with identical autocorrelation, they disprove any theory of perception based on autocorrelation. While the textures with identical autocorrelation might consist of dual micropatterns with different autocorrelation (that become identical only when summed over all possible orientations), it should be stressed that the 'figure of merit' defined by the autocorrelation (Uttal 1975) is the same for the micropattern duals in figure 5 in spite of the fact that the textures generated by them yield strong discrimination. So, Uttal's autocorrelation theory cannot explain effortless texture perception.

We have devoted a section to drawing parallels between textures as defined by their statistics and as defined by their distribution over spatial frequency channels. We noted that the essence of the Julesz conjecture in the spatial Fourier domain is that the discrimination of two spatial gratings is independent of phase, if their spatial frequencies differ by a factor of three or more; this is in agreement with the findings of Graham & Nachmias (1971). We also noted that only limited patches of gratings have terminators, and without them no other counterexamples exist to my quasi-linear conjecture. So, the present theory of grating detection is a quasi-linear theory, useful but as trivial as the original texture conjecture.

In summary, the demarcation criterion – to look for effortlessly discriminable textures with identical power spectra – seems to yield the local nonlinear (feature) extractors of the preattentive visual system. If, instead, some other criterion had been used to explain the processing of random-dot textures, these 'perceptual quarks' could have been easily missed. For instance, in a provocative paper, Barlow (1978) studied the discrimination of random-dot arrays with different first-order statistics, using 'efficiency of detection' as a criterion. (He defined this as a ratio between actual performance and the performance of an ideal observer.) He found no evidence for elongated bar detectors in this detection task. This is not surprising, since for most of the random-dot textures tried by myself and my coworkers (Julesz *et al.* 1973; Julesz 1975) no discrimination was found, even when the micropatterns (dot configurations) were selected so that they would differentially stimulate some known neural feature extractors. Only with very atypical dot-textures (shown in figure 4*a*, *b*, *c*) that contained mainly a certain local dot-configuration, were we able to show the presence of *pools* of 'perceptual quarks'. The distance between these quarks (or *textons*, as I started to call them recently), their number and extent are crucial parameters in texture discrimination. Only after the perceptual significance of these parameters is clarified can we hope for a deeper understanding of texture perception. Some of the experiments reported here are the first steps toward this goal.

This lecture was prepared during my 1979 sabbatical visit in the Biology Department, California Institute of Technology, Pasadena, where I served as a Sherman Fairchild Distinguished Scholar. I thank the Managements of Bell Laboratories, the California Institute of Technology, and the Sherman Fairchild Foundation for their support.

References (Julesz)

Barlow, H. B. 1978 The efficiency of detecting changes of density in random dot patterns. *Vision Res.* **18**, 637–650.

Caelli, T. M. & Julesz, B. 1978 On perceptual analyzers underlying visual texture discrimination: part I. *Biol. Cybernet.* **28**, 167–175.

Caelli, T. M. & Julesz, B. 1979 Psychophysical evidence for global feature processing in visual texture perception. *J. opt. Soc. Am.* **69**, 675–678.

Caelli, T. M., Julesz, B. & Gilbert, E. N. 1978 On perceptual analyzers underlying visual texture discrimination: part II. *Biol. Cybernet.* **29**, 201–214.

Campbell, F. W. & Robson, J. G. 1968 Application of Fourier analysis to the visibility of gratings. *J. Physiol., Lond.* **197**, 551–566.

Enroth-Cugel, C. & Robson, J. G. 1966 The contrast sensitivity of retinal ganglion cells of the cat. *J. Physiol., Lond.* **187**, 517–552.

Graham, N. & Nachmias, J. 1971 Detection of grating patterns containing two spatial frequencies: a comparison of single channel and multichannel models. *Vision Res.* **11**, 251–259.

Hubel, D. H. & Wiesel, T. N. 1962 Receptive fields, binocular interaction and functional architecture in the cat's visual cortex. *J. Physiol., Lond.* **160**, 106–154.

Hubel, D. H. & Wiesel, T. N. 1968 Receptive fields and functional architecture of monkey striate cortex. *J. Physiol., Lond.* **195**, 215–243.

Julesz, B. 1962 Visual pattern discrimination. *I.R.E. Trans. Information Theory* **IT-8**, 84–92.

Julesz, B. 1965 Texture and visual perception. *Scient. Am.* **212** (2), 38–48.

Julesz, B. 1971 *Foundations of cyclopean perception.* Chicago: University of Chicago Press.

Julesz, B. 1975 Experiments in the visual perception of texture. *Scient. Am.* **232** (4), 34–43.

Julesz, B. 1978 Visual texture discrimination using random-dot patterns: comment. *J. opt. Soc. Am.* **68**, 268–270.

Julesz, B. & Caelli, T. M. 1979 On the limits of Fourier decompositions in visual texture perception. *Perception* **8**, 69–73.

Julesz, B., Frisch, H. L., Gilbert, E, N. & Shepp, L. A. 1973 Inability of humans to discriminate between visual textures that agree in second-order statistics – revisited. *Perception* **2**, 391–405.

Julesz, B., Gilbert, E. N. & Victor, J. D. 1978 Visual discrimination of textures with identical third-order statistics. *Biol. Cybernet.* **31**, 137–140.

Marr, D. 1976 Early processing of visual information. *Phil. Trans. R. Soc. Lond.* B **275**, 483–524.

Pratt. W. K., Faugeras, O. D. & Gagalowicz, A. 1978 Visual discrimination of stochastic texture fields. *IEEE Trans. Syst. Managemt Cybernet.* **SMC-8** (11), 796–804.

Schatz, B. 1978 The computation of immediate texture discrimination. *Computer Sci. Dept. Report*, no. 152. Carnegie-Mellon University, Pittsburgh, Pa.

Uttal, W. R. 1975 *An autocorrelation theory of form detection.* Hillsdale, New Jersey: Lawrence Erlbaum Associates.

Victor, J. D. & Brodie, S. E. 1978 Discriminable textures with identical Buffon-needle statistics. *Biol. Cybernet.* **31**, 231–234.

Phil. Trans. R. Soc. Lond. B **290**, 95–116 (1980)
Printed in Great Britain

95

Spatial frequency tuned channels: implications for structure and function from psychophysical and computational studies of stereopsis

By J. P. Frisby and J. E. W. Mayhew
Department of Psychology, University of Sheffield, Sheffield S10 2TN, U.K.

Various psychophysical experiments investigating the role of spatial frequency tuned channels in stereopsis are reviewed and a computational model of stereopsis deriving from these studies is described. The distinctive features of the model are: (1) it identifies edge locations in each monocular field by searching for zero crossings in non-orientated centre–surround convolution profiles; (2) it selects among all possible binocular point-for-point combinations of edge locations only those which satisfy a (quasi-) collinear figural grouping rule; (3) it presents a concept of the orientated and spatial frequency tuned channel as a nonlinear grouping operator. The success of the model is demonstrated both on a stereo pair of a natural scene and on a random-dot stereogram.

1. Introduction

One of the most impressive achievements of the last 15 years or so of vision research has been the psychophysical and neurophysiological investigation of the spatial frequency (s.f.) tuned 'channel' (for reviews, see the paper in this symposium by Campbell, one of the originators of this work). The evidence is now overwhelming that s.f. channels exist in the visual system of many species, including man, and we know a good deal about such things as channel tuning (see, for example, Mostafavi & Sakrison 1976; Wilson & Giese 1977; Wilson & Bergen 1979). Curiously, however, relatively little attention has been given to the question of what functional roles the s.f. channels might serve (Marr's (1976) paper is seminal exception), and even less to empirical tests of such ideas as have been formulated. The channels exist, but what do they do? We have considered how s.f. channels might contribute to texture discrimination (Mayhew & Frisby 1978c), but here we review our work on the possible roles served by s.f. channels in stereopsis.

The problem solved by the visual system in achieving stereopsis is easily summarized: it is to compute descriptions from the left and right retinal images, match them correctly binocularly, measure the associated disparities, and thereby build up a depth map of the visual scene. In principle, relatively high-level descriptions such as object (and/or surface) boundaries could be computed and matched. In this case, the visual system might achieve the goal of correct matching by taking advantage of the constraint that an object usually presents roughly similar boundary shapes in the two retinal images. Of course, use of object boundaries could not provide an entirely satisfactory basis for stereopsis because we easily see the depth variations that frequently occur within such boundaries. Moreover, the random-dot stereogram (Julesz 1960) demonstrates conclusively that object contours are not necessary for the stereopsis computation because no objects can be seen in either random-dot stereo half before fusion. Whether monocularly discriminable object contours are nevertheless a *sufficient* basis for at least a limited form of stereopsis remains a controversial question (Ramachandran *et al.* 1973; Mayhew & Frisby 1976; Frisby & Mayhew 1977a; Mayhew *et al.* 1977; Frisby & Mayhew 1978), although there is no doubt that monocular cues can play a valuable role in guiding the eye movements required for fusion in certain circumstances (e.g. when disparities larger than those covered by Panum's fusional area are presented; Saye & Frisby (1976); Kidd *et al.* (1979); see also Julesz & Oswald (1978)).

Given the finding that high-level descriptions are not necessary for stereopsis, it is natural to propose that disparity measurements begin with the matching of low-level left/right 'point' descriptions (Julesz 1960). This suggestion, however, immediately provokes the follow-up question: what exactly is a 'point' for stereo combination? Grey level points are intrinsically unsatisfactory because a grey level description does not reliably define a point on a physical surface (Marr & Poggio 1976). Hence, what are required are point descriptions that make explicit changes in reflectance. Of course, given the wide range of textures that can serve as carriers of stereopsis (Julesz 1971), there is almost certainly no single definition of a 'point' that could cope with all of the many different types of reflectance changes that can serve as stereo inputs. In this paper, we review some psychophysical studies that have helped to define what point descriptions are in fact used by the visual system for computing stereopsis, and we describe a computational model of stereopsis whose design has been guided by this psychophysical work.

2. SPATIAL FREQUENCY TUNED POINT DESCRIPTIONS FOR STEREOPSIS

Julesz & Miller (1975) investigated spatial frequency (s.f.) selective processes in stereopsis by exploring the effects of adding masking noise of carefully controlled spectral composition to bandpass filtered random-dot stereograms. They found that if the spectral content of the noise lay more than two octaves distant from the spectral content of the stereoscopic image, then stereopsis was unaffected. That is, a stereoscopic percept 'drawn' in one s.f. could be seen quite clearly despite the presence of noise from another s.f. band. If, however, the s.f. of the noise overlapped that of the stereoscopic image, then stereopsis was destroyed. They concluded from this result that 'the global stereopsis mechanism (which processes the binocular fusion of random-dot stereograms) utilizes frequency-tuned analyzers, thus these analysers must reside prior to the stage (or at the stage) of global stereopsis'.

Julesz & Miller's ideas were developed in greater detail by Frisby & Mayhew (1977*a*) who were concerned to apply them to the theoretical problems posed by 'rivalrous texture stereograms' (see also Mayhew & Frisby 1976). Figure 1 illustrates this development and makes clear exactly what Frisby & Mayhew meant by an 'independent s.f.-tuned stereopsis channel'. Each such channel receives its inputs from monocular s.f.-tuned analysers which filter the retinal images for particular bands of spectral content. High and low s.f. channels only are depicted in figure 1, but the dotted lines between boxes represent channels tuned to intermediate frequencies. Each monocular s.f. channel can be thought of as a 2D array of analysers, each of which possesses a receptive field whose shape (see profiles in the centre of the figure) determines the s.f. selectivity of the channel. The row of dots within the monocular boxes of figure 1 represent a 1D slice of each 2D array. The 'activity profile' of the analysers in the slice is shown when they are responding to a pattern with a luminance profile as depicted in the retinal image boxes. These activity profiles were obtained from a computer simulation which convolved the input retinal waveform with the high and low s.f. receptive field profiles shown. In neurophysiological terms, excursions of the activity profile above the row of dots is to be interpreted as above-threshold activity in on-centre units, excursions below as activity in off-centre units. Thus each dot can be thought of as representing a pair of cells, one selective for 'brightness' and one for 'darkness' (Jung 1973). The left and right activity profiles for a given s.f. are combined separately for the purposes of both local and global stereopsis – hence the phrase 'independent s.f.-tuned stereopsis channels'.

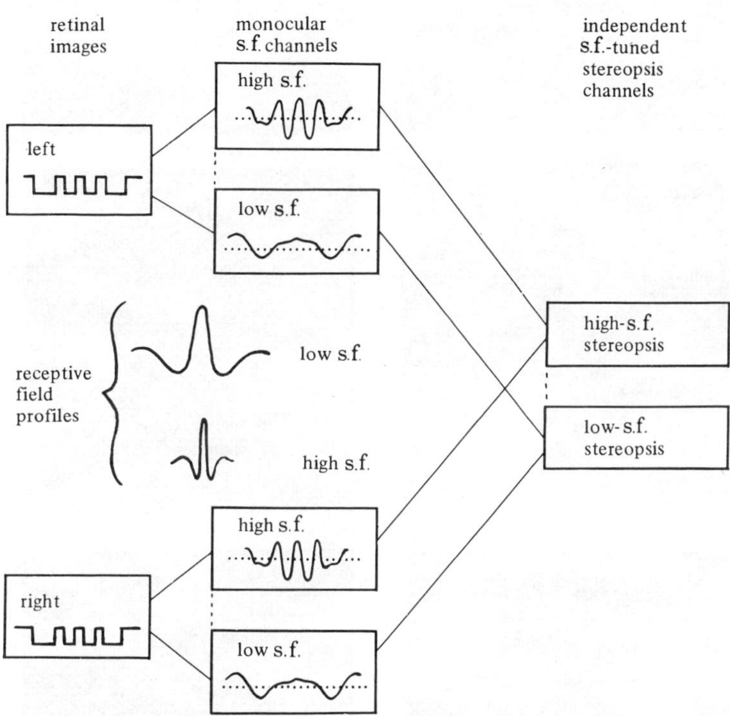

FIGURE 1. The independent s.f.-tuned channels model of stereopsis. The stereopsis boxes represent processes mediating both local and global stereopsis (see text for details). Reproduced from Frisby & Mayhew (1978a) by courtesy of Pion Limited.

The stereopsis model depicted in figure 1 does not specify what aspects of the s.f. filtered profiles are used for making left–right local matches. Frisby & Mayhew (1977a; see also Mayhew *et al.* 1977) implied a scheme whereby any 'left white point' could fuse with any 'right white point' (given the usual constraint imposed by Panum's fusional area); *mutatis mutandis* for left–right 'black point' matches. However, it would be equally possible and almost certainly preferable to use left–right peak and/or zero crossing matches (see later and also Marr & Poggio 1979). Thus the key feature of the model is simply that whatever local matches are made, they are effected between left–right convolution profiles separately for the different s.f. tuned channels, and with separate resolution of the ambiguity problem posed by false local fusions (i.e. separate s.f.-tuned global processes as well as local ones).

Given the independent channels model illustrated in figure 1, it becomes of interest to compare stereopsis contrast thresholds for 'complex' stereograms composed of multiple s.f. components, with similar thresholds for 'simple' stereograms composed of a single s.f. The independent channels model would predict that the threshold for stereopsis of a complex stimulus containing widely separated (two octaves different) s.f. components should be reached when the most sensitive channel reaches its own contrast threshold and that the presence of another s.f.

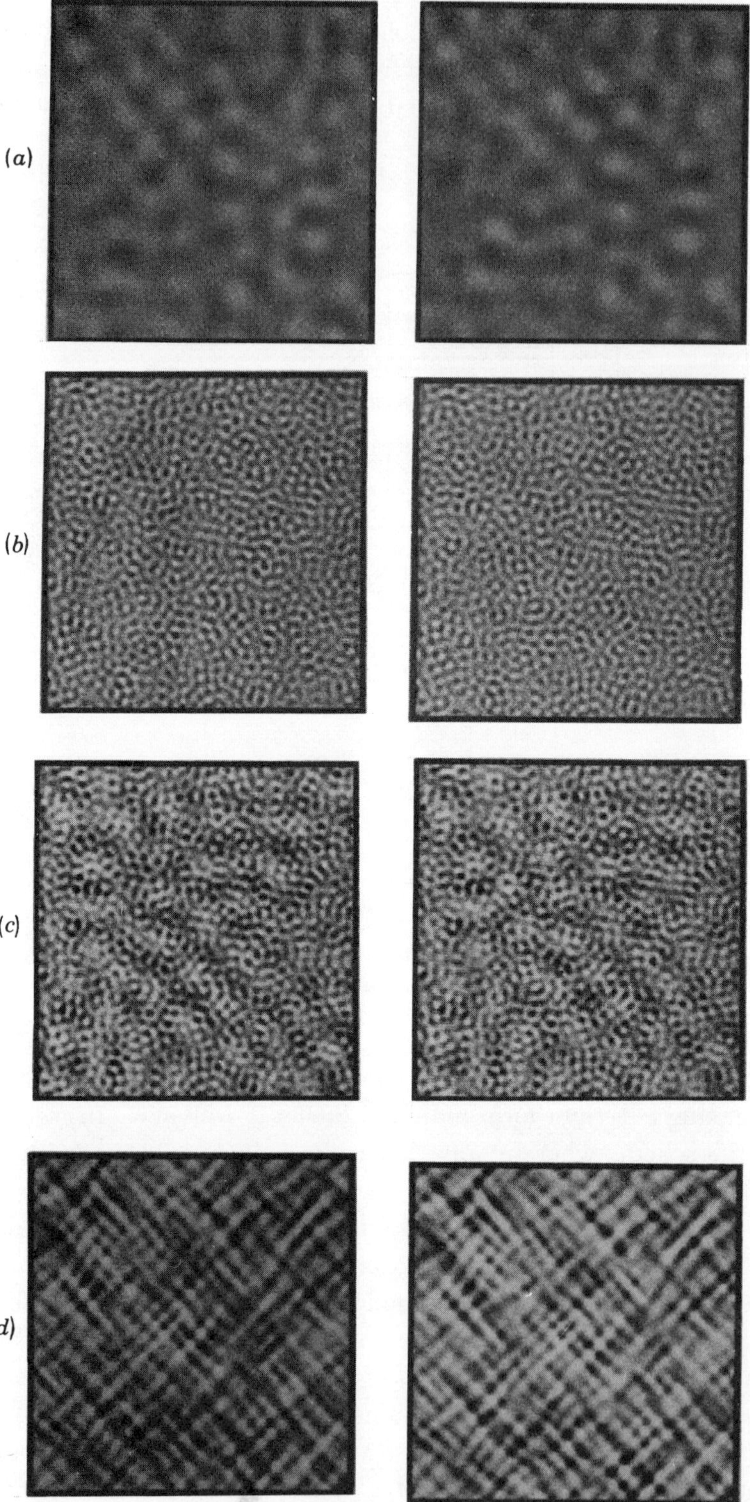

FIGURE 2. For legend see facing page.

component should not play an important role (given due allowance for probability summation). Mayhew & Frisby (1978 a) reported several experiments testing this prediction, using both circularly filtered and orientated stimuli (figure 2). Contrast thresholds for stereopsis were always considerably lower than the independent s.f. channels model predicted and a variety of ways of saving the model from this falsification were tried out but found wanting. As a result, Mayhew & Frisby advanced the so-called SLUG model of stereopsis (several local unitary global) shown in figure 3, in which local matches remain s.f.-tuned (and thus capable of providing a locus for the Julesz–Miller masking effects) but with these feeding a single global stereopsis mechanism (cf. Marr & Poggio's $2\frac{1}{2}$ D sketch) for the resolution of local ambiguities and the build-up of surface descriptions.

At this point we asked: should SLUG be equipped with circularly symmetric local filters, or orientated ones, or both? Julesz & Miller (1975) used circular filtering for their demonstrations but the extensive psychophysical literature supporting the existence of orientated s.f channels (see, for example, Mostafavi & Sakrison 1976), when coupled with the finding that

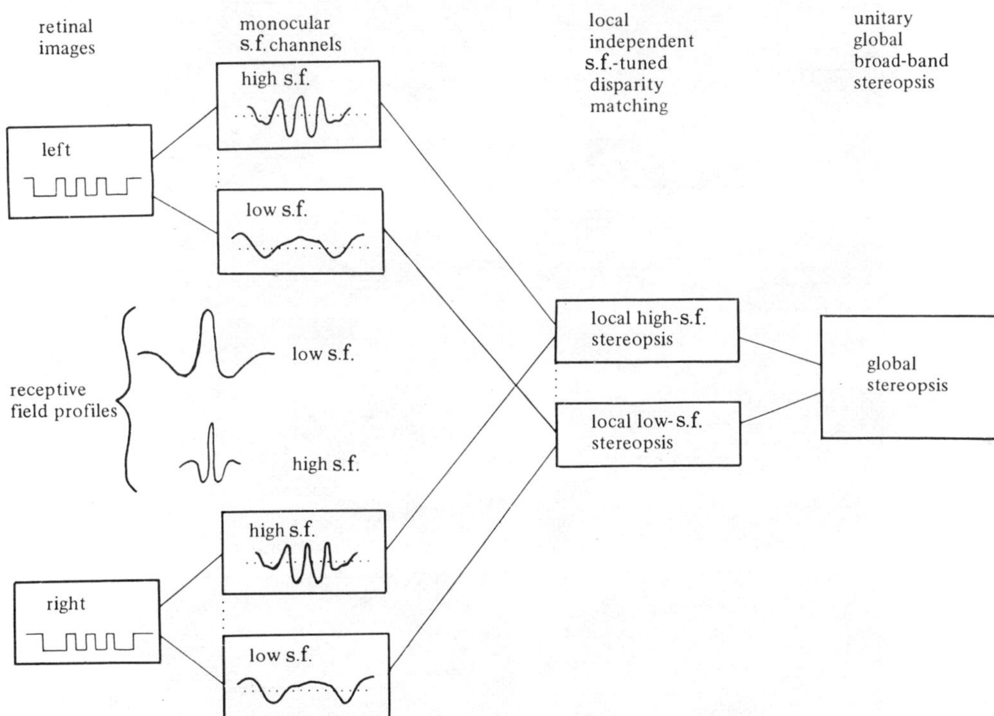

FIGURE 3. The SLUG model of stereopsis: Several local independent disparity-matching processes feed a Unitary Global stereopsis mechanism. Reproduced from Frisby & Mayhew (1978 a) by courtesy of Pion Limited.

FIGURE 2. Contrast summation effects for stereopsis from complex stereograms containing two widely differing spectral components. (a) Low s.f. stereo pair (2.5 cycles/deg); (b) high s.f. stereo pair (10 cycles/deg); (c) complex s.f. stereo pair (2.5 and 10 cycles/deg combined in the contrast ratio of 1:3): this stereogram has a lower contrast threshold for stereopsis than predicted by the independent channels model of figure 1; (d) complex stereo pair made up of two oblique components: as for (c), stereopsis contrast threshold for this complex stimulus is lower than that predicted if its components were processed wholly independently for stereopsis. Note that these contrast summation effects do not hold for contrast thresholds for simple detection of these complex textures. All s.f. values hold (approximately) if the stereo pairs are viewed from about 10 × picture height. In all three stereo pairs, crossed eye fusion produces the percept of a central square floating above its surround. Reproduced from Mayhew & Frisby (1978 a) by courtesy of Pion Limited.

cortical disparity units always seem to be orientated (see, for example, Poggio & Fischer 1977), encourages the belief in at least parallel provision of orientated disparity filters. We have conducted two psychophysical studies on this issue.

The first (Mayhew & Frisby 1978*b*) was an orientational equivalent of the Julesz–Miller masking study in which we discovered that if stereopsis from an orientated texture was masked by adding similarly orientated noise to one field, then rotation of the masking noise so that it would no longer interfere with orientated local matches did not succeed in releasing the stereopsis from the effects of the mask (figure 4). This is difficult to understand if local matches are made on orientated s.f. filtered profiles, although it might just be that the rotated noise, while freeing

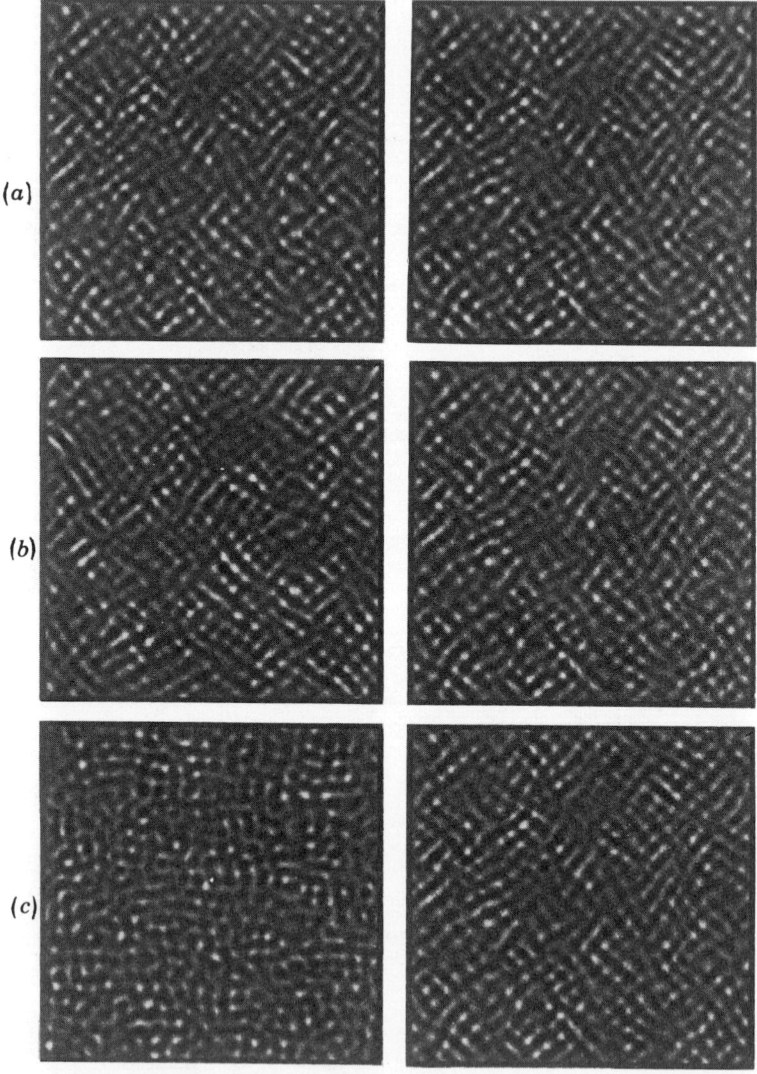

FIGURE 4. Stereopsis masking and orientational tuning. (*a*) Orientated-texture stereo pair: crossed-eye fusion produces the percept of a central square floating above its surround. (*b*) Same stereo pair as in (*a*) but masking noise of similar orientation and s.f. to that of the stereopsis signal has been added to the left half. Stereopsis is severely impaired and probably impossible for most observers. (*c*) Same stereo pair as in (*b*) but with the noise component of left field rotated by 45°. The quality of stereopsis is not improved by this rotation, even though the noise would now be stimulating different orientated s.f. channels from those triggered by the stereo signal. Reproduced from Mayhew & Frisby (1978*b*) by courtesy of Pion Limited.

the orientated matches, nevertheless produces interference at a global level from *ad hoc* spurious matches set up by non-orientationally tuned units. This possibility seems to us doubtful, however, in view of the known resistance of stereopsis to masking stimuli in many circumstances (see, for example, the many illustrations in Julesz (1971) to this effect).

Secondly, we have pointed out that orientated s.f. filters are in principle very poor devices for dealing with certain disparity cues, namely those from a surface with rapidly changing depths

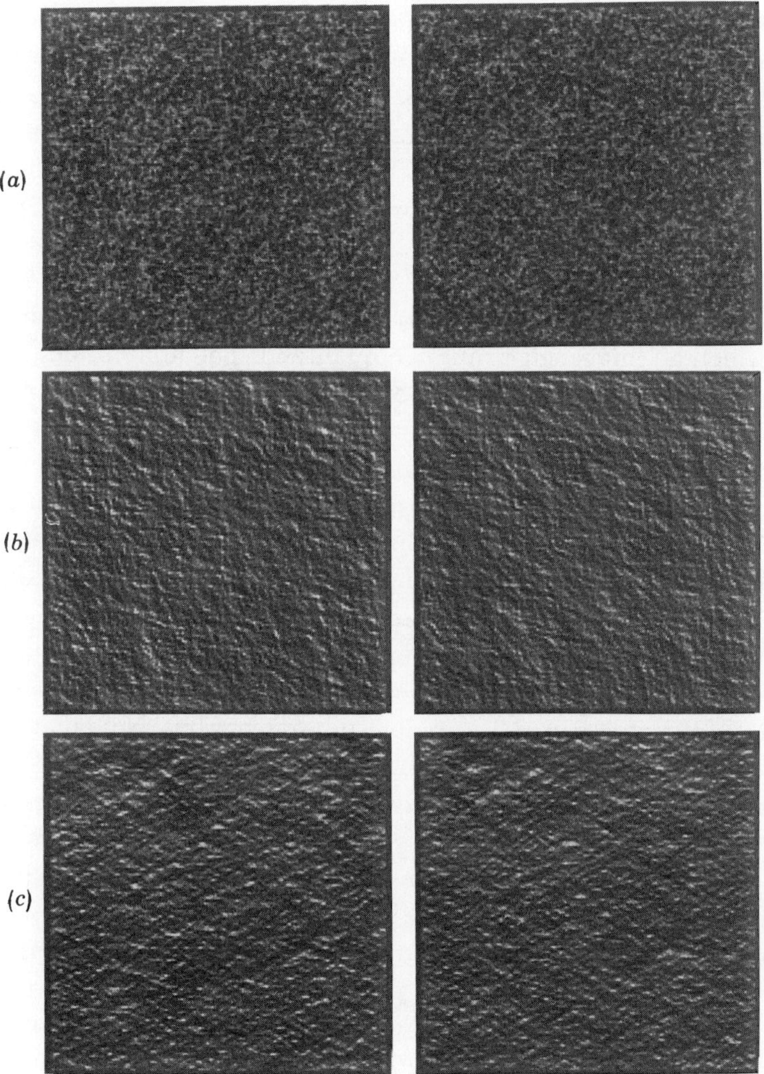

FIGURE 5. The processing of rapidly changing disparities is problematic for orientated s.f. channels. (*a*) Stereogram portraying a surface with near-horizontal corrugations. (*b*) Vertical filtering of (*a*) (orientation bandpass = vertical ± 45°) renders stereopsis impossible. (*c*) Horizontal filtering of (*a*) (orientation bandpass = horizontal ± 45°) severely impairs stereopsis.

(Mayhew & Frisby 1979*a*). Consider, for example, the stereogram shown in figure 5 which depicts a series of horizontal corrugations (as though the observer were looking down on a corrugated roof). Vertically tuned s.f. filters could not *in principle* extract the depth information from this figure: they would inevitably have receptive fields spreading over several 'disparity rasters' and so smear the disparity cues hopelessly. It might be argued that the depth could be mediated by horizontally tuned units in these circumstances but the poor quality of stereopsis deriving from a horizontally filtered version of the corrugated stereogram (figure 5c) suggests otherwise, as does the fact that many naïve subjects cannot obtain any depth whatsoever from this horizontally filtered stereo pair, whereas they can do so easily for the unfiltered original.

We conclude from these two studies that orientated s.f. filters do not seem to be used in the human visual system for establishing disparity matches. If valid, this conclusion would seem to demand a revision of Marr & Poggio's (1979) model of stereopsis which uses just such filters, although the revision required on this score may not be very fundamental (e.g. the simple substitution of circular for orientated filters may be enough). Of course, our rejection of orientated s.f. filters for stereopsis does not preclude other types of orientational selectivity embedded in the stereopsis mechanism. For a discussion of one alternative form of orientational tuning, we turn now to our computational model of stereopsis, called STEREOEDGE, which was designed with the foregoing psychophysical work in mind.

3. STEREOEDGE: A MODEL FOR THE COMPUTATION OF BINOCULAR EDGES

For STEREOEDGE (Mayhew & Frisby 1979a), a 'point' for stereo combination is an image location through which an image edge runs. To qualify for potential fusion, a pair of left and right edge points must possess roughly similar orientation and the same contrast polarity (e.g. a point that is part of a white-to-black edge in one field can fuse only with a white-to-black point in the other field, and not with one whose polarity is black-to-white). All possible local point-by-point combinations satisfying these requirements (and also that of falling within a realistically sized Panum's fusional area) are listed and a selection is then made of just those that conform to certain rules of figural grouping. In this way, STEREOEDGE takes advantage of the constraint that correct points for stereo fusion will be embedded in roughly similar contours in the two retinal images. Or course, these contours need not be object contours: they could be contours defining local elements within an object boundary and hence the constraint is applicable to a wide range of textures used for random-dot stereograms. Note that this constraint is quite different from either of those employed by Marr & Poggio (1976), i.e. the constraints of 'uniqueness of matches' (of suspect validity anyway, given Panum's limiting case) and 'depth continuity'.

By using rules of figural grouping for disambiguating local matches, the processing of disparity information by STEREOEDGE is intimately incorporated in those early visual computations contributing to figure-ground separation (Marr 1976). Thus STEREOEDGE represents an implementation of our earlier speculation that 'the processing of global disparity occurs in parallel with (rather than after) the very first stages of the computation of the symbolic descriptions of the visual scene . . ., the two processes sharing the same neural elements' (Mayhew & Frisby 1978a).

STEREOEDGE has two main parts, one monocular (called ZEROPOINT) and one binocular (called MATCH), and these will be described briefly in separate sections.

3.1. *ZEROPOINT: A procedure for finding monocular edge locations*

STEREOEDGE's first procedure, called ZEROPOINT, begins by convolving a grey level description of each monocular input image with a centre-surround operator (Laplacian). It then locates the points within each two-dimensional convolution profile through which contours pass. Left and right images are dealt with independently at this stage.

3.1.1. *The centre–surround convolution*

The design of the centre–surround operator can be varied at will so that it models a spatial frequency (s.f.) tuned channel of any desired characteristics. For example, figure 6a shows an input stereo pair portraying a teddy bear and figure 6c provides samples of the left and right convolution 'images' obtained by ZEROPOINT when its centre–surround operator is modelled approximately on the human contrast sensitivity function reported by Blakemore & Campbell (1969), i.e. when the centre–surround operator is equivalent to the broad-band channel shown in figure 7. Note that in a biological visual system, the whitish areas of figure 6c might be encoded in on-centre units and the blackish areas of off-centre units. Note also that in this particular case, the large areas of mid-grey do not signify zero convolution counts: the low-pass characteristics of the channel ensure that some response is made even to near-uniform areas of luminance (some retinal ganglion cells respond to overall level of luminance; Robson 1975). This feature has an advantage when ZEROPOINT proceeds to locate contours, as will become clear shortly.

Of course, given the work reviewed earlier implicating s.f.-tuned mechanisms in stereopsis, it is necessary to build in at some stage greater s.f.-selectivity than that of the broad-band channel of figure 7. This is an important issue to which we return later, having described STEREOEDGE's basic structure in terms of operations on a broad-band convolution profile. However, note that in view of our conclusion about the absence of orientated s.f.-tuned disparity processes, all convolutions used by STEREOEDGE are provided by circularly symmetric filters.

3.1.2. *Locating points on contours*

Contour boundaries in convolution images such as those of figure 6b are marked by positive–negative cross-overs (for figure 6c, white–black transitions), and ZEROPOINT is designed to obtain a description of where these zero crossings (z.cs) occur. Thus ZEROPOINT records the location of each z.c. (figure 6d) and ties to each one a description of:

(a) contour polarity (i.e. which side of the z.c. positive or negative);

(b) contour orientation (obtained by measuring the positive–negative gradient in eight orientations around each z.c. and then taking the contour orientation as that of the orientation providing the minimum gradient);

(c) contour gradient perpendicular to contour orientation.

Note that it is necessary to avoid logging positive-to-zero and negative-to-zero returns on either side of a contour boundary as 'genuine' z.cs: obviously they are not. In fact, such 'returns-to-zero' are infrequent for a broad-band operator with a low-pass characteristic of the kind shown in figure 7: usually, in such cases, convolution counts each side of a boundary stay either slightly positive or slightly negative, a fact that helps avoid logging 'spurious' z.cs. However, a few returns-to-zero are to be expected even in a broad-band channel and ZEROPOINT deals with them by eliminating any cross-overs that fall below a certain threshold gradient size. In narrow-band channels, returns-to-zero are much more common and also need a different approach for their elimination, the best one probably being to select as genuine z.cs only those cross-overs that occur in the same location in more than one channel (see later).

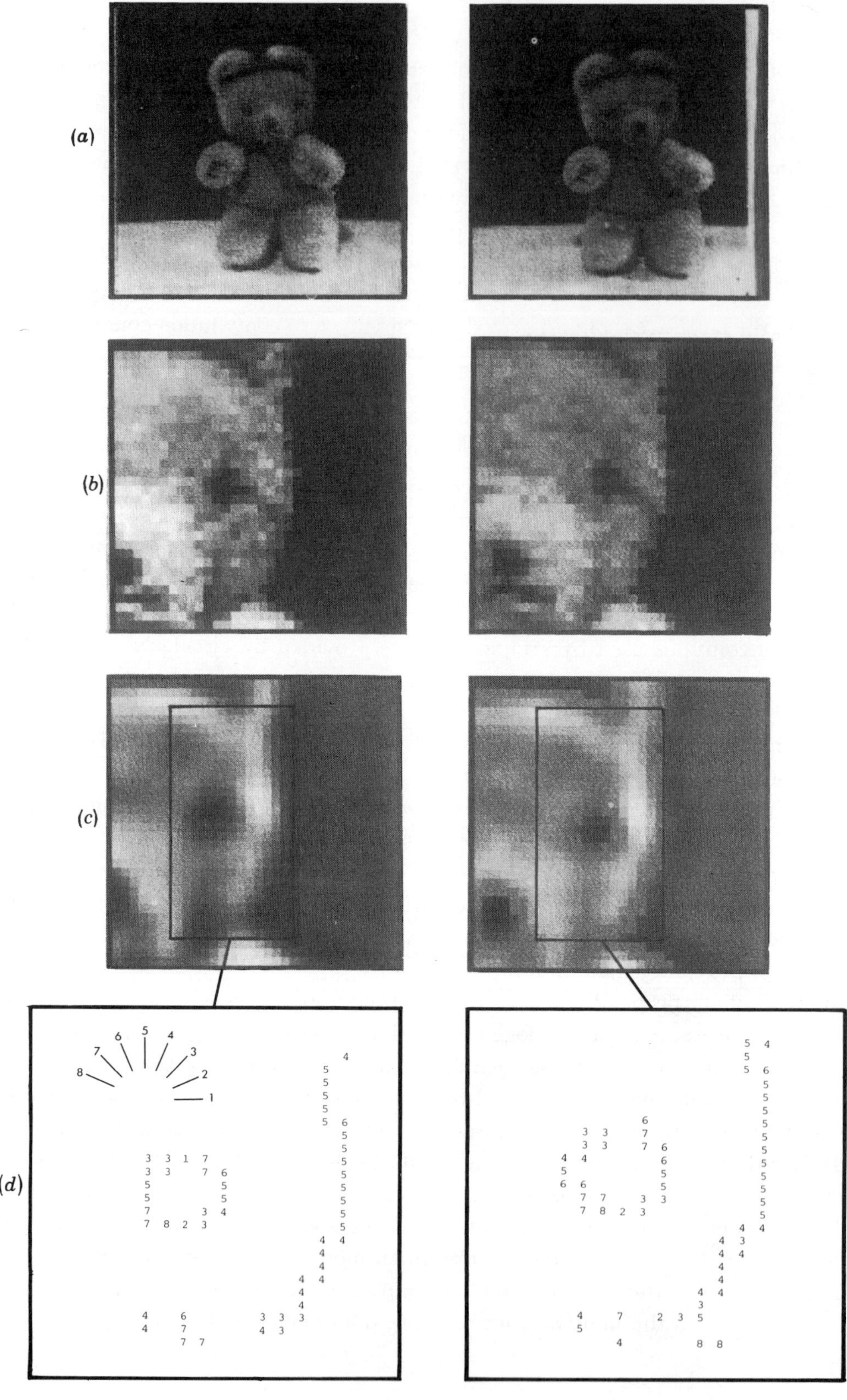

FIGURE 6 *a–d*. For legend see page 107.

3.2. *Match: A procedure for the binocular combination of edge locations*

Monocular 'points' used by MATCH for binocular combination are z.c. locations of similar contour polarity and orientation discovered by applying ZEROPOINT separately to each monocular image. However, similar left and right z.cs are combined (Panum's fusional area = ± 3 pixels horizontally, ± 1 pixel vertically) only if certain neighbourhood constraints are met around each potential z.c. fusion. The procedures applying these constraints embed certain principles of

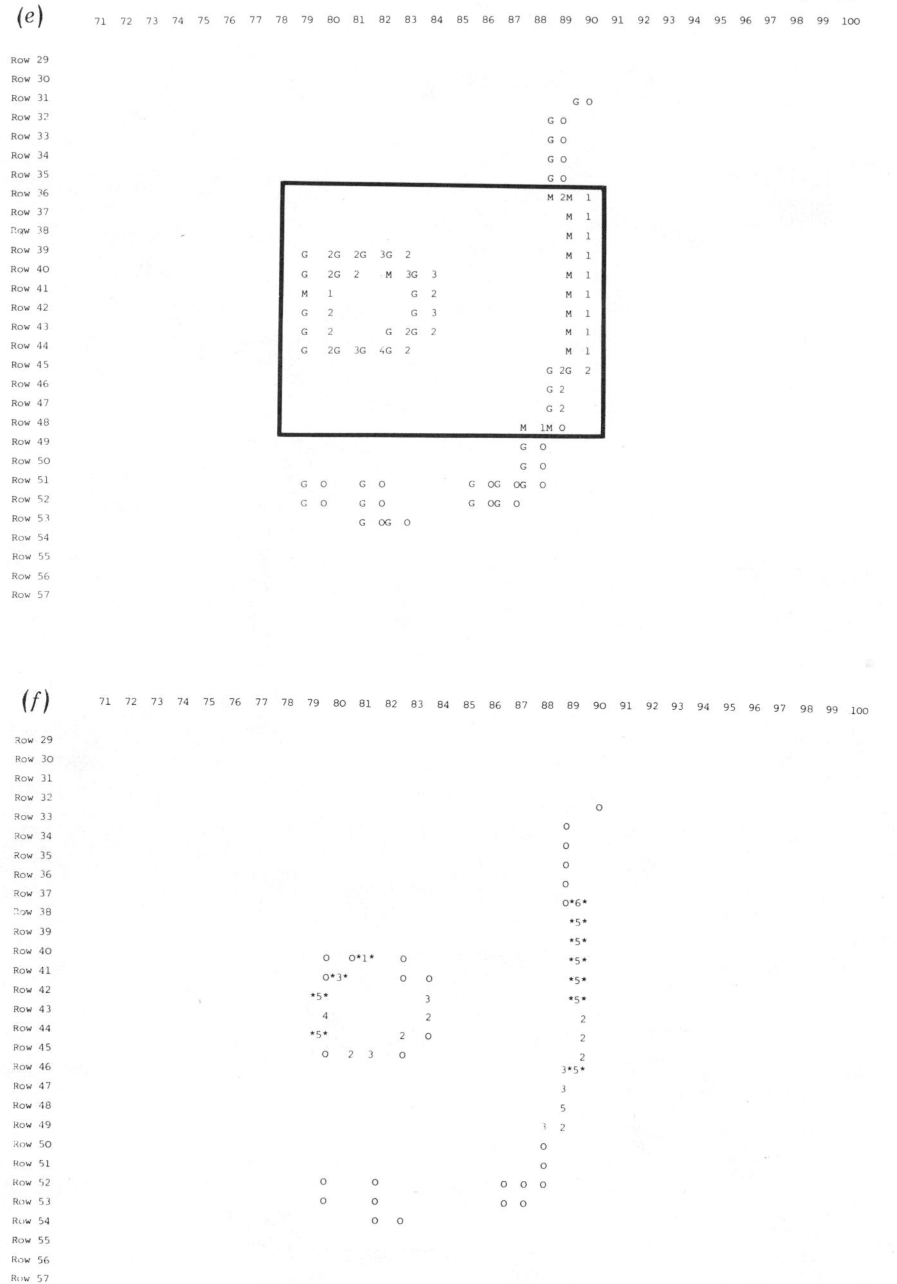

FIGURE 6*e–f*. For legend see page 107.

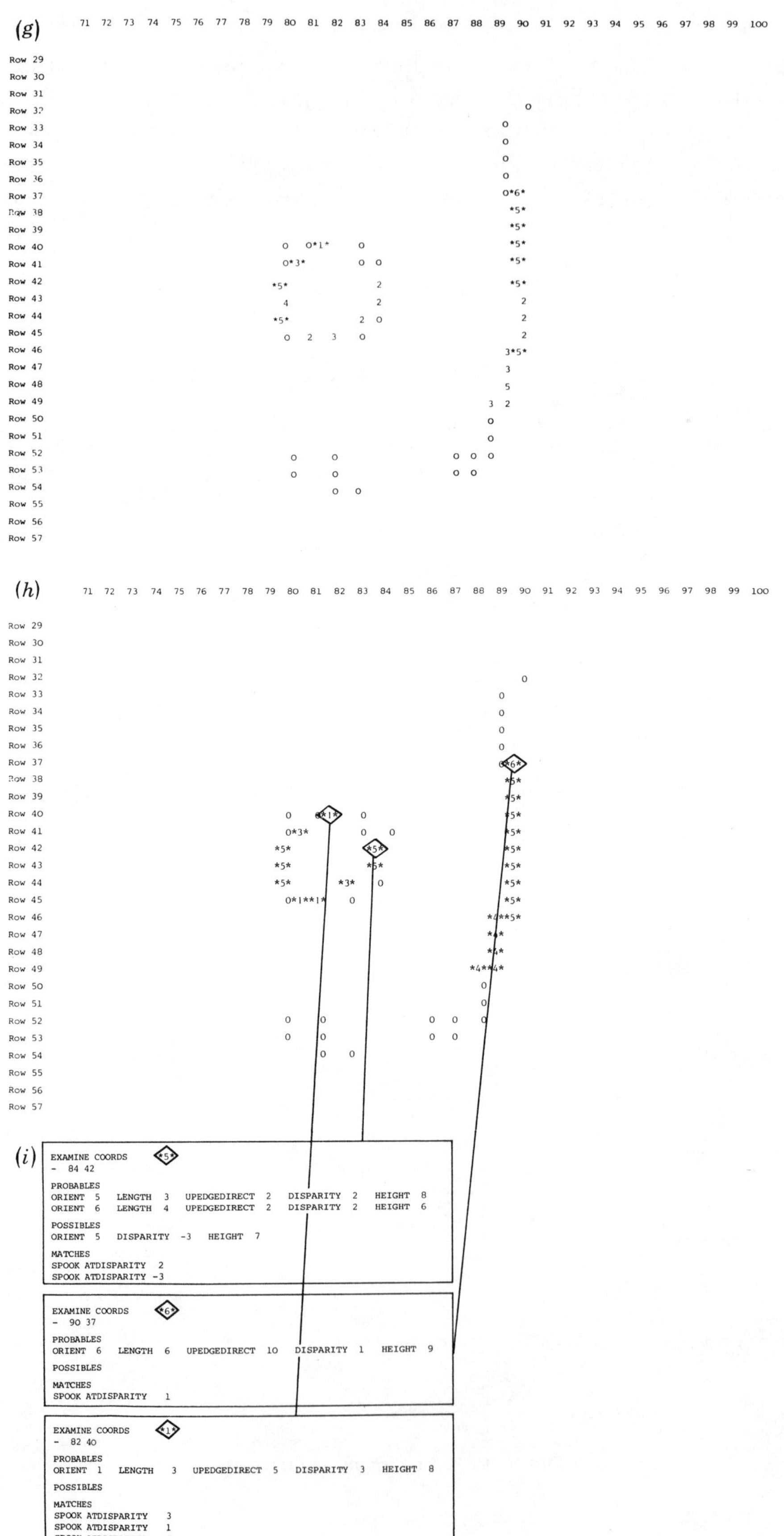

FIGURE 6 *g–i*. For legend see opposite.

figural grouping, and in this way ambiguity resolution among all possible local z.c. matches is achieved.

The strategy used by MATCH for constraining which z.c. combinations are finally utilized is to allow only these z.c. matches that are collinear (or quasi-collinear) in any particular depth plane. (In fact, we have explored extending the general scheme by allowing collinearity across depth planes, i.e. allowing collinear tilts, and there seem to be no difficulties in principle with this extension.) MATCH employs its collinear stratagem at various levels to select from a complete list of all possible z.c. matches (figure 6e) only those z.c. matches that reflect 'correct' edge fusions.

(a) First, a list is generated of all possible cyclopean assertions about short edge sections. Each such section is called a MICROEDGE and each one must be composed of at least three (quasi-) collinear matching z.cs in each eye's image spanning a distance of up to 7 pixels. Gaps of up to 2 pixels are allowed within each MICROEDGE and, as mentioned earlier, z.c. matches must share the same polarity and similar orientation ($\pm 45°$ seems satisfactory and matches

---

FIGURE 6. STEREOEDGE dealing with a stero pair of a natural scene (see text). (a) Grey level images (128×128 pixels) of the stereo halves so arranged that crossed-eyed fusion produces appropriate depth effects (i.e. right stereo half on the left hand side of figure). (b) Grey levels (32×32 pixels) in the region of the teddy bear's left eye and enlarged to illustrate details of STEREOEDGE's operation in subsequent figures. (c) Convolution outputs obtained from using the filter described in figure 7. (d) Zero crossing (z.c.) locations discovered in the right and left convolution outputs of (c) in the regions demarcated by the boxes. The numbers of each z.c. location indicate the orientation associated with that z.c. (number code for orientations inset in the left half). Note that equivalent right–left contours are represented by collections of z.cs that differ in their details, a fact that reflects faithfully the grey level images from whence they came. Any competent stereopsis processor must be able to deal with such left–right image differences. (e) Potential z.c. matches obtained by combining the two halves of (d). Computer storage limitations necessitate that a restricted region is dealt with at any one time, shown here by the inset window. The search for potential z.c. matches begins with the right eye (in a sense, therefore, treated as the 'dominant eye'). Thus for each z.c. in the right eye, a search is made along the same horizontal raster in the left eye (Panum's fusional area $= \pm 3$ pixels) for a suitable z.c. for matching. Requirements for a match are (i) same contrast polarity and (ii) roughly similar orientation ($\pm 45°$). If no suitable left z.c. is found, then the vertical extent of Panum's area is relaxed to ± 1 pixel of vertical disparity. If only one match is found, then this is coded with an M plus a number which represents the disparity of the match (± 3 pixels disparity, equivalent to about $\pm 8'$ disparity if the stereo pair is viewed from about $10 \times$ picture height. If more than one match is found, then this is shown with a G plus a number which gives the number of potential matches (G because the number includes ghosts). (f) Iteration 1 of the filtering algorithm. If a z.c. location is found to have just one possible match, then its orientation is given as a number code (see orientation code inset in (d)) and an asterisk is bound to it on either side. If a z.c. location has more than one possible match, then asterisks are absent and only a number is given which shows the number of possibilities. Z.c. locations with no possible matches according to the point reached by the algorithm at this stage are shown with a zero. (g) Iteration 3 of the filtering algorithm. Note that little change has occurred since iteration 1 for this particular region of the scene, the first iteration having done virtually all the work possible given the filtering constraints embedded in the algorithm. Coding as for (f). (h) Final 'best bet', achieved by resolving any ambiguity left over from the filtering algorithm by selecting the 'strongest' z.c. match at any ambiguous location, i.e. selecting that z.c. match with the largest weighting function. Note the successful resolution of ambiguities recorded in (e), (f) and (g). Coding as for (f). (i) Details of the data base provided by STEREOEDGE. Specimen print-outs are shown for just three of the z.c. locations given in (h). 'Probables' are a list of z.c. matches that survive right up to the 'best bet' stage; 'possibles' are those z.cs that have been excluded at some stage but might later be resuscitated and so are kept in store. The parameters tied to each entry are: ORIENT, orientation given as a number (code shown inset in (d)); LENGTH, the number of z.cs contributing to the MICROEDGE in which the z.c. in question is embedded; UPEDGEDIRECT, the direction of the maximum gradient at the z.c. expressed on a 16 point scale that gives information about contrast polarity; DISPARITY, ± 3 pixels; WEIGHT, weighting function as described in text. The list of MATCHES records ghosts that have been eliminated. Note the successful location of the edges of the eye in depth planes in front of the edge of the head. Note also that although STEREOEDGE prints out individually its matched z.cs, it would be a trivial matter to group these into larger-scale edge assertions.

involving horizontal z.cs seem to cause few problems). Tied to each possible MICROEDGE assertion is the disparity and orientation of points along its length, and a weighting. The latter is a crude evaluation function: the longer and straighter the MICROEDGE the better; gaps in the MICROEDGE reduce the weight. Figure 6*f* illustrates the kind of output available at this stage.

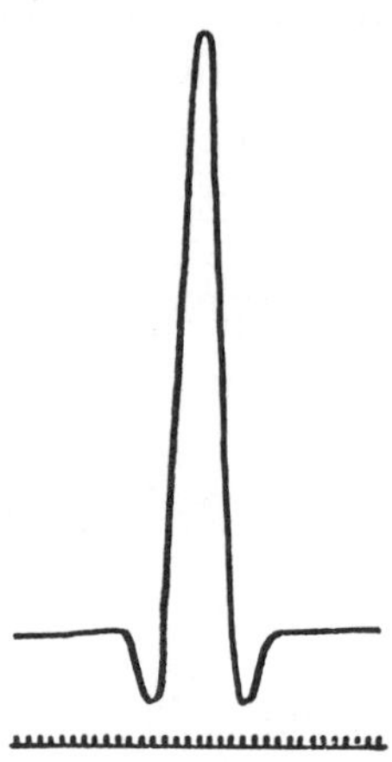

FIGURE 7. Receptive field profile used for producing the convolution images shown in figure 6*c*. The scale below the profile is in image pixels. The receptive field is roughly equivalent to a broad-band channel that would produce the contrast sensitivity function described by Blakemore & Campbell (1969).

(*b*) Next, the list of possible MICROEDGE assertions is pruned down by taking into account certain wider neighbourhood relationships. To stay in the list, a MICROEDGE must be either very strong (large weighting), or the only one in its vicinity, or else supported at one or other end by a neighbouring MICROEDGE that shares a similar orientation and disparity. (In a monocular curvilinear aggregator of the same general type, we have included the capability for allowing support at bends and corners to generate angle assertions. This extension is, however, too demanding of computer storage to be run in binocular mode on our machine at present.) The general elimination procedure is a parallel iterative Waltz-type filtering algorithm (Waltz 1975) in which MICROEDGE assertions without neighbourhood support (cf. incompatible blocks–world line labelling in Waltz 1975) are removed from the current list. MICROEDGES that are eliminated in this way, however, are not completely discarded but instead entered in a list of 'possibles'. Such MICROEDGES are no longer considered in successive iterations of the algorithm but they are recovered should the algorithm remove all MICROEDGE candidates in a given vicinity. (This latter eventuality often happens with z.cs towards the end of an edge, and particularly at the end of thin lines where the terminal z.c. has an orientation perpendicular to the z.cs forming the body of the line, so rendering it ineligible for support from these neighbours). The algorithm typically needs only three iterations to converge (figure 6*f*, *g*).

(*c*) As will be apparent from the foregoing, the constraints embedded in the curvilinear filtering algorithm often fail to force a unique interpretation, an outcome which contrasts with the blocks–world situation where the available constraints are so much stonger. Here, quantization fuzz spawns a blur of similar, mutually supporting and essentially equivalent MICROEDGE assertions so that it is necessary to have an additional step to determine which MICROEDGES are to be allowed to survive to the end. It turns out that it is sufficient simply to use the weighting function to select the 'best' of any competing group (figure 6*h*).

3.3. *The need for s.f. information*

For the purpose of computing primal sketch assertions, Marr (1976) used linear orientated s.f. channels as the measurement devices whose outputs were parsed both for descriptions of the orientations of contours in the input and for descriptions of contour type. S.f. information proved essential for the latter objective, e.g. for assertions of EDGES of various degrees of fuzziness. As will be clear from the foregoing account of STEREOEDGE, we have found it computationally convenient (as well as psychophysically sensible) to extract the orientation structure of an input image by using nonlinear orientated grouping processes operating upon non-orientated convolution profiles. We now turn to the question of whether our general scheme can be expanded to incorporate s.f. information essential to descriptions of edge type.

First, we note that as far as edges are concerned, s.f. channels with different tuning produce z.cs that all tend to fall in the same location (figure 8). As a result, z.cs in Laplacian convolution profiles seem ideal candidates for building up a good 'skeleton' around which to integrate

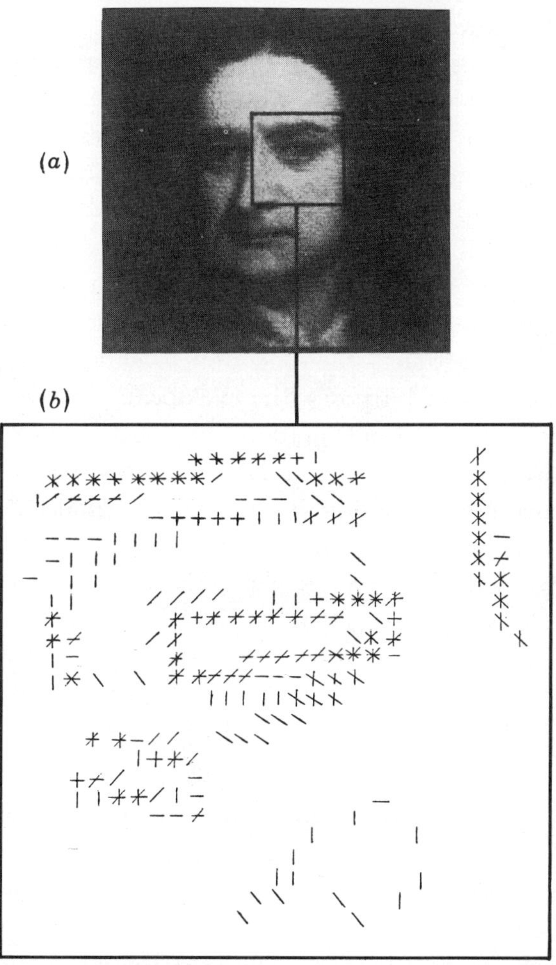

FIGURE 8. (*a*) Grey level input image (128 × 128 pixels) of Sir Isaac Newton. (*b*) Z.cs found by four differently tuned s.f. channels (all non-orientated) on a 32 × 32 pixel section of figure 8*a*: z.cs found by the 2.6 cycles/deg channel are shown with \ , by the 3.6 cycles/deg channel with |, by the 5.2 cycles/deg channel with —, and by the 7.2 cycles/deg channel with /. All s.fs apply for a viewing distance of figure 8*a* of about 10 × picture height. Note that z.cs in different channels show quite good alignment.

s.f.-tuned information relating to edge type. In contrast, peaks in Laplacian profiles from edges fall on either side of the edge's location, with their exact separation depending strongly on the s.f. tuning of the Laplacian and the slope of the edge with which it is dealing.

Secondly, note that the situation is the other way round for lines, where the *peaks* in the Laplacian profiles show convenient alignment, with the z.cs spread out on either side of the line centre. Consequently, a search for peaks showing similar locations in different channel outputs seem a sensible strategy for locating lines. In fact, we have already written a program that uses the nonlinear grouping of peaks to obtain MICROLINE assertions and it is planned to extend this monocular program to one capable of describing binocular lines. The difference between the peaks–z.cs situation for edges and lines follows from the fact that the Fourier components for an edge tend to be in sine phase whereas those for a line are in cosine phase.

Thirdly, the gradient of a z.c. is related to the contrast and frequency of the input. Indeed, because the gradient of a z.c. is directly proportional to input frequency, it is tempting to think that the human system contains an implicit compensation for the high frequency cut of the contrast sensitivity threshold function (Georgeson & Sullivan 1975).

Fourthly, Marr (1976) showed how the local spectrum of peaks delivered by a collection of different s.f.-tuned convolutions could be parsed into a description of edge type (i.e. fuzzy edge, sharp edge, etc.). The same objective can be attained in much the same way working not from peak information (as did Marr (1976)) but from the spectrum of z.c. gradients produced by s.f. channels for any given edge. Indeed, Marr now uses this approach himself (see his paper in this symposium.)

Summarizing the above points regarding edge descriptions and s.f. channels, it seems that a nonlinear orientated grouping of z.c. locations, taking into account z.c. gradients provided by several (say three or four) non-orientated s.f.-tuned channels, is a convenient and sufficient basis for computing edge descriptions – their location, orientation, type and contrast. Moreover, and most importantly for present purposes, the cyclopean grouping processes implemented in STEREOEDGE, for utilizing disparity information given by a broad-band channel, need little extension to be able to cope with the extra information provided by several monocular s.f.-tuned inputs. We are currently extending STEREOEDGE to explore the idea that the description of edge type takes place at one and the same time as the utilization of disparity information. In this way, STEREOEDGE will exhibit a degree of s.f. selectivity which, we expect, will model the Julesz–Miller stereopsis masking effects with which we began our programme of research.

4. LIMITATIONS: THE NEED FOR POST-CYCLOPEAN AND OTHER PROCESSES

4.1 *Higher order grouping processes*

The binocular edge descriptions returned by STEREOEDGE are local assertions characterizing the properties of an edge along its length (i.e. the orientations, polarities and disparities of its constituent points). Obviously, such descriptions can contribute substantially to the rich data base of low-level assertions needed by such processes as texture discrimination, region finding, large-scale curvilinear aggregation for object boundaries, etc. (Marr 1976). Indeed, we have implemented a program (called FRECKLES because it computes BLOB descriptions of various types) that applies higher-order grouping processes to the 'pointillist' output delivered by STEREOEDGE. This program will be described elsewhere (Mayhew & Frisby 1980).

4.2 *The problem of global stereopsis*

Mention was made earlier of the distinctions between *local stereopsis* (individual point-by-point matches) and *global stereopsis* (a resolution of the ambiguity existing within the pool of potential local point-for-point matches, i.e. a selection of correct local fusions at the expense of false local fusions or 'ghosts'). STEREOEDGE, however, reduces virtually to zero the scale of the global problem by insisting that potential local matches must be made only from points with identical polarity and roughly similar orientation. Given these restrictions, and a sensible (realistically small) Panum's fusional area, very few ghosts appear when potential local fusions are listed for the teddy bear stereogram (see figure 6*e*). To be sure, some ghosts do appear but these are usually produced by horizontal edge sections i.e. by intrinsically ambiguous regions of an image as far as depth from disparity is concerned, an ambiguity which can only be sorted out by later stages 'filling in' between correct depth locations assigned to edge ends (see § 4.3). Other ghosts can appear as a result of quantization fuzz and a certain sloppiness at corners due to the ± 1 pixel of vertical disparity which is allowed. Of course, it is of considerable interest to see that such ghosts as do appear in figure 6*e* are eliminated by the simple principle of figural grouping embedded in STEREOEDGE, but the key feature to note is that the global stereopsis problem as such hardly exists when potential point-for-point matches are restricted by a sensible definition of what constitutes a point-for-point match.

It might be asked, however, whether the situation would be as straightforward as this for a random-dot stereogram, which is normally thought to be a type of stereo input which presents a global problem in an especially acute form. The answer for a type of random-dot texture that suits STEREOEDGE's requirements for edges is given in figure 9. Somewhat surprisingly, ghosts are relatively rare here also and present no more problems than for the teddy bear stereogram. Of course, it might be that certain random-dot textures (such as those composed of myriad small dots) might not fall so readily to the present strategy, although it is interesting to observe that such textures often create severe difficulties for human subjects anyway and can produce very long stereopsis latencies (Frisby & Clatworthy 1975). Also, of course, stereo inputs can always be devised that create ghosts that are as numerous and strong as correct fusions (e.g. those with repeating sub-patterns). However, multiple stable states would then be just as characteristic of an artificial stereo system based on STEREOEDGE as they are of the visual system itself (*vide* the wallpaper illusion).

4.3. *The need for a* $2\frac{1}{2}D$ *sketch*

STEREOEDGE delivers a description of edge locations and their relative depths, but it takes no account of the areas of image intervening between edges. Clearly, what is required is for the depth information tied to edges to be integrated with depth information tied to other image features (e.g. lines), and the whole used to build up a complete depth map of surfaces in the scene being viewed. In short, a computation of the kind envisaged by Marr for arriving at the $2\frac{1}{2}D$ sketch seems the obvious next step (see Marr's paper in this symposium). Perhaps one component part of this computation could be 'filling in' the depth assigned to areas between edge locations, conceivably with the use of a minimum curvature algorithm of the type proposed by Ullman (1978) in connection with illusory contours.

Given that STEREOEDGE can fuse successfully patches of texture that are viewed with an appropriate vergence angle (i.e. the correct fusions falling within the allowable window defined by Panum's fusional area), a further requirement is to devise a mechanism that can shift the two eyes' inputs with respect to one another when zero or imperfect combination is discovered (cf. Marr & Poggio 1979). Given that the filtering algorithm used by MATCH measures neighbourhood support by way of selecting correct local fusions, it also seems possible in principle to use the output of this algorithm to drive 'vergence' movements if it records poorly matched inputs (i.e. weak neighbourhood support found). Thus the algorithm seems to lend itself naturally to a 'rivalry-driven' form of vergence movement control, the rivalry signal being terminated when computations embedded in the $2\frac{1}{2}$D sketch find a good fit between left and right descriptions for each part of the field of view. We are currently developing a stereo system of this kind.

A further factor to note as far as eye movement control is concerned is that we have recently

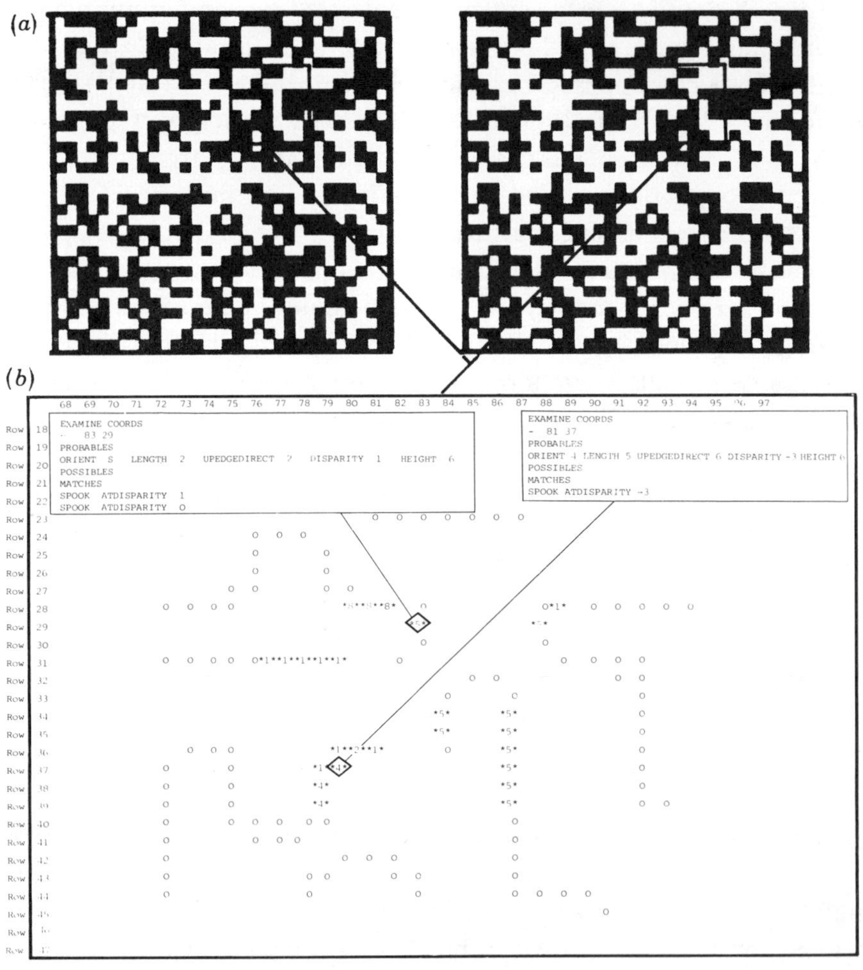

FIGURE 9. STEREOEDGE dealing with a random-dot stereo pair (see text). (*a*) Grey levels (128 × 128 pixels) of the stereo halves. Crossed-eye fusion produces a central protruding square of $+4$ pixels (roughly equivalent to a convergent disparity of 11′ for a viewing distance of about 10 × picture height). (*b*) Final output of STEREO-EDGE: see figure 6*h* for details. Note the successful location in depth of the disparate square with respect to its surround. Thus one of the two z.cs that are picked out with full print-outs comes from the disparate square and has a -3 disparity (STEREOEDGE dealt with the stereo pair as though the square was receding, i.e. the left half of figure 6*a* was treated as the left stereo half). The other picked-out z.c. comes from the surround and has a disparity of $+1$ (because the stereo halves were shifted laterally with respect to one another by 1 pixel so that the 4 pixel disparity would fall within STEREOEDGE's ± 3 pixel Panum's fusional area – a kind of 'eye movement' allowance). Thus the square – surround disparity difference is $+1/-3$ pixels disparity, so faithfully capturing the 4 pixel shift built into the random-dot stereogram.

discovered (Kidd *et al.* 1979) that texture contours (i.e. boundaries between image regions differing, say, in their orientational structure) can facilitate stereopsis and that they do so by guiding vergence eye movements. Accordingly, this kind of capability needs to be incorporated in a reasonably complete model of human stereopsis. Certainly any attempt to limit eye movement control to s.f. filters whose s.f. tuning determines their disparity selectively (Marr & Poggio 1979) seems doomed to failure in the light of our finding that texture contours which present no suitable s.f. signals of this kind can control vergence.

5. Conclusions

An important conclusion to be drawn from STEREOEDGE is that it is quite feasible to utilize disparity cues in the very early stages of the computation of edges. Indeed, the computation of binocular edges is no different in principle from the computation of monocular ones; it is simply somewhat easier because the use of disparity cues helps to distinguish various possibilities for joining up monocular edge points into higher structures. This conclusion nicely complements our psychophysical studies, referred to earlier, which led us to speculate that this is indeed the kind of computational strategy used by the visual system itself (Mayhew & Frisby 1978*a*).

Of greater interest, however, is the rather different perspective offered by our work for the concept of the orientationally selective 's.f.-tuned' channel. Instead of regarding these as providing a linear filtering stage of the kind used by Marr (1976), we find it convenient to view them as nonlinear grouping operators working to find orientated structures in the convolution profiles provided by several s.f.-tuned centre–surround channels. Marr has arrived at a similar conception independently (see his paper in this symposium) and we share his view that at least some of the units presently designated by as 'simple cells' by the neurophysiologists are in fact mediating the nonlinear grouping of zero crossings by way of representing contour assertions. Be that as it may, the concept of the 'orientation-tuned channel' as a nonlinear grouping operator is, we believe, consistent with a great deal of psychophysical evidence, particularly that on stereopsis as reviewed here, and at the same time it makes such channels the embodiment of an eminently sensible computational strategy.

We should like to thank Dr C. Brown for his help with computing equipment and Mr P. Stenton for the many hours of careful evaluation and testing that he has contributed to the 'debugging' of STEREOEDGE. The research was supported by Science Research Council Grant GR/A/50894.

References (Frisby & Mayhew)

Blakemore, C. & Campbell, F. W. 1969 On the existence of neurons in the human visual system selectively sensitive to the orientation and size of retinal images. *J. Physiol., Lond.* **203**, 237–260.

Frisby, J. P. & Clatworthy, J. L. 1975 Learning to see complex random-dot stereograms. *Perception* **4**, 173–178.

Frisby, J. P. & Mayhew, J. E. W. 1977*a* Global processes in stereopsis: some comments on Ramachandran and Nelson (1976). *Perception* **6**, 195–206.

Frisby, J. P. & Mayhew, J. E. W. 1978 The relationship between apparent depth and disparity in rivalrous-texture stereograms. *Perception* **7**, 661–678.

Georgeson, M. A. & Sullivan, G. D. 1975 Contrast constancy: deblurring in human vision by spatial frequency channels. *J. Physiol., Lond.* **252**, 627–656.

Julesz, B. 1960 Binocular depth perception of computer-generated patterns. *Bell Syst. Tech. J.* **39**, 1125–1162.

Julesz, B. 1971 *Foundations of cyclopean perception.* Chicago: University of Chicago Press.

Julesz, B. & Miller, J. 1975 Independent spatial-frequency-tuned channels in binocular fusion and rivalry *Perception* **4**, 125–143.

Julesz, B. & Oswald, H. P. 1979 Binocular utilisation of monocular cues that are undetectable monocularly. *Perception* **7**, 315–322.

Jung, R. 1973 *Handbook of Sensory Physiology*, vol. III, part iii A (ed. R. Jung), pp. 3–152. Berlin: Springer-Verlag.

Kidd, A. L., Frisby, J. P. & Mayhew, J. E. W. 1979 Texture contours can facilitate stereopsis by control of vergence movements. *Nature, Lond.* **280**, 829–832.

Marr, D. 1976 Early processing of visual information. *Phil. Trans. R. Soc. Lond.* B **275**, 483–524.

Marr, D. & Nishihara, H. K. 1978 Visual information processing: artificial intelligence and the sensorium of sight. *Technol. Rev.* **81**, 2–23.

Marr, D. & Poggio, T. 1976 Co-operative computation of stereo disparity. *Science, N.Y.* **194**, 283–287.

Marr, D. & Poggio, T. 1979 A computational theory of human stereo vision. *Proc. R. Soc. Lond.* B **204**, 301–328.

Mayhew, J. E. W. & Frisby, J. P. 1976 Rivalrous texture stereograms. *Nature, Lond.* **264**, 53–56.

Mayhew, J. E. W. & Frisby, J. P. 1978a Contrast summation effects and stereopsis. *Perception* **7**, 537–550.

Mayhew, J. E. W. & Frisby, J. P. 1978b Convergent disparity discriminations in narrowband filtered random-dot stereograms. *Vision Res.* **19**, 63–71.

Mayhew, J. E. W. & Frisby, J. P. 1978c Texture discrimination and fourier analysis in human vision. *Nature, Lond.* **275**, 438–439.

Mayhew, J. E. W. & Frisby, J. P. 1979a Surfaces with steep variations in depth pose difficulties for orientationally tuned disparity-filters. *Perception* **8**, 691–698.

Mayhew, J. E. W. & Frisby, J. P. 1979b The computation of binocular edges. *Perception* **9**. (In the press.)

Mayhew, J. E. W. & Frisby, J. P. 1980 Computational and psychophysical studies towards a theory of human stereopsis. *Artificial Intelligence* (submitted).

Mayhew, J. E. W., Frisby, J. P. & Gale, P. 1977 Computation of stereo disparity from rivalrous texture stereograms. *Perception* **6**, 207–208.

Mostafavi, M. & Sakrison, D. J. 1976 Structure and properties of a single channel in the human visual system. *Vision Res.* **16**, 957–968.

Poggio, G. F. & Fischer, B. 1977 Binocular interaction and depth sensitivity in striate and prestriate cortex of behaving rhesus monkey. *J. Neurophysiol.* **40**, 1392–1405.

Ramachandran, V. S., Madhusudan Rao, V. & Vidyasagar, T. R. 1973 The role of contours in stereopsis. *Nature, Lond.* **242**, 412–414.

Robson, J. G. 1975 Receptive fields: neural representation of the spatial and intensive attributes of the visual image. In *Handbook of perception*, vol. 5: *Seeing* (ed. E. D. Corterette & M. P. Friedman), pp. 81–116. New York: Academic Press.

Saye, A. & Frisby, J. P. 1975 The role of monocularly conspicuous features in facilitating stereopsis from random-dot stereograms. *Perception* **4**, 159–171.

Ullman, S. 1976 Filling-in the gaps: the shape of subjective contours and a model for their generation. *A. I. Memo* no. 367 Artificial Intelligence Laboratory, Massachusetts Institute of Technology.

Waltz, D. 1975 Understanding line drawings of scenes with shadows. In *The Psychology of computer vision* (ed. P. H. Winston), pp. 19–91. New York: McGraw-Hill.

Wilson, H. R. & Bergen, J. R. B. 1979 A four mechanism model for threshold vision. *Vision Res.* **19**, 19–32.

Wilson, H. R. & Giese, S. C. 1977 Threshold visibility of frequency gradient patterns. *Vision Res.* **17**, 1177–1190

Discussion

P. E. KING-SMITH (*Ophthalmic Optics Department, U.M.I.S.T., P.O. Box* 88, *Manchester M*60 1*QD, U.K.*). The authors demonstrate that there is no instantaneous perception of orientation in a pattern derived from superposing two narrow-band, perpendicularly filtered images of a random dot pattern, and suggest that this indicates that the output from orientation specific channels is not available for instaneous perception. Could an alternative explanation be that the bright and dark 'blobs' formed by superposing the two filtered images may stimulate *non-orientated* channels which, in turn, inhibit orientation-specific channels?

J. P. FRISBY AND J. E. W. MAYHEW. The key question about orientated and non-orientated channels as far as we are concerned is: what are they doing? Until they have been assigned some functional role in a computational theory (see Marr's contribution to this symposium), it is difficult to evaluate how plausible any *ad hoc* putative inhibitory interactions between channels might be. The important point about our texture discrimination demonstrations is that they seem difficult to reconcile with any straightforward Fourier analysis theory of low-level visual function for which the linear orientated spatial frequency tuned channel was supposed to provide the physiological underpinning.

D. MARR (*Artificial Intelligence Laboratory, M.I.T., Cambridge, Massachusetts* 02139, *U.S.A.*). The idea that collinear grouping ('curvilinear aggregation'; Marr 1976) may be used to help solve the matching problem in human stereopsis is an interesting one. It is, however, not necessary to involve grouping at this stage (Marr & Poggio 1979). If an ambiguous match arises, the two candidates will almost always have disparities of opposite signs, and to remove ambiguity it is necessary only to consult the *signs* of neighbouring, unambiguous matches. In other respects, Frisby & Mayhew's program is equivalent to Marr & Poggio's theory, recently implemented by Grimson & Marr (1979).

Reference

Grimson, W. E. L. & Marr, D. 1979 A computer implementation of a theory of human stereo vision. Image Understanding Workshop, April 1979, A.l.lab., M.I.T., Cambridge, Massachusetts.

J. P. FRISBY AND J. E. W. MAYHEW. We had not seen a report of Grimson & Marr's program, but now that we have we agree that there are some similarities between that implementation of Marr & Poggio's theory and our own program. Despite some common features, however, the differences seem to us to be more fundamental and important. Our program has been guided by psychophysical results suggesting that disparity processing is intimately integrated with the computation of symbolic descriptions of edges, blobs, lines, etc. Marr & Poggio, on the other hand, regard the extraction of disparity information as taking place within its own separate visual processing module. These different starting points have led to certain key differences between the programs in their use of orientated processes and in the role that they give to spatial frequency tuned channels.

Considering the orientation domain first, it is an important aspect of our approach that the computation of disparity and the extraction of local orientation structures are mediated by interrelated and mutually supporting processes. Our psychophysical results, however, indicated that orientated filters were not involved and so we turned to using orientated collinear grouping processes to guide the removal of ambiguity of zero crossings discovered in circularly filtered left–right images. STEREOEDGE was written, therefore, as a computational test of the idea that a nonlinear grouping process could have the dual function of extracting orientation structure and disparity information, and at the same time resolve any ambiguous matches that might arise. Interestingly, and significantly as far as the question of general approach is concerned, Grimson & Marr also chose to use circular filters rather than the orientated filters employed originally by Marr & Poggio, but they did so for the elegant computational reasons described by Marr & Hildreth (see Marr's paper in this symposium) rather than to make their program more psychophysically plausible.

Of course, we agree with Dr Marr when he says that Grimson & Marr's program demonstrates that it is not necessary to solve the stereopsis ambiguity problem by building in collinear grouping processes – but this is so at the expense of the strong assumptions made by Marr & Poggio about the relation between disparity processing and spatial frequency tuned channels. Thus Marr & Poggio develop the idea that disparities of different magnitudes are processed independently by different spatial frequency channels. Their theory holds that large disparities are dealt with by low spatial frequency units, with vergence movements initiated to bring into correspondence high spatial frequency channels dealing with small disparities. By limiting the size of the disparity that can be processed by any one channel to around plus or minus the width of the central region of the receptive fields of the units composing the channel, the theory avoids the problem of having to choose between many ambiguous matches. The key question here, however, is whether wholly independent disparity processing within different spatial frequency tuned channels actually takes place within the human visual system. The psycho-physical evidence on this point is not yet clear and although we have contributed to the development of this kind of proposal ourselves (Mayhew & Frisby 1976; Frisby & Mayhew 1977a), our more recent work has found little support for it (Frisby & Mayhew 1977b; Mayhew & Frisby 1979c). Consequently, in our own theory we do not ascribe to spatial frequency tuned channels the role accorded to them by Marr & Poggio. Rather, as we note in our paper, it is a natural development of our program to take advantage of the contraints and correspondences between spatial frequency channel measurements that can be used for the computation of primitive assertions (Marr 1976), to force unique disparity assignments in most cases. Thus in our development of STEREOEDGE, local disparity matches will remain s.f.-tuned (as in a SLUG-type model: see our paper) but global processing to resolve ambiguities will utilize cross-s.f.-channel correspondences. Moreover, by taking advantage of these correspondences, together with those referred to above within the orientation domain, a much greater disparity range for local s.f.-tuned matches will be possible than in Marr & Poggio's model. Pilot work to date suggests that this approach is promising and it certainly fits in with our overall conceptual framework, namely to embed disparity processing intimately within the very first stages of the computation of primitive symbolic descriptions of edges, blobs and lines.

References

Frisby, J. P. & Mayhew, J. E. W. 1977b Spatial frequency tuned channels and stereopsis. Paper delivered to the Experimental Psychology Society, March 1977, University of Sheffield.
Mayhew, J. E. W. & Frisby, J. P. 1979c Convergent disparity discriminations in narrow-band-filtered random-dot stereograms. *Vision Res.* **19**, 63–71.

K. H. RUDDOCK (*Biophysics Section, Physics Department, Imperial College, London SW7 2BZ, U.K.*). In the authors' analysis of early visual processing, they postulate Laplacian operators, with non-orientated spatial response characteristics, that feed into orientation selective response units. Experiments with patterns containing two-dimensional spatial structure show that there are two classes of adaptation mechanism, one sensitive to symmetric 'spot-shaped' targets and the other to elongated, 'bar-shaped' targets (Naghshineh & Ruddock 1978). The former are monocularly and the latter binocularly driven, as is the case in the Frisby–Mayhew model. Both the adaptation data and independent threshold detection data (Burton 1976) indicate, however, that the non-orientation selective units operate both in parallel and in series with the orientation selective units. Have the authors considered the possibility of parallel operation of their two classes of response unit, perhaps as a means of incorporating additional stimulus characteristics such as colour and movement?

References

Burton, G. J. 1976 Visual detection of patterns periodic in two-dimensions. *Vision Res.* **16**, 991–998.
Naghshineh, S & Ruddock, K. H. 1978 Properties of length-selective adaptation mechanisms in human vision. *Biol. Cybernet.* **31**, 37–47.

J. P. FRISBY AND J. E. W. MAYHEW. The short answer is no. While it might well be that other processes acting on the outputs of 'our units' might make explicit additional stimulus characteristics, our present concern is simply to develop a model capable of dealing with the early processing of monochromatic static three-dimensional scenes.

Phil. Trans. R. Soc. Lond. B **290**, 117–135 (1980)
Printed in Great Britain

Analogue models of motion perception

By M. J. Morgan

Department of Psychology, University of Durham, Science Laboratories,
South Road, Durham, DH1 3LE, U.K.

An object moving in discrete spatial jumps is difficult to distinguish from a continuously moving object, provided the time between jumps is not too great. The extent of this perceived continuity may be measured by probing the perceived spatial location at times between the target jumps, by either a vernier alignment or a stereoscopic technique. As the time between jumps increases the accuracy of spatial interpolation falls, until finally the object is seen only at its actual spatial locations. These results can be analysed in the frequency domain by treating the signal for apparent motion as the analogue of a periodic waveform containing relatively low frequencies (the continuous motion) and higher frequencies giving rise to the discreteness of the motion. If such an input has the higher frequencies progressively removed by physical filtering, it is perceived as increasingly continuous. The fact that such filtering is not necessary for perceived continuity when the discrete jumps occur at rates greater than about 30 Hz suggests that frequencies greater than that limit are removed by the visual system itself.

1. Introduction

Vision is characterized by spatial representations, but we do not know what it is that gives these representations their tremendous power, coupled with their deceptive phenomenal simplicity. For example, a computer can easily be programmed to play the game of 'noughts and crosses' (tic-tac-toe) but in a numerical form that makes the strategy virtually inscrutable to the ordinary person. Even a child, however, can play the game skilfully when the problem is given a spatial form in which the underlying strategy of making the symbols form straight lines becomes intuitively evident. Vision is useful not just for seeing, but for many different kinds of problem solving. Very difficult problems can be solved by giving them a spatial form of representation, and allowing the innate skills of vision to do the rest.

Although we do not know exactly what characterizes spatial representations, certain obvious remarks can be made. Perhaps the most obvious is that spatial representation allows for the possibility of movement, and thereby links our perception of the world to the motility of our bodies. We can be confident that visual representation allows for movement because in the absence of the latter it would not possess its fundamentally metrical character. A metric is not defined until congruence definitions have been stated, and as Russell and others have pointed out, the notion of congruence depends upon operations such as translation and rotation, under which shapes are defined as remaining invariant. To establish congruence relations, we need a method with which to compare the sizes of lines and angles in different places, and it is difficult to see how we could give meaning to this unless we could in some way internalize the concept of moving an object around in space.

Motion, then, is basic to the representation of space. But what, in turn, characterizes movement in the phenomenal domain? This has been a philosophical puzzle ever since Zeno's terse remark to the effect that 'An arrow is where it is'. What Zeno claimed is that the distinctive attribute of motion is lost as soon as we try to pin down the spatial position of an object at an instant of time. The invention of the calculus seems to have resolved this problem to the satisfaction of the physicist by making motion mathematically tractable, but it is not obvious that it clears it up completely from the psychologist's point of view. The momentary position of a moving object can certainly be predicted by vision with sufficient accuracy for, say, a fielder to intercept a rapidly moving cricket ball. But what does this imply for the phenomenal location of a moving object at an instant of time? We know from experiments on flicker fusion threshold that the visual system is relatively sluggish in its response to temporal change. How is this related to the phenomenal continuity of movement; and how does the visual system cope, if it does in fact cope at all, with the problem of localizing a moving target in space?

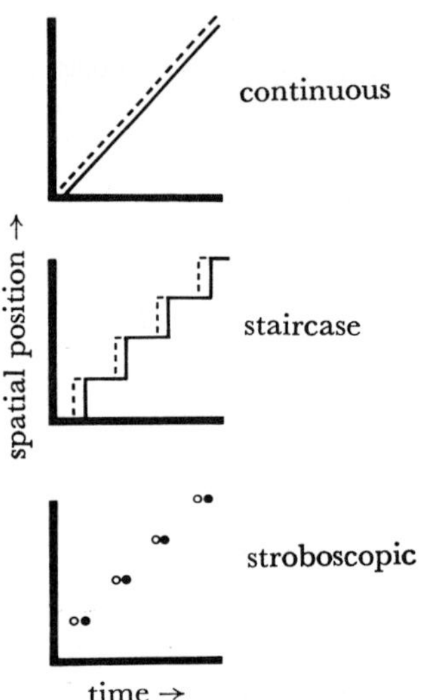

FIGURE 1. In each graph, the two lines or sets of dots represent the changes in spatial position over time of two targets in a dynamic vernier acuity task. Only the spatial positions in the direction of motion are plotted; in addition the targets are assumed to be slightly separated in the orthogonal spatial dimension as in a typical static vernier task. In the continuous case (top), both targets are in continuous motion with a constant spatial separation. In the two kinds of apparent motion (staircase and stroboscopic), the two targets are presented in exactly aligned spatial positions with a temporal displacement. Such targets appear to the observer as if they were spatially misaligned, provided that the motion is phenomenally continuous.

Several lines of evidence suggest that the phenomenal spatial location of a moving target is not determined solely by its instantaneous spatial position. In the phenomenon of 'apparent motion', for example, a target is seen as if it is changing its spatial location continuously, when in reality it is making discrete spatial jumps. One way of measuring this phenomenal continuity rather precisely is by attempting to make a vernier alignment of two moving targets. Consider the situations shown diagrammatically in figure 1. The graphs in this figure represent changes over time of the spatial location of the targets in the direction of motion. In continuous motion, the spatial location of one of the targets lags continuously behind that of the other. Not surprisingly, this is perceived by the subject as a spatial misalignment between the targets. But consider now the two kinds of apparent motion illustrated in figure 1. In 'staircase' motion the targets make discrete spatial jumps separated by periods of rest. Stroboscopic motion is similar except that the targets are flashed briefly after each jump. In both of these kinds of motion we can arrange that the targets occupy identical spatial locations, but that they occupy these positions at slightly different times, as shown in figure 1. It turns out that this temporal phase lag appears to the subject as a *spatial* offset between the stimuli, even though the spatial positions are actually aligned (Morgan 1976; Burr 1979). If the observer is asked to make a spatial adjustment to align the stimuli, he advances the spatial position of the temporally lagging stimulus in the direction of motion (figure 2).

We can refer to this descriptively as an 'interpolation' effect in apparent motion, since the observer is acting as if the phenomenal location of a discretely moving target were in between its actual spatial locations. The same effect is seen in a stereoscopic version of the alignment task. If the targets are presented to corresponding retinal points in the two eyes but with a small temporal delay, the phenomenal spatial misalignment is now detected as a depth shift as if the stimuli had a retinal disparity (Lee 1970; Morgan & Thompson 1975; Ross & Hogben 1975; Morgan 1979*a*; Burr & Ross 1979).

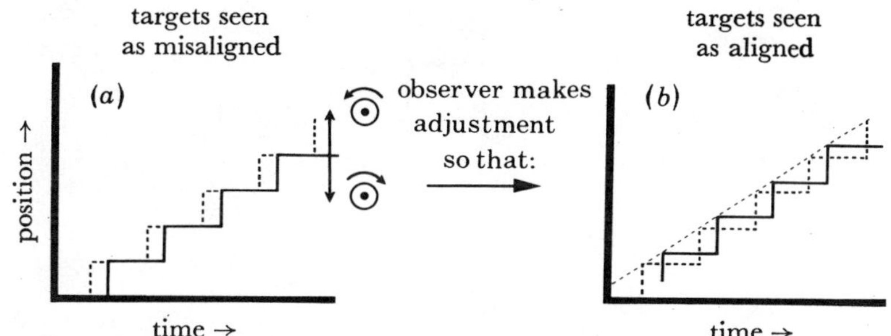

FIGURE 2. This figure explains how the observer can make a spatial adjustment so as to make temporally staggered 'staircase' targets (see figure 1) appear as if they were spatially aligned in a vernier task.

It is initially tempting to consider the interpolation effect as yet another example of the ability of the visual system to make intelligent deductions from limited sensory information. The naturally occurring analogue of the apparent movement situation would be one in which a target moves behind a picket fence (Burr & Ross 1979), or a prey is glimpsed fleetingly as it moves through a thicket. In the alignment situation, the visual system could be considered to be making a deduction in the following propositional form: 'target A arrives at the same place as target B, but at a later time; therefore, target B must be spatially ahead of target A'.

Although this idea is plausible, it is probably not the correct account of interpolation. The basic objection to the 'hypothesis formation' account is that it fails to explain the temporal constraints upon the effect. Both the vernier alignment interpolation and stroboscopic Pulfrich effect disappear when the interstimulus interval (i.s.i.) exceeds about 50 ms. At an i.s.i. of 200 ms, for example, the targets appear aligned when their actual physical positions are in alignment. This is despite the fact that such targets are still seen as moving. It would seem, then, that we must make a clear distinction between stimuli that produce an impression of movement, and stimuli that produce an impression of *continuous* movement.

An alternative to the idea that interpolation is a kind of visual 'hypothesis' is that it is a fact forced upon the visual system at a relatively peripheral level by physiological constraints. We can begin the search for these constraints by asking two theoretical questions. First, how would one set about building a physical device to assign a momentary position to a moving target? Secondly, why does a continuously moving target not appear to the visual system as a shapeless blur? I shall argue that answers to these two questions are closely related.

Any device that is attempting to represent the spatial position of a moving target will have to cope with the problem that worried Zeno, namely, that the position is constantly changing, and is thus indefinite inside any finite period of time. Only if the system could change its own state in no time at all could it respond to an instantaneous target position. Any physically realizable system will have a finite speed of response that will limit the precision with which it can assign a location to the moving target. It will be an inevitable property of any such system that is unable to distinguish between continuous and discontinuous motion when the jumps of the latter occur sufficiently rapidly in time. The critical i.s.i. at which this occurs can be used to measure the time constants of the system under investigation.

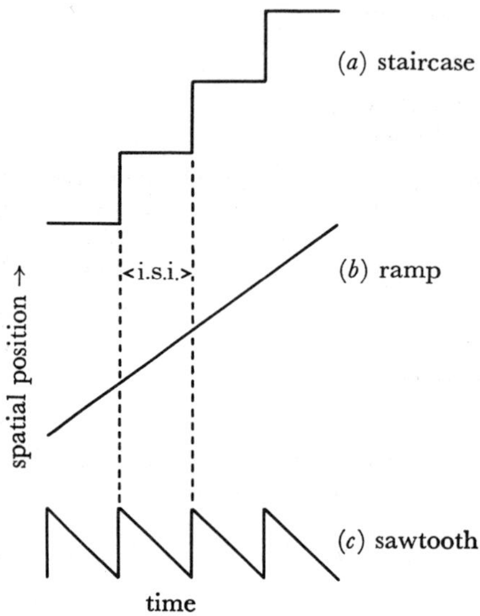

FIGURE 3. This figure shows how 'staircase' motion (a) can be synthesized from continuous motion (ramp) (b) and a higher frequency modulation of spatial position (sawtooth) (c). For further explanation see text.

Before describing experiments based upon this idea, it is necessary to show in slightly greater detail how a discretely moving target can be considered to contain within it different spatio-temporal frequency components. Consider the staircase representation of apparent motion shown in figure 3a. As well as representing the trajectory of an apparently moving target, this staircase could be taken to represent a signal used to produce a discretely moving target, such as a voltage applied to a spot on an oscilloscope screen. If we wished to synthesize such a signal, we could do so by a combination of the signals shown in figure 3b and c. The first of these is a ramp, which by itself would correspond to a target in continuous movement. The second is a high frequency modulation of the target in a sawtooth pattern.

We can therefore characterize a staircase signal in the spatio-temporal frequency domain as a mixture of different components, with lower frequencies corresponding exactly to a continuously moving target, and higher frequencies being responsible for the discontinuous features of the motion. This is further illustrated in figure 4 which shows the superimposed power spectra of three different staircases, of differing i.s.is. Each of these staircases has the same low frequency components, corresponding to a continuous triangular wave. The higher frequency components differ between the staircases. For example, a staircase of i.s.i. 128 ms has a fundamental at

7.8 Hz and harmonics at 15.6 Hz, 23 Hz, and so on. The 32 ms staircase, on the other hand, has no frequency component below 31 Hz to distinguish it from continuous motion.

Given this way of describing discontinuously moving targets, the suggestion can now be made that the phenomenal continuity of a staircase may be due to the inability of the visual system to represent its higher frequency components. For example, it will be shown below that a staircase of i.s.i. 32 ms has a very high degree of phenomenal continuity. This can be explained by supposing that the frequency components distinguishing it from a continuously moving

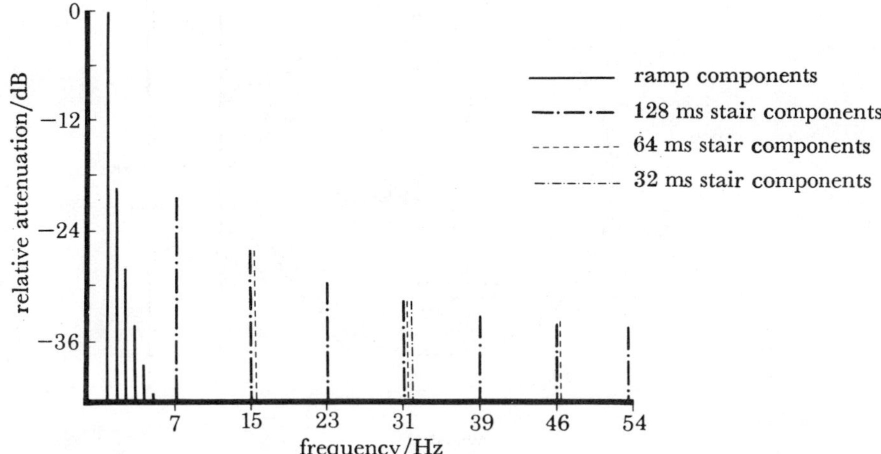

Figure 4. The figure shows how 'staircase' motion (see figure 3) can be broken down into different frequency components. The power spectra of three different staircases with differing i.s.is (see figure 3 for explanation) have been superimposed to illustrate their different frequency composition. The three staircases have the same ramp components, which define a low frequency triangular wave, but differ in the higher frequency components making up the added sawtooth modulation (see figure 3). The data were obtained from a fast Fourier transform of actual staircase stimuli.

target are effectively not represented at the level of the visual system where the analysis of visual direction takes place. According to this argument, the 'interpolation effect' ceases to be a paradox and becomes a simple consequence of the relatively sluggish response of the visual system. The seeming paradox was that temporally staggered targets could be seen as spatially out-of-phase even though their physical positions were the same. However, we now see that it is in an important sense misleading to say that their 'physical positions are in alignment'. This statement refers to the *instantaneous* physical positions of the targets: for example, the discrete space–time coordinates of a stroboscopic target. But if the visual system cannot respond quickly enough to analyse these discrete positions independently, it will necessarily be averaging the target position over finite periods of time. In these circumstances, a temporal delay between the targets would have an identical result to a spatial offset.

2. Frequency components above 25 Hz have little effect upon phenomenal continuity

In this experiment the observers carried out a vernier alignment between two moving stimuli. The experimental arrangement is illustrated in figure 5 for the case where the two bars were in staircase motion with an i.s.i. of 128 ms. The display was generated on an oscilloscope screen with fast decay P15 phosphor. There was a temporal delay in the plotting of the two bars

122   M. J. MORGAN

such that one was lagging by a constant fraction (0.25) of the i.s.i. The observer's task was to
adjust the spatial position of the lagging stimulus so that it appeared to be in alignment with the
leading stimulus (figure 2), and from the chosen setting a motion continuity index was calculated
as explained in figure 6. A central fixation point was provided and a closed-circuit television
picture of the eye was examined to check that no tracking took place. Further details of the

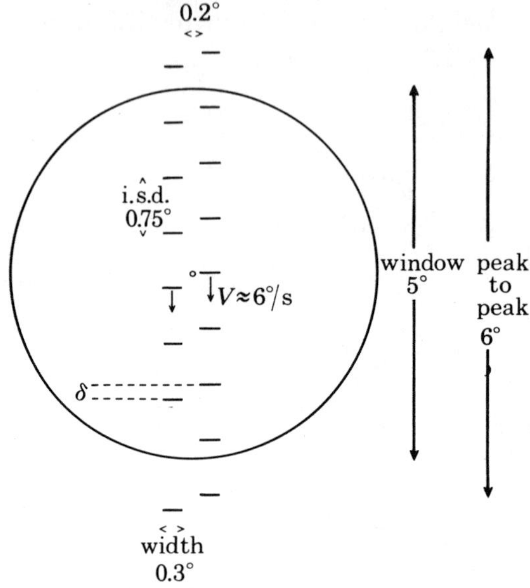

FIGURE 5. Schematic representation of the display used for experiments on vernier alignment of stimuli in staircase
motion. The two bars were in vertical motion, and the observer had to adjust the spatial separation (δ) so
that they appeared to be in alignment. In this illustration the i.s.i. was 128 ms, there were therefore eight
steps from peak to peak with an interstep distance of 0.75°. With an i.s.i. of 64 ms the number of steps would
be doubled and the inter-step distance halved, and so on for other i.s.is.

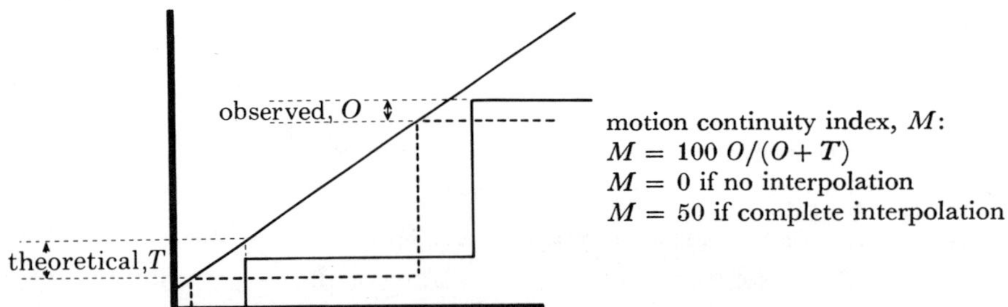

FIGURE 6. This figure explains the calculation of the motion continuity index, which measures the interpolation
effect in vernier or stereoscopic alignment of apparently moving targets. The observer sets the spatial position
ordinate of the temporally lagging target (lag $= 0.25 \times$ i.s.i.) to make it appear in alignment with the leading
target. The theoretical value for complete interpolation assumes that the presentations of the lagging target
will be placed on the continuous trajectory joining the discrete space–time positions of the leading target.

experimental procedure are available (Morgan 1979b). The temporal frequency composition
of the stimuli was manipulated in two ways. First, three different staircases were used, with
i.s.is of 128, 64 and 32 ms respectively. As shown in figure 4, these staircases have different
frequency components distinguishing them from a continuously moving target. Secondly,
before being used to move the targets on the display, the various staircase signals were passed
through an analogue filter to remove frequency components above a specified frequency. In

other words, they were subjected to low-pass filtering. For example, with the low-pass corner frequency set at 12 Hz, a staircase of i.s.i. 128 ms would be physically distinguished from a continuously moving target only by the presence of an added sinusoidal modulation of frequency 7.8 Hz.

The mean data collected from four observers are illustrated in figure 7. There are three main points to note. First, there is much more of an interpolation effect with the 32 ms staircase than with one of i.s.i. 128 ms. The 64 ms staircase is intermediate. The 32 ms staircase produced

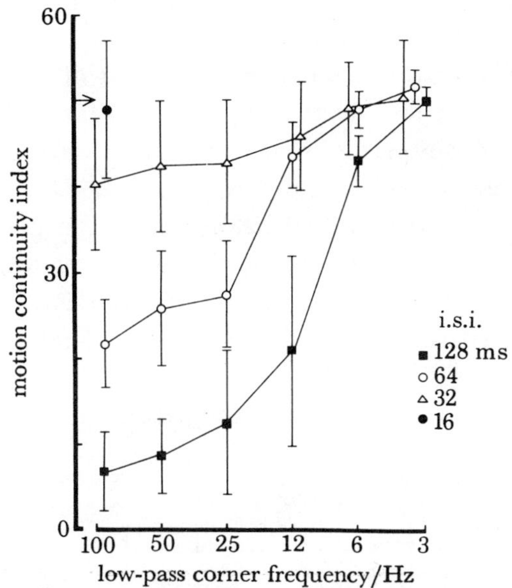

Figure 7. Results from an experiment in which observers carried out vernier alignment between staircase-moving targets as illustrated in figure 5. The staircase signals were subjected to various degrees of low-pass analogue filtering (abscissa) before being used to move the targets on the c.r.o. screen. For explanation of the motion continuity index (ordinate) see figures 2 and 6. The points are means over four observers and the vertical bars represent standard deviations. For further explanation see the text.

almost complete interpolation even when it was virtually unfiltered (low-pass frequency 100 Hz), whereas in the same circumstances the 128 ms staircase produced no interpolation effect. The second obvious point is that as the staircases had more of their higher frequency components removed by filtering, the motion continuity index rose. Even the 128 ms staircase produced a large interpolation effect when filtered to remove frequencies higher than 6 Hz. Finally, the results suggest that there is relatively little effect of filtering until frequencies below 25 Hz are removed.

These results can all be put together if we assume that frequencies in the signal higher than about 25 Hz are not represented as spatial movements at the level of the visual system where the visual directions of the targets are compared. The staircase of i.s.i. 32 ms contains no component below 31 Hz to distinguish it from continuous motion, and will thus have a high degree of motion continuity. A 128 ms staircase filtered at 12 Hz will still have a component at 7.8 Hz to distinguish it from a continuous target, and thus will not show a high degree of motion continuity. There is a steep rise in the continuity of the 64 ms staircase when the low pass frequency changes from 25 Hz to 12 Hz because this staircase has a fundamental at 15 Hz (figure 4).

The results therefore suggest that modulations of the target position at frequencies greater than about 25 Hz have little influence upon its phenomenal location, as measured by the alignment technique. A prediction from this is that the phase of such modulations relative to the continuous low frequency components will be of little importance. This was verified in the next experiment.

3. Mirror image equivalence between high frequency components

As explained diagrammatically in figure 3, a staircase signal can by synthesized by addition of a ramp and a sawtooth in which the local velocity is equal and opposite to the ramp. If the sawtooth is mirror-imaged and then added to the ramp, we have the signal illustrated in figure 8a. The local velocity of this stimulus is now twice that of the ramp, and the instantaneous jumps are in the reverse direction of the ramp. Despite the physical differences between this signal and the staircase, we can predict that they will have equivalent perceptual effects if the fundamental frequency of the sawtooth exceeds about 25 Hz. This was verified in the same vernier alignment situation that was used in the previous experiment. The two stimuli to be aligned were presented either as staircases with an i.s.i. of 32 ms, or as the mirror-imaged versions shown in figure 8. The results for two observers conformed to expectations in that both kinds of stimulus produced the same degree of interpolation, as measured by the motion continuity index. Phenomenally, the two kinds of stimulus were difficult to distinguish. In particular, the 'reverse jumps' of the mirror-imaged stimulus were not perceptible.

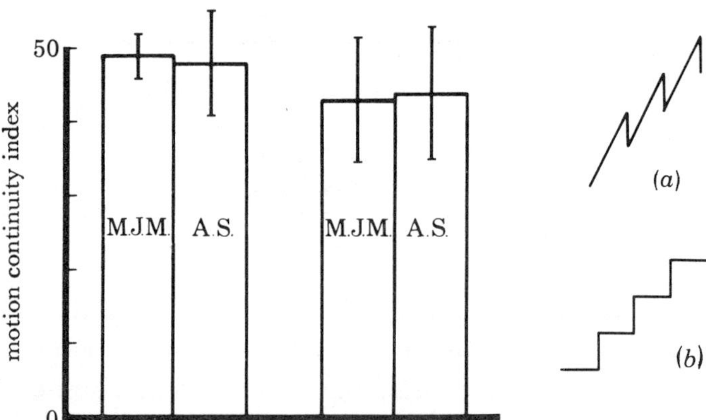

Figure 8. The figure shows the results of an experiment comparing the motion continuity of two kinds of moving stimuli. One of these (b) was a staircase, synthesized from a ramp and a sawtooth modulation as in figure 3. The second (a) was identical except that the sawtooth was mirror-imaged. Motion continuity was assessed by the interpolation effect in vernier alignment with a delay of $0.25 \times$ i.s.i. Other details as in figure 5. Results are shown separately for two observers (M.J.M. and A.S.). For further explanation see the text (§3).

4. Effects of light adaptation state upon interpolation

It has been argued above that the interpolation effect depends upon the relatively sluggish nature of the visual response, which forces an averaging of visual direction over time, and thus a confusion between a temporal and a spatial offset. If this is so, it might be possible to manipulate the extent of the interpolation by controlling the speed of the visual response. A possible means that suggests itself is the control of light adaptation level. It is a well established finding that as the eye becomes more dark adapted, its time constants are increased. Thus, visual persistence increases with dark adaptation (Mollon 1969) and the flicker fusion threshold is reduced at lower frequencies (Kelly 1961). It is therefore possible that in the apparent movement situation, an effect of adaptation state upon interpolation might be found. This result has been reported in the stroboscopic stereophenomenon (Morgan 1979a). This experiment first of all verified the influence of the i.s.i. upon the interpolation effect. It was found in this case that interpolation was complete with an i.s.i. of 20 ms, but absent with an i.s.i. of 50 ms. Results with an i.s.i. of 30 ms showed an intermediate degree of interpolation. The luminance of the display and the surround was then decreased by 2 logarithmic units. This had no effect upon the extent of interpolation with the two extreme i.s.is (20 and 50 ms) but interpolation with the intermediate i.s.i. of 30 ms became complete. The prediction was therefore verified.

5. DEMONSTRATIONS OF SPATIAL AVERAGING WITH MOVING TARGETS

The experiments reported so far suggest that there is some form of filtering involved in the interpolation phenomenon, but they have had little to say about the mechanism of such filtering. One hypothesis is as follows. We know that even very brief visual inputs can give rise to a considerably more protracted visual response; this is the phenomenon of visual persistence. It follows that a target sweeping along a retinal array is going to provide information not only about its current position, but about previous positions as well, depending upon target velocity and the length of persistence. Thus at any one time there will not be a single retinal image corresponding to the target, but rather a range of different images. If this is so, how could two such targets be compared, either in the vernier or in the stereo situation? One possibility would be to compare just the leading edges, that is, the most recently available information about direction. However, this would not explain the interpolation effect, since it postulates a comparison between targets based upon their momentary actual physical position. An alternative is that the distribution of visual directions from persisting signals is sharpened in some way, perhaps by an inhibitory process, to assign a mean position to the target. This averaging process would have the required property of acting as a low-pass filter for spatio-temporal modulation, and of explaining the interpolation effect. Some further experiments will now be described supporting the view that there is such an averaging process.

Suppose a horizontally moving target is viewed binocularly. If the signal could be made to persist for longer in one eye than the other, the account just given would predict that there would be a depth shift, as if the more persistent signal were spatially lagging. Greater persistence in one eye could be arranged by covering that eye with a neutral density filter, it being well established that *decreases* in intensity of the target cause *increases* in persistence (Mollon 1969). The depth shift with one eye covered by a filter is just the Pulfrich effect (Pulfrich 1922), which is hardly a novel prediction. But we now see that the traditional 'transmission lag' interpretation of the Pulfrich stereophenomenon has an alternative, which stresses the effects of the light reduction upon persistence, rather than latency, of the visual response. One way to test the persistence hypothesis is to cause physically greater persistence of the signal in one eye, and to pit this against the effects of a filter over the other eye. In one experiment (Morgan 1975) a stroboscopically moving target was presented separately to the two eyes. Every time the target flashed in a certain place in one eye it was flashed not only in the exactly corresponding place in the other eye, but was also presented at its previous position. Thus, at every time the target was presented at the nth position in one eye, it was flashed simultaneously at the nth and the

$(n-1)$th position in the other eye. As predicted this produced a depth shift, as if the signal in the 'more persistent' eye were lagging. Moreover, this effect could be cancelled out by placing a suitable neutral density filter over the 'less persistent' eye. The second experiment (Morgan 1977) was a continuous version of the previous one. One eye viewed a horizontally moving vertical bar target, and the other eye viewed an identically moving but slightly wider bar. When the leading edges of the two bars were in physical alignment, the observer saw a depth effect as if the wider bar were spatially lagging. This depth could be cancelled by placing a filter over the eye seeing the thinner bar. When the thinner bar was physically aligned with the exact geometrical centre of the wider bar, there was no depth effect. This result suggests that the averaging process was remarkably linear.

6. Similarities between staircase and stroboscopic motion

One advantage of relating the interpolation effect to visual persistence is that we are now able to explain why the effect applies to both staircase and to stroboscopic motion. In staircase motion the stimulus remains physically present on the retina in the intervals between its jumps, whereas in stroboscopic motion it is flashed briefly at each position. However, if each presentation of the target gives rise to a persisting impression, the physical difference between the stimuli may not entail an important phenomenal difference. To check on this point, an experiment was carried out in which the duration of the target at each of its positions was systematically varied, and apparent alignment was measured as in the first experiment. At one extreme condition, only a single 2 ms flash of the target was presented, corresponding to stroboscopic motion. At

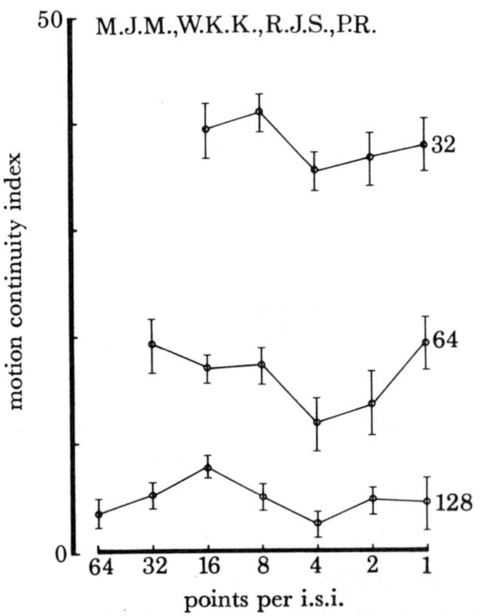

FIGURE 9. Results of an experiment investigating effects upon motion continuity of the length of time for which the target was physically present during the i.s.i. The three sets of points show results for different i.s.is (values in milliseconds). Target duration was manipulated by the number of times it was plotted during the i.s.i. (abscissa), each plot taking 2 ms. The points plotted during the i.s.i. were in identical spatial locations. Motion continuity was assessed by the interpolation effect in vernier alignment with a delay of $0.25 \times$ i.s.i. The points are means over four observers and the vertical lines represent standard deviations. For further explanation see the text (§6).

the other extreme, the target was flashed every 2 ms until the i.s.i. was complete. Between these two extremes, an intermediate number of equally spaced 2 ms flashes were plotted. The experiment was carried out with three different i.s.is and the results are plotted in figure 9. First of all, the experiment confirms the effect of i.s.i. found in previous experiments. Secondly, it is apparent that there is little systematic effect of the target duration (number of points per i.s.i.) upon the motion continuity index. In particular, there is little difference between the limiting stroboscopic case of a single flash and the staircase situation in which the target duration fills the i.s.i. There are some interesting aspects of the data that require further investigation. With all three i.s.is there is a small but systematic tendency for the continuity index to reach a minimum when 4 points were plotted in each i.s.i., that is, when the cumulative target duration was 8 ms. There is no obvious explanation of this phenomenon.

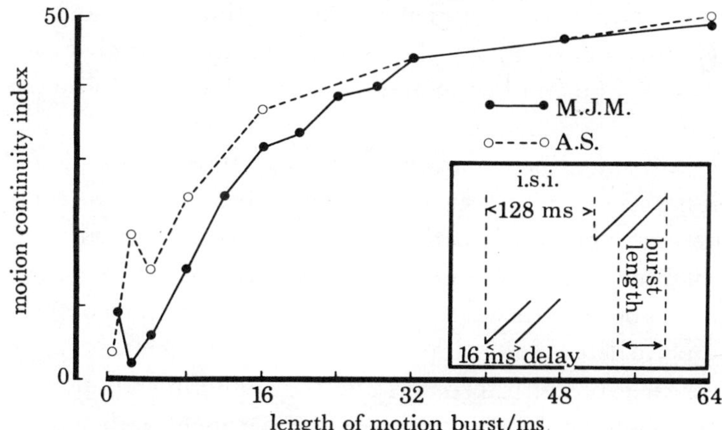

FIGURE 10. Results of an experiment investigating effects upon motion continiuty of the length of time for which the targets were continuously moved during the i.s.i. The observer performed a vernier alignment between two targets with the spatial and temporal relations shown in the inset panel. Other details as in figure 5. For further explanation see the text (§7).

7. A HYBRID BETWEEN CONTINUOUS AND STROBOSCOPIC MOTION

We have seen that with an i.s.i. of 128 ms, targets are aligned by their physical positions, irrespective of the temporal delay between them. The interpretation of this finding in terms of the spatial averaging hypothesis is that the temporal period over which integration occurs must be less than 128 ms. Inside any shorter period, the mean spatial position of the temporally staggered staircases will generally be zero. By the same argument, the integration period must be greater than 32 ms, or we should not get such a high interpolation figure when the staircases have an i.s.i. of 32 ms. Suppose we now manipulate the average spatial position of the targets within the i.s.i. by subjecting them to continuous movement. This gives rise to a hybrid between continuous and stroboscopic motion as illustrated in figure 10. The two temporally staggered targets are presented for the duration of a 'motion burst' and then disappear until the next burst of motion. We now ask how long the burst must be for the observer to cancel out the temporal delay by an appropriate spatial offset. The experiment was carried out with two observers, using a vernier alignment task as in experiment 1. The results (figure 10) show that a motion burst of 64 ms was sufficient to produce completely accurate alignment. We can therefore conclude that assignment of target position takes place within an integration period no greater than 64 ms, and probably not much greater than 32 ms. This agrees well with the finding of the first experiment, that spatial modulations of frequency greater than 25 Hz are phenomenally attenuated.

It is also interesting to compare the present result with Ross & Hogben's (1974) finding of a 50 ms 'short-term' memory in stereopsis, which suggested that inputs to the two eyes are integrated provided they do not occur more than 50 ms apart.

8. Threshold for the interpolation effect

Supposing the visual direction of a moving target to be determined by some averaging process, how precise are the judgements involved? If a moving target simply becomes a shapeless blur, we should not expect judgements of vernier alignment and stereoscopic depth to be carried out with any precision. However, work by Westheimer & McKee (1975, 1978) has shown that vernier acuity and stereoscopic depth judgements for continuously moving targets remain accurate, even when the presentation time is too short to permit pursuit eye movements. In the following experiment, Walia Kani and I compared vernier and stereoscopic acuity in a situation where the targets were in staircase motion with an i.s.i. of 20 ms.

The two targets were presented on separate oscilloscope screens (Hewlett-Packard 1333A with P15 phosphor). In the stereo task the two screens were fused with a mirror stereoscope, and in the vernier task they were optically superimposed with a half-silvered mirror. The targets were bars whose width subtended $0.25°$ of visual angle. In the vernier alignment task the separation between the ends of the bars was $1'$. The velocity of the ramp component in the staircase was $4.8°/s$. The temporal delay in the plotting of the two staircases was varied over trials in a randomized psychophysical procedure to determine the minimum temporal separation that could be detected by the observer. In the stereoscopic experiment, either the right or the left eye was delayed, and the observer had to report the direction of target motion in depth ('clockwise' or 'anticlockwise'). In the vernier alignment task, either the top or the bottom target was delayed, and the observer reported which target appeared to be spatially lagging ('top' or 'bottom'). The display was generated at a rate of 1 frame every 290 µs.

Results are shown in figure 11. In presenting these data, the temporal delays have been converted into a notional spatial equivalent, by calculating the distance the target would have moved during the delay if had been in actual continuous motion. For example, at a velocity of $4.8°/s$ a temporal delay of 1 ms corresponds to a notional spatial offset of $17''$. It should be remembered, however, that the targets were actually in staircase rather than continuous motion, so that the calculated spatial offset refers to the *mean* separation between the targets rather than their instantaneous offset, which is at most times zero.

If we take the threshold as the point of 75% detection, the results for two observers in figure 12 show that stereoacuity for the staircase targets was in the region $10–20''$. This corresponds to a temporal delay of approximately 1 ms. Thresholds for the vernier alignment situation were twice as great as this for one subject (M.J.M.) and one and a half times as great for the other (W.K.K.). To see if vernier acuity would be improved by allowing the observers to track the target, the experiment was repeated with instructions to follow the target with the eyes rather than fixating on a stationary mark as in the previous condition. Results (figure 11) showed an improvement in both observers to an acuity of about $10''$.

Under ideal conditions, the threshold for stereoacuity and vernier acuity is as little as $2''$. With stationary targets and a 1 min gap, McKee & Westheimer (1978) have recently reported

improvements with practice from 10 to 5″. With targets moving up to 3.5°/s, Westheimer &
McKee (1975) found vernier thresholds of between 6 and 10″. It is apparent that the acuity in
the present situation is quite a bit worse than these values, although it is still impressive when it
is considered that the stimuli were in discontinuous motion, and that the temporal separation
was only 1 or 2 ms. It is not clear whether the difference in acuity between our study and that
of Westheimer & McKee (1975) was due to the difference in the kind of motion, or to the higher
velocity used in our experiment. It is of interest that the motion used by Westheimer & McKee
was in fact a staircase with an i.s.i. of as long as 10 ms, but the offset between the stimuli was
spatial rather than temporal.

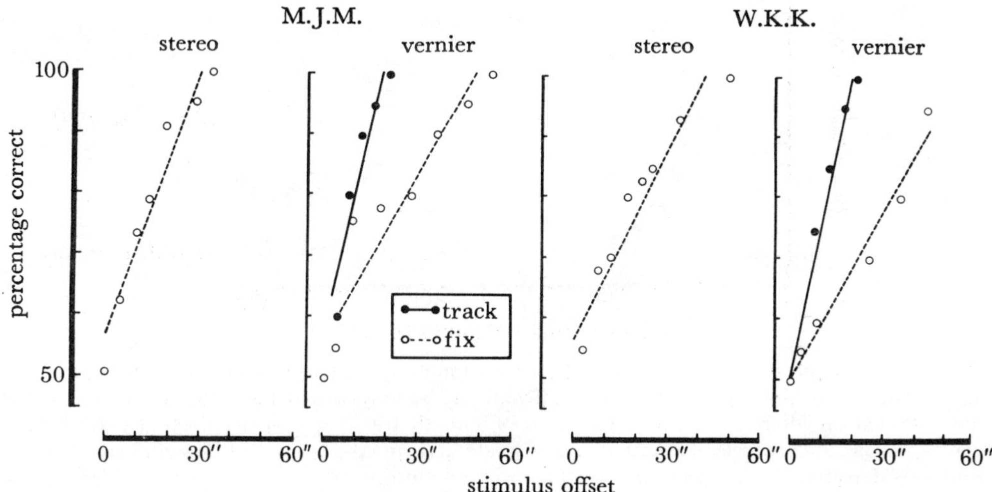

FIGURE 11. Results of an experiment on vernier and stereoscopic acuity with targets in staircase motion (i.s.i. =
20 ms). The number of correct identifications of depth (stereo) or left–right alignment (vernier) is shown as a
function of the virtual spatial separation between the staircases. A virtual separation of 17″ corresponds
to a delay between the staircases of 1 ms. Results are shown separately for two observers (M.J.M., emmetropic; W.K.K., myopic corrected to 6/3). For further explanation see the text (§8).

9. THE ROLE OF EYE MOVEMENTS IN INTERPOLATION

The finding in the previous experiment, that vernier acuity was improved by tracking the
target, raises the question of whether the interpolation effect might depend entirely upon eye
movements. If the eyes track the apparently moving targets, any temporal delay between them will
be automatically converted into a spatial offset on the retina, and there would be no need to
invoke an interpolation process. A very similar question about the role of eye movements has
been extensively discussed in relation to a phenomenon first described by Zöllner (1862). A
shape such as a triangle is moved behind a very narrow slit, so that only a very small fraction
of the shape is visible at any time. If the observer is instructed to maintain careful fixation on the
slit, all the parts of the shape ought to fall on the same part of the retina, yet despite this, a
spatially extended image of the shape can sometimes be seen. The shape is frequently compressed
in the direction of its motion. There is an intriguing analogy here with the interpolation effect in
apparent motion, in that spatial perception is apparently resulting from purely temporal
information. But as Helmholtz pointed out (see Southall 1962), Zöllner's effect is very easily
explained if the observer makes tracking eye movements so as to 'paint' the temporally successive
parts of the shape on to different retinal points. Despite much argument in the literature

(reviewed by Anstis & Atkinson 1967), it seems that Helmholtz was probably right about the role of eye movements. For example, if the display is switched off when the subject starts to track, or if tracking is prevented by the barbiturate drug sodium amytal, then the subject's ability to identify the moving shapes is considerably impaired (McManus & Morgan 1978). The results of this experiment are illustrated in figure 12.

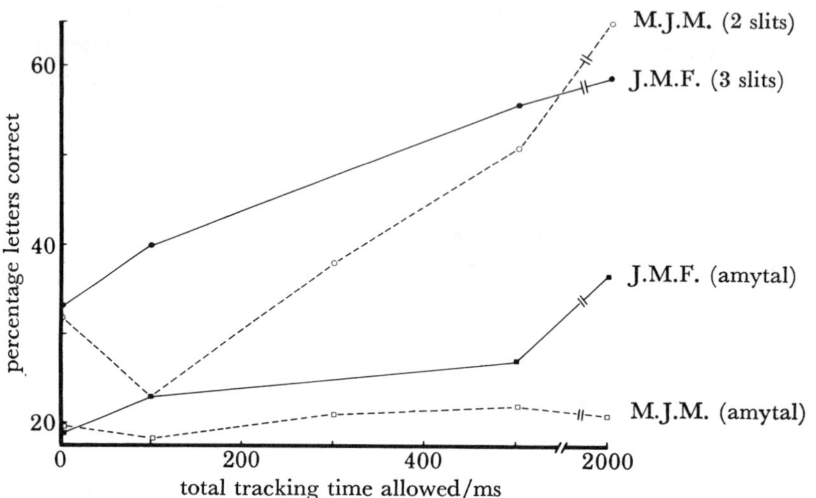

FIGURE 12. Results of an experiment in which the observer attempted to identify alphanumeric characters as they were moved rapidly behind narrow slits. Eye movements were recorded by a computer, and the stimulus could be switched off after a controlled duration of smooth tracking had occurred. In the zero tracking condition (abscissa) the observer was instructed to fixate and the display would be switched off immediately if tracking was detected by the computer. In the amytal condition the two observers (M.J.M. and J.M.F.) took an oral dose of 240 mg sodium amytal before the experiment, to block eye tracking. For further details see text (§9).

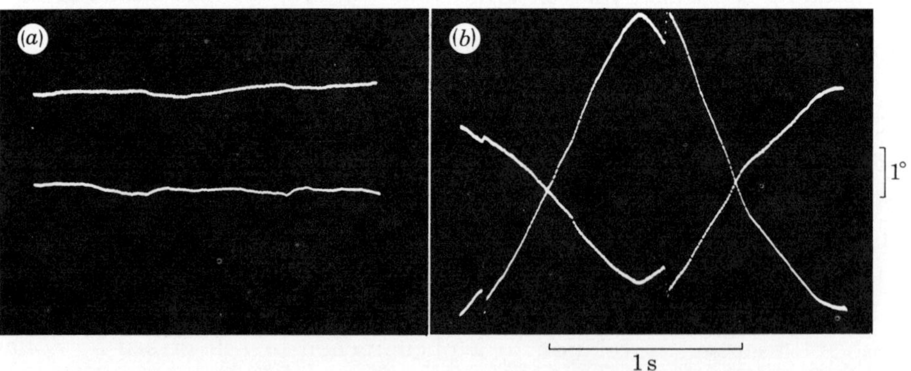

FIGURE 13. Binocular eye movement recordings from a subject (M.J.M.) engaged in a stereoacuity task (see figure 11). One of each pair of records represents movements of the left eye and the other the right eye. Record (a) was taken when the subject was instructed to fixate; record (b) when he tracked the moving targets. Records from the left eye are phase-inverted relative to the right because for both eyes records were taken from the temporal margin of the limbus.

However, it seems unlikely that tracking eye movements are responsible for the interpolation effect in vernier and stereoscopic alignment. In an elegant experiment, Burr (1979) has shown that the interpolation effect is still observed when the display is presented within the latency period for instituting smooth pursuit movements. To investigate this matter further, binocular eye movement records were taken from a subject engaged in the acuity task previously described. The recorder consisted of a fibre optic Y guide for locating the limbus in each eye (Findlay 1974). The limit of resolution of this device was 2′, and it was sufficiently sensitive to detect microsaccades. A typical example of a record when the subject was attempting to fixate is shown in figure 13a, and it reveals no systematic pursuit movements. In contrast, figure 13b shows a record when the subject was instructed to track the moving target, which was a staircase with an i.s.i. of 20 ms and an interocular delay of 4 ms.

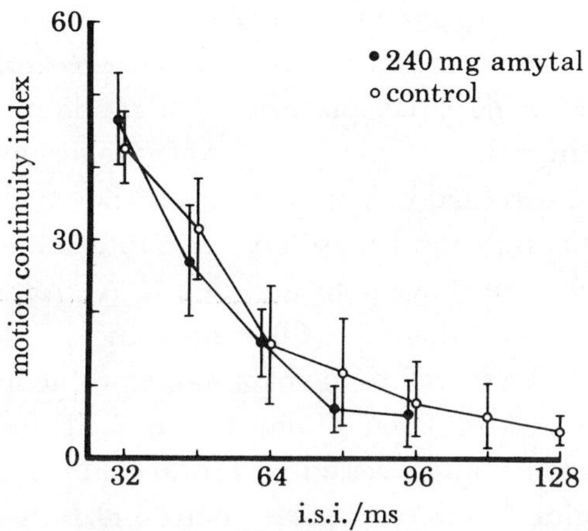

FIGURE 14. The figure shows results of an experiment on effects of sodium amytal (240 mg) on the vernier interpolation effect in one subject (J.M.F.). The severely disruptive effects of the drug upon smooth pursuit movements are shown in figure 15. Despite this disruption, the drug has no effect on the motion continuity index at any of the i.s.is.

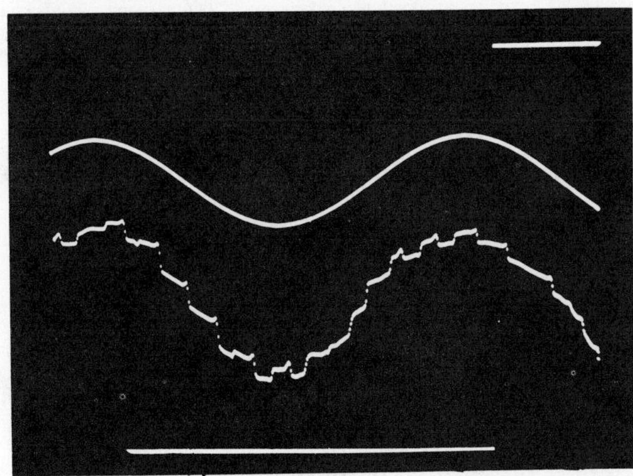

FIGURE 15. The record shows an example of the way in which sodium amytal (240 mg) disrupts smooth pursuit movements. The top record shows movement of the target (1 Hz), the bottom movement of the eye. Note the continual interruption of pursuit by saccadic eye movements. (Subject J.M.F.)

In another experiment on this problem, a subject carried out the vernier task before and after a dose of sodium amytal sufficient (240 mg) to disrupt smooth tracking. The results showed no effect of the drug upon the motion continuity index over a large range of i.s.is (figure 14). Eye movement records confirmed that the ability to track moving targets was severely impaired (figure 15) (Rashbass 1961).

These experiments do not prove that interpolation would occur in the absence of small involuntary drifts and tremors of the eye, but they have shown that large-scale pursuit movements are not necessary. The problem of the role of very small eye movements is one shared with studies of 'static' acuity (Westheimer & McKee 1975).

10. The dynamic visual noise stereo effect

If dynamic visual noise (d.v.n.), which resembles the electronic snowstorm on a detuned television, is viewed with a filter over one eye, an effect similar to the Pulfrich stereophenomenon is seen: the noise takes on a coherent rather than a random movement, and rotates in depth. (The motion is clockwise with a filter over the left eye and anticlockwise with a filter over the right eye). Tyler (1974; 1977) has put forward a 'random spatial disparity hypothesis', according to which the filter introduces a delay so as to cause fusion of random dots in different frames, thereby giving rise to a retinal disparity. Only horizontally separated dots in different frames will give rise to depth shifts, and these give rise to a monocular movement cue, thus explaining the correlation between movement and depth. A problem with this explanation is that the effect can be seen even when the filter introduces a far smaller delay than the television inter-frame interval. We therefore have the same problem as in explaining the stroboscopic Pulfrich effect (Lee 1970; Morgan & Thompson 1975). Tyler (1977) suggests an explanation based upon visual persistence and averaging. His account is similar to the one suggested here, except that the averaging involves disparity detectors rather than spatial position and movement.

The d.v.n.-Pulfrich effect is often considered to be the same as an effect described earlier by Ross (1974) in which a square of d.v.n. stood out in depth from a d.v.n. background if the latter were presented with an inter-ocular delay. However, this effect was only seen if the delay was greater than 70 ms, so it is rather hard to relate it to effects produced by neutral density filters. According to the findings of Ross & Hogben (1974), stereo fusion breaks down with delays greater than 50 ms, so perhaps the Ross (1974) effect was due to a depth difference between monocularly and binocularly seen parts of the noise field (Wist, 1969). The observation that d.v.n. can sustain smooth tracking eye movements (Ward & Morgan 1978) may also be relevant to depth effects in d.v.n.

11. Discussion

There has been considerable discussion recently in the cognitive psychology literature of a role for an 'analogue' process in visual perception (Shepard 1978). The idea of a more holistic or analogical representation of visual events contrasts strongly with prevailing neurophysiological and computational approaches, both of which favour more discrete, symbolic or propositional representations. One of the key notions in the analogue approach is that when a subject attempts to imagine a visual transformation such as a rotation in space, he constructs a continuous, or almost continuous, series of intermediate spatial representations. Thus the time taken to imagine the transformation will rise linearly with the spatial separation between the initial and final figures. (Shepard (1978) may be consulted for a review of the experimental evidence.)

Robins & Shepard (1977) have specifically attempted to implicate a form of analogue processing in the perception of apparent motion. They claim that in the apparent movement situation, the subject constructs intermediate spatial representations corresponding to a target in continuous or near-continuous motion. They attempted to verify this claim by asking subjects to decide whether a dot flashed at a point on the phenomenal trajectory of the apparently moving target occurred before or after the target reached that position in space. The further along the phenomenal trajectory the point was flashed, the longer it had to be delayed relative to the start of the i.s.i. to be judged 'after'. Robins & Shepard concluded that their results are 'in agreement with the idea that subjects based their judgements in the experimental condition on the comparison between the probe and an internal representation of a bar rotating back and forth'.

At first sight, this finding is compatible with the 'interpolation' effect in apparent motion. However, further examination shows that the relation is superficial. Robins & Shepard used a display consisting of two bars only, with an onset–onset interval of 380 ms and an offset–onset interval of 180 ms. Since these figures greatly exceed even the longest i.s.i. used in the 'interpolation' experiments it is very unlikely indeed that true interpolation occurred in the Robins & Shepard study. Their findings can perhaps be explained in a completely different way. Robins & Shepard were apparently unaware of earlier studies of interpolation in vernier alignment and stereopsis, so they took no account of the importance of eye movements. Their subjects were not instructed to fixate, so they may have tracked the movement, probably by a saccade rather than smooth pursuit (Morgan & Turnbull 1978). This means that the 'before–after' judgement could have been made entirely by retinal location of the probe flash, the subjects responding 'before' if the flash was to one side of the fovea and 'after' if it was to the other side. Since relative visual direction of flashes presented before and during a saccade depend primarily on their relative retinal locations, with little compensation for eye movement (Matin & Matin 1969), this interpretation would explain the data.

The idea that apparent motion involves the active construction of intermediate representation is somewhat implausible given the very small time intervals involved. It is relevant here to point out that the times taken for an imaginary 'mental rotation' are at least an order of magnitude greater than the critical i.s.is for apparent movement (Shepard & Judd 1976). It begs the question to put this difference down to 'the generally greater speed of imagery when it is driven externally than when it has to be programmed and generated internally' (Shepard & Podgorny 1978, p. 224), since this is a description of the phenomenon rather than an explanation of it. Another problem with the 'intermediate representation' idea in apparent motion is that it appears to ignore the existence of phenomenal persistence. If intermediates are constructed, how are they combined with the persisting signals from earlier physical presentations? The argument that I have attempted to put forward is that the 'intermediates' *are* in fact the set of persisting images, with a phenomenal location depending upon a spatial averaging process. If this is accepted, there is no need for an active process to construct intermediates.

There are at least two senses that one could give to the idea of an analogue process in perception. The first is that in respect to the 'primary qualities' of space, time and motion we generally ascribe the same set of properties both to physical events and to perception. Thus it is meaningful to speak of the duration of an experience, and of the physical event that caused that experience. Although the durations may differ numerically, they are both durations. This contrasts sharply with 'secondary qualities' like colours and smells, where we draw a rigid distinction between the *conceptual* properties of the physical event (e.g. wavelength) and the *perceptual* properties of the phenomenal event (e.g. colour).

There is thus a certain sense in which we treat spatial and temporal aspects of our experience as being 'analogues' of the physical world, rather than being merely arbitrary representations. This often seems to have been what is meant by calling perception a 'model' of the external world. For example, Hertz spoke of perception as giving us 'the actual dynamical relations' between things, and this would hardly make sense unless we could apply the concepts of dynamics both to the phenomenal and physical domain.

Spatial and temporal representations (and therefore movement) are thus analogical representations simply in the Kantian sense that, with respect to them, our concepts and our sensory intuitions are in some sort of agreement. This point is not particularly controversial.

The other meaning of 'analogue' processing is much more controversial. It implies that the neural code for an event must bear a resemblance, either to the event itself, or to the phenomenal event, or to both. Again, if this merely implies that neural events occur in time and space, it is not controversial, but usually more than this is implied; the idea is that the brain contains something like moving pictures of the outside world. A perception of continuous movement, for example, would involve something moving continuously in the brain, as in the Gestalt isomorphist theory. Shepard makes it quite clear that this is not what he has in mind when he invokes 'analogical' representations. The claim is rather of the first kind, namely, that perceived motion resembles motion (for example, in being continuous). There is little reason to dispute this very weak version of the claim that the perception of motion is an analogue process.

References (Morgan)

Anstis, S. M. & Atkinson, J. 1967 Distortions in moving figures viewed through a stationary slit. *Am. J. Psychol.* **80**, 572–585.

Burr, D. C. 1979 Acuity for apparent vernier offset. *Vision Res.* **19**, 835–838.

Burr, D. C. & Ross, J. 1979 How binocular delay gives information about depth. *Vision Res.* **19**, 523–532.

Findlay, J. M. 1974 A simple apparatus for recording microsaccades during visual fixation. *Q. Jl. exp. Psychol.* **26**, 167–170.

Kelly, D. H. 1961 Visual responses to time-dependent stimuli. 1. amplitude sensitivity measurements. *J. opt. Soc. Am.* **51**, 422–429.

Lee, D. N. 1970 A stroboscopic stereophenomenon. *Vision Res.* **10**, 587–593.

Matin, L. & Matin, E. 1969 Visual perception of direction when voluntary saccades occur. 1. Relation of visual direction of a fixation target extinguished before a saccade to a flash presented during a saccade. *Percept. Psychophys.* **5**, 65–80.

McKee, S. P. & Westheimer, G. 1978 Improvement of vernier acuity with practice. *Percept. Psychophys.* **24**, 258–262.

McManus, I. C. and Morgan, M. J. 1978 The effect of eye movements on the perception of form and depth of moving targets. Paper presented to meeting of the Experimental Psychology Society, July 1978.

Mollon, J. D. 1969 Temporal factors in perception. D.Phil. thesis, University of Oxford.

Morgan, M. J. 1975 Stereoillusion based on visual persistence. *Nature, Lond.* **256**, 639–40.

Morgan, M. J. 1976 Pulfrich effect and the filling in of apparent motion. *Perception* **5**, 187–195.

Morgan, M. J. 1977 Differential visual persistence between the two eyes: A model of the Fertsch–Pulfrich effect. *J. exp. Psychol.: hum. Percept. and Perform.* **3**, 484–495.

Morgan, M. J. 1979*a* Perception of continuity in stroboscopic motion: a temporal frequency analysis. *Vision Res.* **19**, 491–500.

Morgan, M. J. 1979*b* Spatio-temporal filtering and the interpolation effect in apparent motion. *Perception.* (In the press.)

Morgan, M. J. & Thompson, P. 1975 Apparent motion and the Pulfrich effect. *Perception* **4**, 3–18.

Morgan, M. J. & Turnbull, D. F. 1978 Smooth eye tracking and the perception of motion in the absence of real movement. *Vision Res.* **18**, 1053–1059.

Pulfrich, C. 1922 Die Stereoskopie im Dienst der isochromen und heterochromen Photometrie. *Naturwissenschaften* **10**, 553–564.

Rashbass, C. 1961 The relationship between saccadic and smooth tracking eye movements. *J. Physiol., Lond.* **159**, 326–338.

Robins, C. & Shepard, R. N. 1977 Spatio-temporal probing of apparent rotational movement. *Percept. Psychophys.* **22**, 12–18.

Ross, J. 1974 Stereopsis by binocular delay. *Nature, Lond.* **248**, 363–364.

Ross, J. and Hogben, J. H. 1974 Short term memory in stereopsis. *Vision Res.* **14**, 1195–1201.

Ross, J. & Hogben, J. H. 1975 Pulfrich effect and short-term memory in stereopsis. *Vision Res.* **15**, 1289–1290.

Shepard, R. N. 1978 The mental image. *Am. Psychol.* **33**, 125–137.

Shepard, R. N. & Judd, S. A. 1976 Perceptual illusion of rotation of three dimensional objects. *Science, N.Y.* **191**, 952–954.

Shepard, R. N. & Podgorny, P. 1978 Cognitive processes that resemble perceptual processes. In *Handbook of learning and cognitive processes* (ed. W. K. Estes), pp. 189–237. Hillsdale, N. J.: L. Erlbaum.

Southall, J. P. C. 1962 *Helmholtz's treatise on physiological optics*, vol. 3, p. 251. New York: Dover.

Tyler, C. W. 1974 Stereopsis in dynamic visual noise. *Nature, Lond.* **250**, 781–782.

Tyler, C. W. 1977 Stereomovement from interocular delay in dynamic visual noise: A random spatial disparity hypothesis. *Am. J. Opt. Physiol. Opt.* **54**, 374–386.

Ward, R. & Morgan, M. J. 1978 Perceptual effect of pursuit eye movements in the absence of a target. *Nature, Lond.* **274**, 158–159.

Westheimer, G. & McKee, S. P. 1975 Visual acuity in the presence of retinal image motion. *J. opt. Soc. Am.* **65**, 847–50.

Westheimer, G. & McKee, S. 1978 Stereoscopic acuity for moving retinal images. *J. opt. Soc. Am.* **68**, 450–55.

Wist, E. R. 1970 Do depth shifts resulting from an interocular delay result from a breakdown of binocular fusion? *Percept. Psychophys.* **81**, 15–19.

Zöllner, F. 1862 Über eine neue Art anorthoskopischer Zerrbilder. *Annln Phys.* **117**, 477–484.

Discussion

H. B. BARLOW, F.R.S. (*Physiological Laboratory, Cambridge CB2 3EG, U.K.*). I think that these results are fascinating because they seem to imply something that I did not previously suspect, namely that the visual system performs some kind of integration along a constant velocity path in space and time. That seems to me what is implied by a spatial shift and a temporal delay producing exactly interchangeable effects with regard to the perception of a vernier or stereo misalignment. But to reach this conclusion it is crucial to know that resolution is unimpaired by movement. It would be relatively simple for the visual system to *ignore* evidence of the blurring of moving objects, but the ability to extract high resolution information in spite of movement is quite another matter and a much more interesting one. So my question is: What was the resolution attainable in the task that Professor Morgan showed in figures 7 and 9, and was it affected by the variable filtering imposed; also, what was the velocity of movement?

M. J. MORGAN. The question of acuity is indeed a central one, and I have added some relevant data in the written version of the paper to try to answer this point (§ 8 and figure 11). Briefly, the acuity for a temporal delay was about 1 ms in the stereoacuity task and 2 ms in the vernier offset task. Target velocity was 4.8°/s. These times would correspond to notional distances of 17 and 34″ respectively if the targets had been moving continuously. This acuity is not as good as that reported by Westheimer & McKee for a real spatial offset: they found a threshold of 6–10″ both for stereo and vernier acuity. Therefore, one cannot conclude that resolution is completely unimpaired by discontinuous motion. Moreover, vernier acuity was considerably improved if the observer tracked the target (figure 11). There is therefore loss of acuity, but one has to remember that the real offset is temporal, and that the spatial offset is only an average value. These studies of acuity are not very extensive, and clearly much more has to be done, particularly in comparing continuous and discontinuous movement. I have not yet examined effects of filtering upon acuity.

Phil. Trans. R. Soc. Lond. B **290**, 137–151 (1980)
Printed in Great Britain

Low-level and high-level processes in apparent motion

By O. J. Braddick

Department of Experimental Psychology, University of Cambridge,
Downing Street, Cambridge CB2 3EB, U.K.

When a group of dots within a random-dot array is discontinuously displaced, it appears as a moving region perceptually segregated from its stationary surround. The spatial, temporal and other constraints governing this effect are markedly different from those classically found for the apparent motion of isolated stimulus elements. The random-dot display appears to tap a low-level motion-detecting process, distinct from the more interpretive process elicited by the classical displays.

The distinct contributions of these processes can be identified in 'multi-stable' displays which yield alternative percepts of apparent motion depending on which one or both of the processes is activated. Such experiments illustrate the interaction of relatively stimulus-constrained and relatively autonomous processes in visual perception.

Two contrasting approaches dominate much recent work on visual perception. One is to explore how properties of the stimulus may be decoded in the patterns of activity of neural channels or detectors, each of which has its own selective tuning (Braddick *et al.* 1978). The other approach (exemplified by Gregory 1970) considers perception as a problem-solving process that must interpret the sensory input as evidence for some external object or event, and has tended to cast its explanations in functional terms rather than as hypothetical neural mechanisms.

Generally these two approaches have been adopted to attack rather different problems. However, the perception of smooth continuous motion from discontinuous stimulation (variously called beta apparent motion, stroboscopic motion, or the phi phenomenon) has attracted accounts of both kinds. It may therefore provide an opportunity to consider how selective-detector models and interpretive theories of visual perception conflict or interconnect.

Neural units that respond selectively to a particular direction of motion have been widely studied. Such units can be effectively stimulated by a succession of stationary flashed spots or lines, similar to the stimuli yielding apparent motion for a human observer. In fact, such discontinuous stimulation has been an important means for analysing the mechanism of directional selectivity (Barlow & Levick 1965; Bishop *et al.* 1972; Emerson & Gerstein 1977).

However, perceptual research has given a number of results that would not be expected if stroboscopic motion perception resulted simply from the activation of directionally selective 'movement detectors'. There are reports that the critical parameter is not retinal separation but apparent separation (Attneave & Block 1973), and that apparent movement can occur between stimuli too widely separated to fall in any plausible receptive field (Smith 1948). The occurrence or direction of apparent motion can depend on the subject's attitude (Neuhaus 1930) and past experience (Neff 1936). The interpretation of the pattern as an object can determine the apparent motion (Sigman & Rock 1974) and this can lead to perception of motion in depth between plane figures (Kolers 1972). These last observations in particular would tend to support a view of apparent motion as a 'perceptual hypothesis' to account for the sensory evidence provided by successive images.

Segregation of random-dot patterns by apparent motion

The classical method for studying the parameters that control apparent motion has been for observers to judge whether a sequence of simple stimuli appears simultaneous, in motion, or successive. However, in practice these perceptual categories are not very stable or well defined. In fact, a more complex stimulus can provide a perceptual criterion of apparent motion that is easier to use. This is a 'random-dot kinematogram' (Julesz 1971) consisting of successive matrices of black and white square elements. In any one matrix, the pattern of elements is random, but on successive exposures the elements in a central region of the pattern are all displaced through the same distance, while those in the surrounding area remain in the same positions. The elements in the central region appear to move as a coherent object, with a clearly perceived boundary between this moving zone and the static surround. Now this segregation is not defined in any single random pattern. It can only appear as a result of some visual mechanism that detects the spatio-temporal relation between elements in successive exposures; that is, in some sense, a motion detecting mechanism.

When such perceptual segregation of random dot patterns is used as the criterion for apparent motion, one finds rather different properties and parameters from those obtained in studies of classic apparent movement of isolated stimulus elements. Table 1 summarizes some of the significant differences.

Table 1. Determinants of apparent motion found with two perceptual criteria

criterion of segregation in random-dot display	criterion of smooth apparent motion for isolated element
spatial displacement must be 15′ or less (Braddick 1974)	spatial displacement may be many degrees (see, for example, Neuhaus 1930; Zeeman & Roelofs 1953)
interstimulus interval (i.s.i.) must be less than 80–100 ms (with 100 ms stimulus exposure) (Braddick 1973)	i.s.i. may be up to at least 300 ms (see, for example, Neuhaus 1930)
segregation abolished by bright uniform field in i.s.i. (Braddick 1973)	motion perceived whether i.s.i. is bright or dark
successive stimuli must be delivered to the same eye or to both eyes together (Braddick 1974), as must bright field for effective masking (Braddick 1973)	successive stimuli may be delivered to the same or different eyes (Shipley et al. 1945)
pattern defined by chromatic but not luminance contrast is inadequate (Ramachandran & Gregory 1978)	stimuli may be defined by chromatic contrast alone alone (Ramachandran & Gregory 1978)

The demonstration of the spatial limit (Braddick 1974) requires a slightly different stimulus from that described above. If the displacement is too large, the appearance of coherent motion of the central region breaks down, but this region is still changing from frame to frame; its elements appear to be in random, disconnected motion. It therefore still appears segregated from a static surround. However, if the elements in the surround are uncorrelated from frame to frame (figure 1), centre and surround segregate when the centre is seen to move coherently over small displacements, but they appear as a homogenous area of incoherent motion when the displacement of the centre is large. When a range of element sizes is used, the displacement at which the breakdown of segregation occurs is a constant visual angle, not a constant distance in terms of the pattern elements (figure 2). This suggests that the limit is genuinely spatial rather than a consequence of some statistical limitation in the matching of element positions between successive exposures.

Note that in this, as in the other results in the left column of table 1, the criterion was strictly one of segregation rather than of the appearance of motion. Even when segregation is abolished because of the size of displacement or the duration or luminance of the i.s.i., individual elements or clusters of elements may be observed to move appropriately. The difference between the criteria of segregation and of perceived motion or displacement may account for the differences

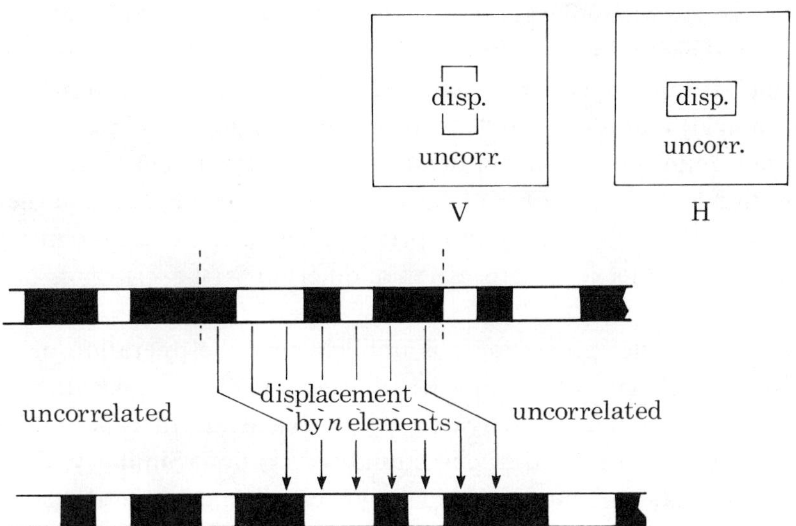

FIGURE 1. Displays used to investigate spatial limits on apparent motion in random-dot patterns. A single row of each pattern of a pair is illustrated. Outside the central rectangle (boundary indicated by dotted lines) the two patterns are uncorrelated; inside the central rectangle the dots are displaced horizontally in one pattern relative to their positions in the other. The two patterns were alternated repetitively with 75 ms exposure and 10 ms inter-stimulus interval (i.s.i.). Top right: the arrangement of the rectangular displaced region could be vertical or horizontal within the overall square $9° \times 9°$ pattern. Subjects were required to report the rectangle's orientation. (From Braddick 1974.)

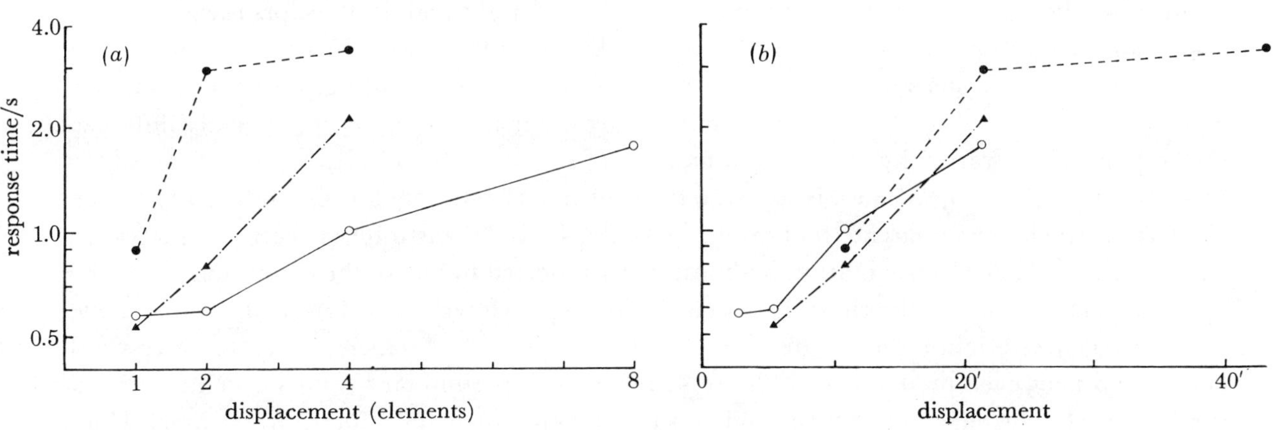

FIGURE 2. Response time for the report of orientation of the displaced rectangle in displays of the type shown in figure 1. The three plots are for different element sizes: ○, 2.7′; ▲, 5.4′; ●, 10.8′. Data are the mean of the logarithm of the response time for five subjects. The same data are plotted (a) in terms of displacement expressed in units of the pattern element width, and (b) in terms of displacement expressed as a visual angle. Long response times indicated poor segregation, evidenced also by high variability of response times, low rated clarity of the rectangle's boundaries, and frequent errors in the reported orientation. These measures, like the plots of response time shown here, coincided for different element sizes if displacements were expressed as visual angles rather than as multiples of the element dimension. (From Braddick 1974.)

between the results of Braddick (1974) and those of Bell & Lappin (1973) using random-dot patterns.

TWO-PROCESS THEORY OF APPARENT MOTION

I have proposed (Braddick 1974) that the differences listed in table 1 arise because the two perceptual criteria depend on two distinct processes that extract information about visual displacement. The segregation effect seems to characterize the process that, of the two, occurs at an earlier stage in the visual system. Evidence for this is: the relatively short spatial and temporal range over which it can combine information; its vulnerability to interference from a stimulus (bright uniform field) that is likely to have little effect on high-level pattern processing mechanisms; and its failure to operate dichoptically. This low-level 'short-range' process may tentatively be identified with the response of directionally selective neurons in the visual pathway to discontinuous stimulation. The more interpretive phenomena of apparent motion may then be associated with the higher-level process that determines the criterion of smooth perceived motion.

If there are two distinct processes, it is unlikely that the operation of each one would be restricted to the specific types of stimulus which is used to characterize it in table 1. Presumably the higher-level process can be activated by the elements of random-dot kinematograms, although its activity does not lead to perceptual segregation. Similarly, the classic type of display consisting of isolated elements would be expected to activate the short-range, low-level process if the various constraints in the left column of table 1 were satisfied. It would be surprising if its action was not reflected in some way in the perception of these stimuli.

REVERSAL OF SHORT-RANGE APPARENT MOTION

For example, experiments currently in progress in my laboratory indicate that the interfering effect of a bright i.s.i. can be demonstrated with stimuli other than random dot patterns. Figure 3 illustrates the type of display. An annulus divided into bright and dark sectors is exposed in a succession of positions, each one rotated anticlockwise with respect to the one before. The rotation is always in steps of one-fifth of a period of the annular grating. Of course, this can equally well be described as a clockwise shift through four-fifths of a period. The absolute size of the step can be varied by varying the number of sectors in the circle, but this 1:4 ratio is kept constant. The subject's task is to fixate the centre of the display for 30 s and to record the periods in which the apparent rotation is clockwise. If the 35 ms interval between successive exposures is dark, clockwise rotation is almost never reported in any of the conditions used: the apparent motion follows the shorter, anticlockwise steps. However, if during the interval the annular region is bright (equal in luminance to the bright sectors) clockwise apparent reversal occurs and may even predominate. Figure 4 shows some preliminary results obtained with a single subject. The effect depends strongly on the rate at which the stimuli are exposed. Here the i.s.i. is kept constant at 35 ms, and the duration of the exposures varied: the abcissa in figure 4 is the onset–onset time, which is the sum of exposure time and i.s.i. Each curve is obtained with a particular sector size, and the parameters on the figure are the sizes of the anticlockwise steps, expressed as visual angles. For small steps, the amount of reversed motion perceived increases steeply with increasing onset–onset time, and in the range used approaches 100 % reversal. As the step size increases, this rise occurs at longer onset–onset times. However,

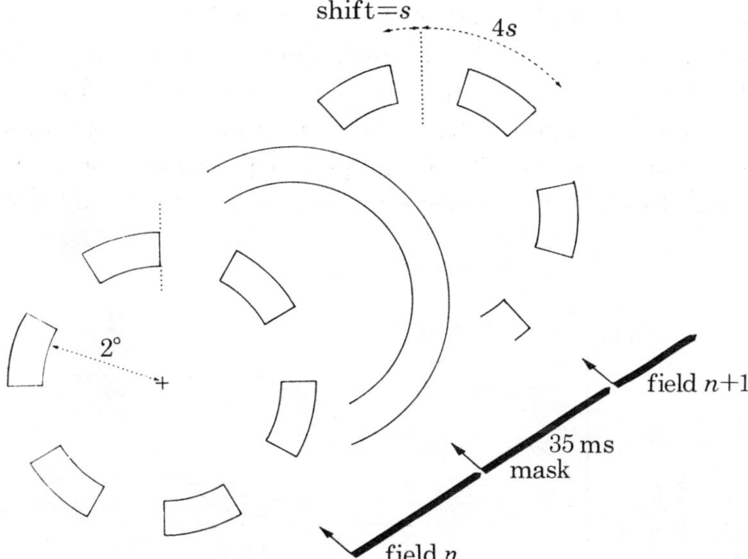

FIGURE 3. Display showing reversal of apparent motion with a bright i.s.i. The three fields shown were exposed superimposed in space and successively in time. The outlined areas were bright on a dark background. Successive exposures of the sectored annulus were rotated anticlockwise by one-fifth of period (i.e. a sector pair). The period shown here is one-sixth of the circle; values used varied from one-third to one-thirtieth of the circle.

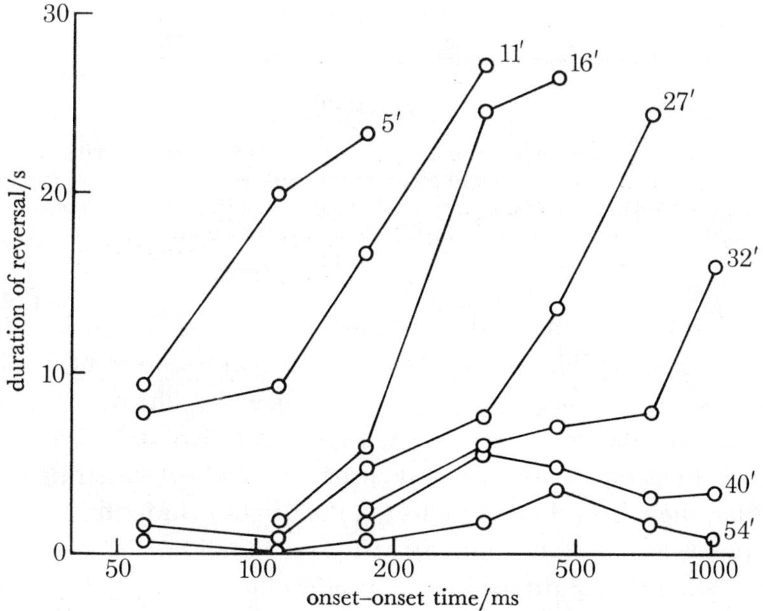

FIGURE 4. Duration of reversed motion (in seconds) seen in 30 s periods of viewing displays of the type shown in figure 3 (each point is the mean of 5–9 observations by one subject). Onset–onset time (plotted logarithmically on the abcissa) is the i.s.i. duration (always 35 ms) plus the exposure of a single field. The parameter on each curve is the shift s between successive exposures of the annulus, expressed as the visual angle subtended at the viewing distance of 2 m. Different values of s were obtained by the use of annuli with different numbers of sectors. Note that with a 35 ms dark i.s.i. all of these points would be below 1 s.

if the steps are greater than about 30′ of visual angle, this rise does not occur: clockwise motion remains at around 10 % or less of the viewing period. One might argue that, following the trend for the smaller displacements, this rise does occur but at onset–onset times longer than those used in the experiment. Figure 5 shows, however, that there is a real difference between the small and large displacements. This figure plots a particular point on the rising curves: the onset–onset time at which reversed motion was seen one-third of the time. For the small shifts,

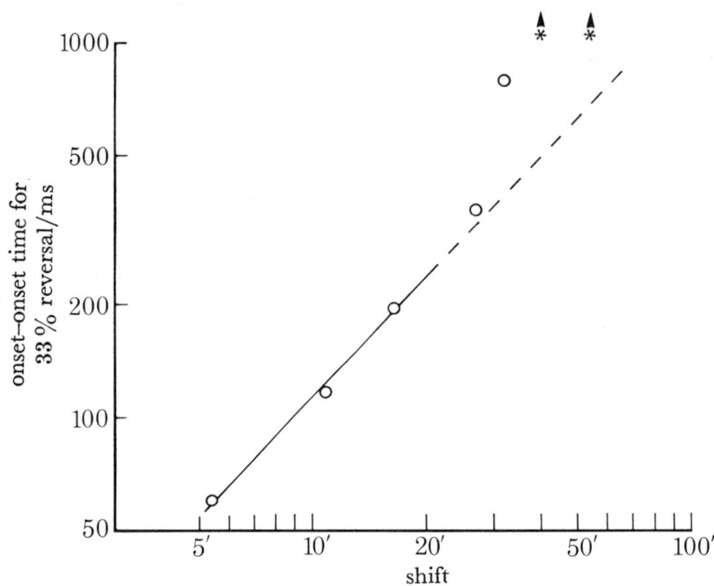

FIGURE 5. Onset–onset time (in milliseconds) producing 10 s reversal of motion in a 30 s viewing period, obtained by interpolation from data in figure 4, as a function of the shift between successive exposures of the sectored annulus. Shifts are expressed as visual angles subtended. Note that both axes are logarithmic. The line drawn has a slope of 1.06. The asterisks indicate large shifts for which 10 s reversal was not obtained in the range of onset–onset time used.

there is a regular relation between this time and the size of the shift. The line drawn has a slope of 1.06 on the log–log plot. This is close to the slope of 1 that would result if a constant reversal fraction occurred at a constant velocity. At a shift of about 30′, the data break away from this straight-line relation. For the two largest shifts, a reversal rate of 33 % is never attained in the range of onset–onset times employed, which it clearly should be if the straight-line relation was followed. Recall that these data show the effect of the bright field in the i.s.i., since with a dark i.s.i. the reversal rate was uniformly approximately zero for all the shifts and onset–onset times. Thus the outcome is that the bright field has a specific effect for small displacements. This is in accord with the idea that bright i.s.is act specifically on the short-range, low-level process responsible for apparent motion. In comparing the 30′ breakpoint in this experiment with the smaller value implied by the random-dot experiments, the position in the visual field should be taken into account: the annular stimulus was 2° from the fixation point. It is plausible that the range of the short-range process, like most other spatial parameters of vision, should increase with retinal eccentricity, although this requires direct confirmation in both types of experiment.

Unfortunately, I cannot yet offer any adequate theory of *why* the bright field in the i.s.i. should induce a reversal of apparent motion from the short-range process. This lack prevents any fully satisfying account of the experiment in terms of the two-process theory of apparent motion.

TWO PROCESSES IN A MULTISTABLE MOTION DISPLAY

A perceptual difference that appears to relate to the dichotomy between the two postulated processes has been studied by Petersik (1975) and Pantle & Picciano (1976). They used a display first described by Ternus (1926), similar to that shown in figure 6a. In this display a set of three elements is shown alternately in two positions, so arranged that the positions of the two rightmost elements in one exposure coincide with the position of the leftmost elements in the alternating exposure. Ternus reported that, even though two of the three elements remain

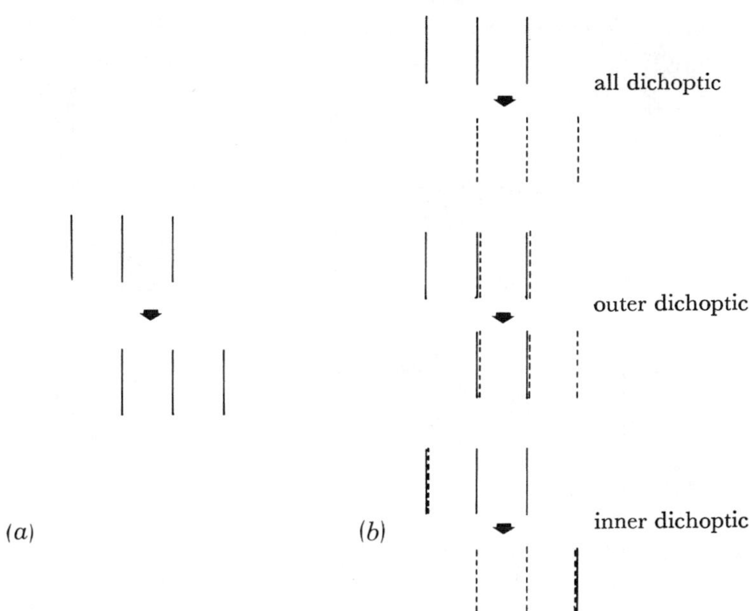

FIGURE 6 (a) The basic display giving group-motion and element-motion percepts. Vertical separation in the diagram is solely to indicate temporal sequence; there was no vertical separation in the display. A complete display sequence consisted of the upper pattern initially visible, followed by a (variable) i.s.i., followed by 200 ms exposure of the lower, with the upper then reappearing after the same i.s.i. (b) Three dichoptic conditions of presentation. Lines presented to the left eye are shown as solid, those presented to the right eye as broken. In the actual displays all lines were solid. Versions of these displays in which left-eye and right-eye images were interchanged were used in half the trials. (From Braddick & Adlard, 1978.)

individually in constant positions, the group of three was seen to move to and fro as a whole. He regarded this as a Gestalt phenomenon; i.e. the perception was determined by the overall organization of the stimulus rather than by its local properties. Petersik and Pantle & Picciano showed that this 'group movement' depended on the temporal parameters of the sequence: it was observed if the i.s.i. was relatively long (80 ms or greater), but for short i.s.is, such as 20 ms the dominant appearance was of 'element motion' in which the central two elements remained static and the outer element jumped to and fro across or around them. Pantle & Picciano (1976) suggest that the two percepts result from two distinct mechanisms and explicitly identify the mechanism yielding element motion with that involved in the segregation of random-dot kinematograms.

This identification is supported by the dependence on i.s.i. (compare the temporal limit on segregation in Table 1) and also by the finding that element motion, like segregation, did not occur when the successive stimuli were presented to different eyes (Pantle & Picciano 1976). The effects of luminance in the i.s.i. provide a further analogy. Figure 7 (Braddick & Adlard 1978) shows data from a display like figure 6a. The i.s.i., which could be either dark or a uniform bright field equal to the background luminance of the patterns, was varied. The subject saw a single displacement and its reversal in a rapid sequence, and had to report whether he perceived group or element movement. (Other responses were permitted but were rarely used.) With dark i.s.is of increasing durations, there is a steady transition from element to group motion as reported by Petersik (1975). With the bright i.s.i. element movement is always more predominant than with dark, and except for the shortest i.s.i. it is close to 100%. (Braddick (1973) found that bright i.s.is had to be greater than 20 ms to abolish segregation in random-dot kinematograms also.) Thus the i.s.i. conditions that are supposed to suppress the short-range process also strongly favour element motion. A similar result has recently been reported by Petersik & Pantle (1979).

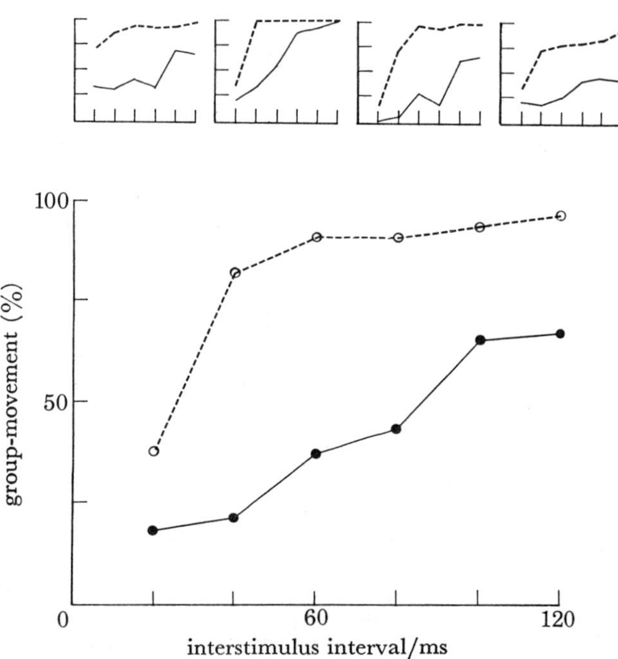

FIGURE 7. Proportion of group-movement responses as a function of i.s.i. duration for the display sequence of figure 6a. The i.s.i. could be either dark (●) or a uniform field of luminance equal to the background of the patterns (○). The main graph shows mean data for four subjects (20 trials each per point); individual data appear in the insets at top. (From Braddick & Adlard 1978.)

There remains a major obstacle to asserting that the short-range process is responsible for element motion in this display. The spatial displacement of the element that is perceived to move is not over a short range. It is three times the inter-element separation, hence three times larger than the displacement in group motion which is presumably to be ascribed to the higher-level, longer-range process, and in our display it is over 3° – at least ten times greater than the limit implied by the segregation experiments (Braddick 1974).

The short-range process signals null motion

However, the outermost element is not the only one involved in the difference between group and element movement. The two inner elements appear stationary in the element movement percept, while in group movement they are seen to move with the group. Perhaps, then, the specific contribution of the short-range process is not to signal the motion of the outer element, but to signal that the inner elements remain stationary. Any system of directionally selective detectors must have a characteristic null response when no movement occurs (Barlow & Hill 1963).

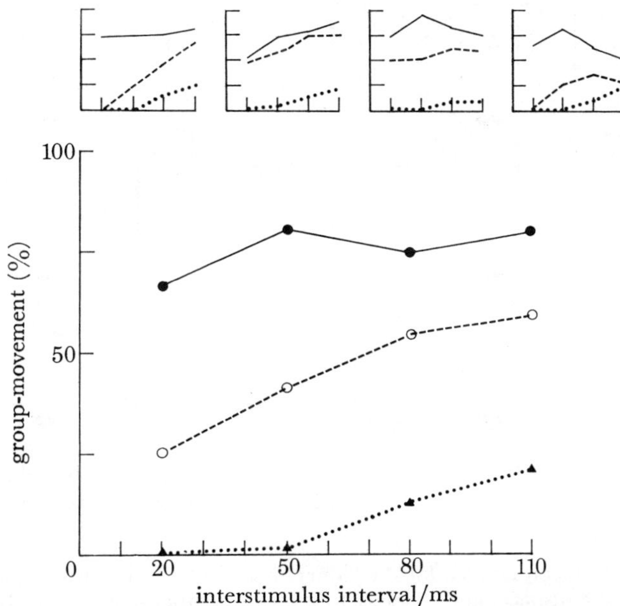

FIGURE 8. Proportion of group-movement responses as a function of i.s.i. for the three dichoptic display sequences of figure 6*b*. ●, All dichoptic; o, inner dichoptic; ▲, outer dichoptic. The main graph shows mean data for four subjects (20 trials each per point); individual data appear in the insets at top. (From Braddick & Adlard 1978.)

To test this possibility, we have taken some of the variables that are presumed to affect the low-level and high-level processes differentially, and applied them selectively to different elements in the pattern (Braddick & Adlard 1978). Figure 6*b* illustrates one way of doing this. Presenting the whole display dichoptically (top) is known to favour group movement (Pantle & Picciano 1976). We could also restrict dichoptic presentation to the outer elements (middle) or the inner elements (lower), with the remaining elements being seen by both eyes together.

Figure 8 presents the results. As Pantle & Picciano found, complete dichoptic presentation produces a uniformly high proportion of group-movement reports. There is also a substantial amount of group movement seen when the inner lines are dichoptic, but there is almost complete element movement, particularly at short i.s.is, when the outer lines are dichoptic. Thus the effect of dichoptic presentation in reducing element movement seems to depend not on dichoptic presentation of the element that apparently moves, but of the elements that appear stationary.

An analogous result comes from the manipulation of the i.s.i. In display sequence *a* illustrated in figure 9, 120 ms (most of which is bright) elapses between the disappearance of the outer line on the left and its reappearance on the right, while only a 20 ms (dark) interval occurs between disappearance and reappearance of the inner lines in their fixed positions. In sequence *b*, the time relations are reversed. Figure 10 shows the proportions of group-movement and element-movement reports obtained with these displays. Recall that for the basic display of figure 6*a*, long, bright i.s.is favour group movement. In this experiment, group movement was seen almost invariably in sequence *b*, when a long, bright i.s.i. intervenes between exposures of the *inner* lines. In sequence *a*, where the outer lines have such an i.s.i. but the inner lines have a short, dark i.s.i., perception of element movement is the rule.

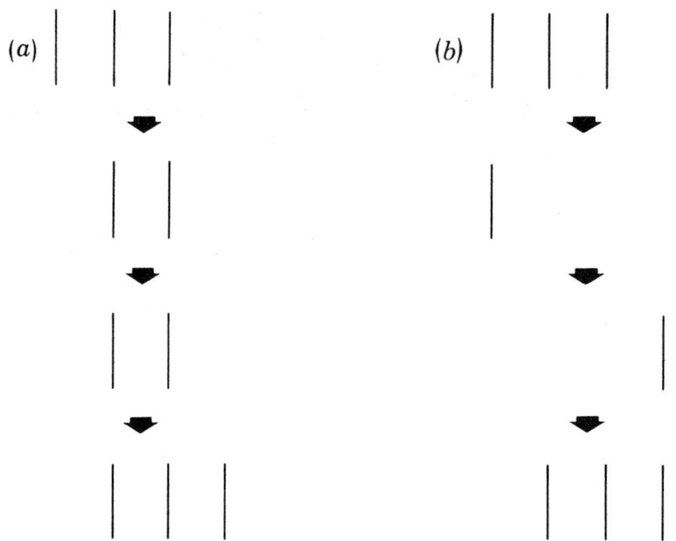

FIGURE 9. Two displays dissociating i.s.i. for the 'inner' and 'outer' elements of the display. Vertical separation was not present in the displays and is solely to indicate temporal sequence. In each case, the top row was visible at the onset of the trial, the second row was exposed for 50 ms, then 20 ms i.s.i., then the third row was exposed for 5 ms, then the fourth row was exposed for 200 ms. The reverse sequence then followed immediately. (From Braddick & Adlard 1978.)

My interpretation of these results is that, when conditions are right for the inner lines to activate the short-range process, element motion of the outer element is perceived; but if the short-range process is not activated, group movement occurs. Now short, dark i.s.is in binocular presentation, while required for the short-range process, do not exclude the higher-level process. This process, I have suggested, is more interpretive in nature. That is, the perceived motion may be selected among alternatives on the basis of complex information derived from the overall configuration, past experience, and so on. However, if the lower-level process – hypothetically, activity of directional detectors quite early in the visual pathway – is signalling that the inner two lines have *not* moved, this signal constrains the interpretations that the higher-level process can select. If those lines are stationary, then the only option is to see the third line as moving between the two outer positions. If because of long, bright i.s.i. or dichoptic presentation of the inner lines, the short-range process is silent, then there is no such constraint and the high-level process can freely operate its own selection rules: these generally favour group movement. Ullman (1979) has provided an elegant analysis of how such selection rules might operate to optimize the perceived motion paths.

Petersik *et al.* (1978) have recently reported an ingenious experiment that fits this account nicely (although it was not conceived with this in mind). They used random-dot kinematograms to create a two-bar display; that is, each bar was seen as a block of dots which remained static while its surround was in random motion, or *vice versa*. This pattern was then switched to a similar one in which the bars were displaced so that the left-hand bar now occupied the former position of the right-hand bar, a two-bar analogue to the sequence of figure 6*a*. The effect was that subjective figures, themselves generated by the segregation effects of the short-range movement process, were seen to move. This perceived movement is presumably a consequence of the longer-range process. The observation therefore implies that figures formed by the short-

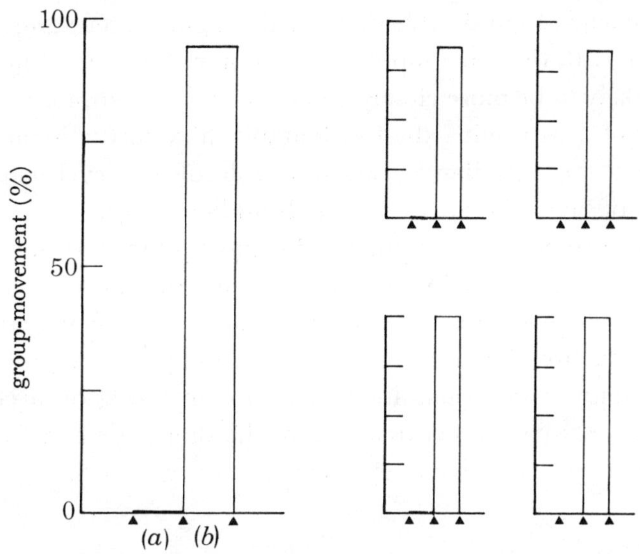

FIGURE 10. Proportion of group-movement responses for the two display sequences illustrated in figure 9. The left diagram shows mean data for four subjects (20 trials per display); individual data appear in the insets on the right. (From Braddick & Adlard 1978.)

range process can serve as an input to the longer-range process, and thus supports the assertion that the short-range process operates earlier in the visual pathway. Further, they compared two alternative versions of this display. In one, the detailed pattern of dots making up the central bar remained the same before and after the switch. In the other, while this bar was created in the same position in the successive kinematograms, the detailed dot structures before and after the switch were uncorrelated. In the former case, the short-range process will yield a signal of 'no movement' for the central bar throughout the whole sequence. In the latter case, the dots change when the switch occurs, so such a signal is not sustained. The account given here would therefore predict that in the former case the short-range process would constrain the perception to element motion, while in the latter case group motion of the bars would be the preferred perception. This is exactly what Petersik *et al.* found.

Interaction of low-level and high-level processes

I believe that this account of the interplay of low-level and high-level processes in the perception of apparent movement may make some general points that are illuminating in considering how specific-detector and interpretive processes contribute to perception. First, even when we know, or believe we know, what information a low-level physiological analyser is transmitting, we should not be too facile in jumping to conclusions about how that information is used in perception. In the Ternus display, I have argued that motion detectors are activated under certain conditions. However, the effect of that activation is not to produce the perception of movement, but the perception of no movement.

Secondly, it is characteristic of the higher-level processes that they operate with a good deal of freedom: all the phenomena of multistable or reversible figures are examples where a variety of perceptions are possible with the same input. The action of lower-level mechanisms wired into the visual pathway is likely to be more closely determined by the stimulus, and this determinate response has the effect of constraining the freedom available to the higher-level 'interpretive' processes. I have argued for a similar constraining role of low-level feature detection in the quite different context of binocular single vision (Braddick 1979).

Those confronting the problems of computer vision have contrasted 'top-down' and 'bottom-up' processes in arriving at an internal representation from the external stimulus (Boden 1977). Undoubtedly both sorts of process are involved in effective human perception. Interpretive processes are likely to have 'top-down' properties, at least in part: the problem of such processes is that their very autonomy makes them inefficient at converging on a correct solution; they have too many options. Low-level processes, such as the short-range motion detector, can constrain the interpretations so as to make the selection of appropriate perceptual hypotheses feasible.

Mr A. Adlard collaborated in several of the experiments described. This work was supported by the Medical Research Council.

References (Braddick)

Attneave, F. & Block, G. 1973 Apparent movement in tridimensional space. *Percept. Psychophys.* **13**, 301–307.

Barlow, H. B. & Hill, R. M. 1963 Evidence for a physiological explanation of the waterfall phenomenon and figural aftereffects. *Nature, Lond.* **200**, 1345–1347.

Barlow, H. B. & Levick, W. R. 1965 The mechanism of directionally selective units in rabbit's retina. *J. Physiol., Lond.* **178**, 447–504.

Bell, H. H. & Lappin, J. S. 1973 Sufficient conditions for the discrimination of motion. *Percept. Psychophys.* **14**, 45–50.

Bishop, P. O., Dreher, B. & Henry, G. H. 1972 Simple striate cells: comparison of responses to stationary and moving stimuli. *J. Physiol., Lond.* **227**, 15P–17P.

Boden, M. 1977 *Artificial intelligence and natural man.* Hassocks, Sussex: Harvester Press.

Braddick, O. 1973 The masking of apparent motion in random-dot patterns. *Vision Res.* **13**, 355–369.

Braddick, O. 1974 A short range process in apparent motion. *Vision Res.* **14**, 519–527.

Braddick, O. J. 1979 Binocular single vision and perceptual processing. *Proc. R. Soc. Lond.* B **204**, 503–512.

Braddick, O. J. & Adlard, A. J. 1978 Apparent motion and the motion detector. In *Visual psychophysics: its physiological basis* (ed. J. Armington, J. Krauskopf & B. R. Wooten), pp. 417–426. New York: Academic Press.

Braddick, O. J., Campbell, F. W. & Atkinson, J. 1978 Channels in vision: basic aspects. In *Handbook of sensory physiology*, vol. 8: *Perception* (ed. R. Held, H. Leibowitz & H. L. Teuber), pp. 3–38. Heidelberg: Springer-Verlag.

Emerson, R. C. & Gerstein, G. L. 1977 Simple striate neurons in the cat. II. Underlying directional asymmetry and directional selectivity. *J. Neurophysiol.* **40**, 136–155.

Gregory, R. L. 1970 *The intelligent eye*. London: Weidenfeld and Nicholson.
Julesz, B. 1971 *Foundations of cyclopean perception*. Chicago: University of Chicago Press.
Kolers, P. A. 1972 *Aspects of motion perception*. Oxford: Pergamon Press.
Neff, W. S. 1936 A critical investigation of the visual apprehension of movement. *Am. J. Psychol.* **48**, 1–42.
Neuhaus, W. 1930 Experimentelle Untersuchung der Scheinbewegung. *Arch. ges. Psychol.* **75**, 315–458.
Pantle, A. J. & Picciano, L. 1976 A multistable movement display: evidence for two separate systems in human vision. *Science, N.Y.* **193**, 500–502.
Petersik, J. T. 1975 Two types of apparent movement in the same visual display. Paper presented at the 16th annual meeting of the Psychonomic Society. Denver, Colorado.
Petersik, J. T., Hicks, K. I. & Pantle, A. 1978 Apparent movement of successively generated subjective figures. *Perception* **7**, 371–383.
Petersik, J. T. & Pantle, A. 1979 Factors controlling the competing sensations produced by a bistable strobo-scopic motion display. *Vision Res.* **19**, 143–154.
Ramachandran, V. S. & Gregory, R. L. 1978 Does colour provide an input to human motion perception? *Nature, Lond.* **275**, 55–56.
Shipley, W. G., Kennedy, F. A. & King, M. E. 1945 Beta-apparent movement under binocular, monocular and interocular stimulation. *Am. J. Psychol.* **58**, 545–549.
Sigman, E. & Rock, I. 1974 Stroboscopic movement based on perceptual intelligence. *Perception* **3**, 9–28.
Smith, K. R. 1948 Visual apparent movement in the absence of neural interaction. *Am. J. Psychol.* **61**, 73–78.
Ternus, J. 1926 Experimentelle Untersuchungen über phänomenale Identität. *Psychol. Forsch.* **7**, 81–136.
Ullman, S. 1979 *The interpretation of visual motion*. Cambridge, Mass.: M.I.T. Press.
Zeeman, W. P. C. & Roelofs, C. O. 1953 Some aspects of apparent motion. *Acta psychol.* **9**, 159–181.

Discussion

K. H. Ruddock (*Biophysics Section, Physics Department, Imperial College, London SW7 2BZ, U.K.*).

(i) Dr Braddick describes the temporal and spatial response characteristics of two mechanisms involved in the detection of apparent motion. In view of the extensive evidence for directionally selective resonses in cortical neurons, would Dr Braddick please explain why he proposes that the central of your two mechanisms is of the 'perceptual hypothesis' forming kind?

(ii) We have found that a hemianopic subject, with severed left optic radiation, is able to detect apparent motion between two bars presented in his 'blind hemifield'. The bars were each $5.5° \times 0.2°$, orientated with long sides parallel and separated by some $3°$, a configuration that should selectively stimulate the central mechanism of Dr Braddick's analysis. The subject reported only the appearance of a dark shadow when the stimulus lines were presented separately, yet he unfailingly identified correctly the direction of apparent motion. How would Dr Braddick interpret this observation?

O. J. Braddick. (i) Tentatively, I would associate the directional selectivity of striate cortical cells with the short-range rather than the higher-level process. Note that many such cells are monocularly driven. The 'more central' mechanism is, I would conjecture, well beyond area 17. I have proposed that it is of a 'hypothesis forming' nature simply because, in the classical kind of display, the perception of apparent notion can be affected by what may be called 'semantic' aspects of the display and by the observer's biases and experience.

(ii) Presumably Dr Ruddock's hemianopic patient is receiving information from his 'blind' hemifield only by a subcortical pathway. Weiskrantz has found that a similar patient can localize stimuli by forced choice although he denies 'seeing' them. I would probably have to interpret Dr Ruddock's observation in terms of such subcortical localization being available to the higher-level motion process I have proposed. (Although conceivably a $3°$ shift might activate the short-range process in peripheral vision.) It is interesting if motion is more directly apparent to the subject than location: this is not entirely clear from the question.

If such a patient showed clear evidence of the *short-range* process in the hemianopic field, that would constrain quite heavily the locus of that process and raise some interesting problems.

M. J. MORGAN (*University of Durham, Department of Psychology, Durham DH1 3LE, U.K.*). I am wondering what the relation might be between Dr Braddick's short-range process and the interpolation effects that I described in my paper. We seem to be in agreement that the classical kind of apparent motion seen with long i.s.is in the order of 200 ms differs markedly from continuous motion. I think that the only reason why apparent motion with long i.s.is was ever called 'continuous' is that this was assessed by verbal report rather than by 'class A' psychophysical procedures. In reality, it is not continuous at all, if it is assessed by the interpolation effect, or by Dr Braddick's perceptual segration phenomenon.

It is interesting that in all the experiments that I have reported on the interpolation effect, the spatial separation corresponding to the i.s.i. at which there was a significant degree of interpolation i.s.is of 32 ms or less) was no greater than 0.2°. When a 64 ms staircase had its inter-step jump reduced from 0.4° to 0.2°, the motion continuity index rose markedly, although this was not true when the jump size of the 128 ms staircase was reduced. In a separate experiment P. Mather showed that the stroboscopic Pulfrich effect broke down entirely when the jump size exceeded 1°. I wonder if Dr Braddick could comment on the relevance of these findings to his short range process? In particular, what role does he think that visual persistence and spatial averaging might play?

O. J. BRADDICK. In speaking of 'smooth apparent motion' over relatively long temporal and spatial intervals, I was referring to succession or alternation of just two stimuli. I was not asserting that smooth *continuous* motion can be perceived from a succession of stimuli such as Professor Morgan uses. Kolers (1972, p. 37) reports that, while a single displacement over $7\frac{1}{2}°$ looks smooth, a succession of displacements appears jerky unless they are 14′ or smaller, which indeed does suggest that only the short-range process can yield continuous perceived motion.

Even with a single jump, Professor Morgan may well be right that displacements with long i.s.is are never perceptually identical to real continuous motion. But apparent motion over large i.s.is and displacements is a real phenomenon, not just a consequence of sloppy criteria: subjects can clearly distinguish alternative organizations of motion, for instance.

It is interesting that the limiting jump size that Professor Morgan mentions for the interpolation effect is comparable with the spatial limit that I have suggested for the short-range process. I presume that he would explain his figure as the range of a spatial averaging process. Spatial and temporal averaging may account for intermediate position judgements in discontinuous displays. However, I do not think that such averaging can explain motion perception, since it would lose information about the temporal ordering of spatial positions. Hence, averaging or summation provides no basis for perceiving the direction of motion: information must be combined over space and time in a more complex (if you like, more nonlinear) way. I do not know whether it is more than coincidence that the spatial ranges of averaging for interpolation and of directional motion detection are so similar.

D. MARR (*The Artificial Intelligence Laboratory, M.I.T., Cambridge, Massachusetts 02139, U.S.A.*).
Computationally, there are two kinds of task associated with motion, which Marr & Ullman (1979) have called tasks of separation and tasks of integration. Tasks of separation are those that can in principle be solved by using only instantaneous measurements, like position and its time

derivatives in the image. They include tasks like the separation of differently moving objects from one another and from the background. Tasks of integration, on the other hand, are those that cannot be solved using only instantaneous measurements, but require the combination of information over time. Ullman (1979, §4) has shown that the recovery of three-dimensional structure from motion is a task of this kind. It seems likely that these two types of task are served by the two mechanisms that Dr Braddick describes. See Marr & Ullman (1979) for a computational account of mechanisms of the first kind, and Ullman (1979), of the second.

References

Marr, D. & Ullman, S. 1979 Directional selectivity and its use in early visual processing. *Proc. R. Soc. Lond.* B. (In the press.)

Ullman, S. 1980 *The interpretation of visual motion.* Cambridge, Mass.: M.I.T. Press.

Phil. Trans. R. Soc. Lond. B **290**, 153–168 (1980)

Printed in Great Britain

153

The perception of apparent movement

By S. M. Anstis

Department of Psychology, York University, 4700 Keele Street, Downsview, Ontario M3J 1P3, Canada

When two similar pictures, overlapping but slightly displaced, were projected on a screen in alternation, apparent movement could be seen. How similar must successive pictures be to give apparent movement? This is the 'correspondence problem'. Manipulations of the local and global correspondences between pictures included motion phenomena such as reversed apparent movement; a four-stroke oscillatory cycle which gave an illusion of continuous motion in one direction; edges defined by texture, stereoscopic depth, or flicker, kinetic edges; and wave motion. It was concluded that human motion perception may comprise two separate mechanisms. Local point-by-point correlations between pictures are detected by a relatively peripheral system, probably based on directionally selective neural units. More subtle global correspondences are analysed by a more cognitive system which extracts edges before it processes motion.

1. Introduction

Motion detection is one of the most ancient and primitive forms of vision (Walls 1942). Perhaps this is because it is so important for survival. For any animal, the most important visual stimuli are other animals, which must be detected and recognized quickly and reliably. Potential mates must be approached, links in the food chain above one's own position are predators to be avoided, and links below are prey to be captured. Colour vision and shape recognition are often effective in finding a mate, because they are aided by, for example, mating plumage. However, these systems alone would frequently fail to detect prey or predators because they would be defeated by natural camouflage. Motion detection is more reliable: prey and predators may freeze in a fixed posture to escape detection, but sooner or later they must make a move, and give themselves away to any eye that is equipped with motion detectors.

For humans too, motion gets attention. To catch the eye of a friend in a crowded airport one could wear a red hat, but it is more effective simply to wave a hand and trigger off his peripheral motion detectors. Motion not only gets attention but holds attention. Most people, given a choice between a photograph or a painting which has colour but not motion, and a black and white television, which has motion but not colour, will find their attention held for far longer by the latter than by the former.

To study motion in the laboratory, the stimulus is often simplified from a continuous movement to a set of discrete stimuli which are flashed in sequence. This gives a convenient and tractable display; moreover, and more importantly, it exposes a discrepancy between the stimulus and the percept. Why does the intermittent stimulus look as though it is moving smoothly? This is the phenomenon of apparent movement (a.m.), which was studied by Wertheimer (1912) and by Korte (1915). These authors mapped out the intervals in time and space that gave optimal apparent movement, and this research tradition has been ably extended by Morgan, whose article elsewhere in this symposium explores the spatial and temporal filtering that are produced by the space and time constants of the visual system.

Wertheimer's classic study used simple dot and line stimuli, and the direction of a.m., if it occurred, could only be between the two positions of his flashed spot. His simple stimulus constrained a simple answer. This constraint, however, has been removed in various recent experiments that looked for a.m. between pairs of complex pictures. Now, the use of these stimuli raises a new question which Wertheimer never asked, namely: How similar must successive pictures be for motion to be seen between them? This will be referred to as the 'correspondence problem', because the visual system has to decide which are the corresponding points in the two pictures, between which motion is to be seen. If two identical pictures are presented in sequence, slightly out of register, the perceptual problem seems easy to solve because there is a simple, one-to-one correspondence between every point in one picture and every similar point in the other. Suppose now, though, that a cluster of ten spots in one picture is followed by a cluster of another ten spots, shifted and slightly disarranged, in a second picture. For each initial spot, the visual system must select one of the spots in the second picture as being the true corresponding target, and reject the other nine as being phantom targets (see Julesz (1971) for a discussion of a similar problem in stereopsis). We confront and solve such perceptual problems every time we go to the cinema. It is only in the most boring movie sequences, such as a slow pan over a static landscape, that successive movie frames are approximately identical. As soon as the real action starts, say when a man runs across the screen, then his limbs flex and his body forms a different geometry on each frame, yet one automatically identifies him as the same visual stimulus or object in each frame, and sees a continuous object in motion. The correspondences between successive frames are sufficient to carry the percept of motion. But if the scene cuts from a man standing by his horse to a new shot of a cactus in the desert, one correctly perceives this as a change of scene; not as a man who jumps across the screen and changes into a cactus. In this case the correspondence or similarity between pictures is not sufficient to give a percept of motion. In what follows I shall attempt to specify the degree, and kind, of similarity that will just give apparent movement; our central problem, then, is the correspondence problem. My main technique is to project in alternation on a screen a pair of 35 mm slides, which are almost but not quite in register. The similarity between the two pictures can be manipulated, and the timing of the alternate exposures can be varied: one may either cut between pictures i.e. switch one picture on and the other off at the same time, or else one may dissolve between them, i.e. fade one picture down as the other fades up, as in the Victorian pastime of dissolving views. Although timing is not our main concern, it will be shown that small alterations in timing can radically alter the perceptual organization of apparent movement in some cases. To anticipate my conclusions, I shall suggest that human visual motion perception involves two quite different systems or mechanisms. (Braddick (1974) was the first person to put forward this idea.) Identical or closely similar pictures, with only a small spatial shift between them, are analysed by a simple point-by-point mechanism (system 1) based on fairly peripheral, hard wired motion detectors. More subtle correspondences between pictures will defeat this simple mechanism, and these are analysed by a more 'cognitive' system (system 2) which extracts edges or forms before it processes motion.

A homely illustration of the notion of perceived object similarity as a prerequisite for one type of perceived motion comes from the old story of Brer Rabbit, who challenged Brer Hedgehog to a five mile race. Both animals started together at the first milestone, and Brer Rabbit ran the first mile as fast as he could. But he found Brer Hedgehog was at the one-mile stone ahead of him. He ran even faster over the second mile, but again Brer Hedgehog was there before him. The same thing happened at every milestone, so Brer Rabbit lost the race. What he did not know was that there were really six hedgehogs: Brer, Mrs, and four little hedgehogs. Brer Rabbit's movement was all too real, but the hedgehog's movement was only apparent, and depended crucially on the fact that all the hedgehogs looked sufficiently alike to be taken for the same individual.

Having drawn attention to the existence of the 'correspondence problem', we shall turn now to consider the logical structure of available models of movement detection, to illustrate the magnitude of the 'correspondence problem' as a threat to theoretical orthodoxy.

2. A SIMPLE MODEL

We shall present a simple analogue model of a motion sensor, and then try to apply it to human visual motion perception. We shall suggest that it successfully models the simpler forms of motion perception which depend upon hard-wired neural motion detectors (see Grüsser & Grüsser-Cornehls (1973) for a review), but it fails, in an instructive way, to explain the subtler, more 'cognitive' forms of motion perception.

The model can be embodied in optical or electronic form. In principle, it could also be expressed as a set of equations, or as a computer simulation, but the hardware analogue forms are easier to understand. We shall start with a simple version which senses change but is non-specific for direction, and then we shall add directional selectivity to the model.

Consider the photograph of a clock in figure 1a. This photograph has been specially reprocessed in figure 1b and c so that in figure 1b the stationary parts – the case and dial – are still visible, but the moving parts – the hands and the gear teeth – have disappeared. Figure 1b is a 'summed picture'. It is a time exposure, in which the static parts of the scene slowly burned themselves into the photographic emulsion, but the moving parts blurred out and disappeared. Conversely, in figure 1c the moving parts are clearly visible, but the static parts have been greatly attenuated or have disappeared. Figure 1c is a 'difference picture' (Mackay 1959). The clock was photographed twice in succession, and the later picture was optically subtracted from the earlier by sandwiching the negative of one picture with the positive of the other. Thus, in figure 1b temporal *summation* accepted static objects and rejected changing or moving objects, whereas in figure 1c temporal *differencing* achieved the opposite. Now, the optical process of temporal differencing can distinguish changes over time, but not the direction of movement. Directional selectivity can be added to the model by a 'shift-and-subtract' process: the procedure here would be to take a negative of a movie frame and spatially shift it around over a positive of its preceding frame until the best match was found. The movement represented by the two frames would be directly given by the direction of the required shift. If different regions of the picture contained movements in different directions, one solution would be to cut the picture up into little pieces and slide them around independently. A practical and flexible method for doing this (in effect) is to examine the scene point by point, using an array of detector pairs with a fixed shift or separation between each pair. Of course, many pairs of detectors would be needed. The operation that compares the two picture samples need not be subtraction: multiplication (correlation) or addition could be used instead, with suitable small modifications to the model.

Barlow & Levick (1965) suggested that a directionally selective neuron in the rabbit retina works along these lines. In their model (see figure 2a), receptors A and B sample adjacent retinal regions. B's output is delayed and then subtracted from A's output. If a stimulus spot moves from B to A (the null direction) then B inhibits A and there is no output. But if a spot moves from A to B (the preferred direction), B's output arrives too late to inhibit A, and there is an output which signals motion.

In principle, the interaction between A and B need not be subtractive. Barlow & Levick pointed out that addition (excitation) would do just as well, but they found direct evidence demonstrating that in fact the rabbit neurons use subtraction (inhibition). Reichardt (1961) proposed a model of motion detection by the beetle's eye, in which B's delayed output, B', was *multiplied* by A's output (see figure 2b). Multiplication measures the correlation between the patterns seen by A and B, and the product AB' reaches a maximum value when the same pattern

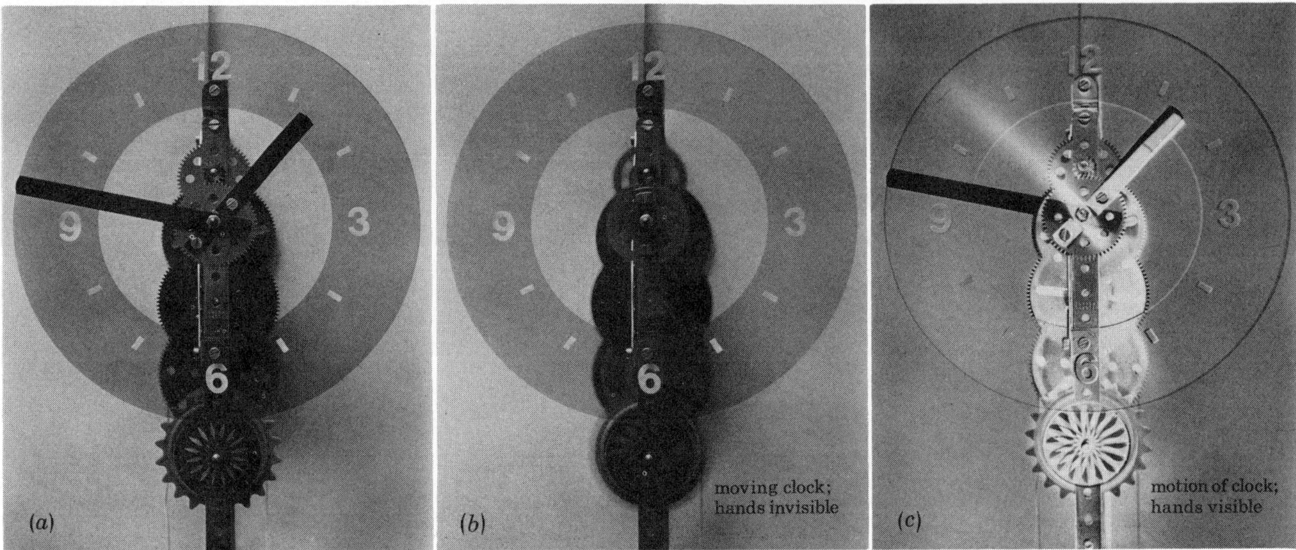

FIGURE 1. Simple model of change (or motion) detector. (a) Original photograph; (b) summed picture: time exposure shows static parts but moving parts blur out and disappear; (c) difference picture made by superimposing negative picture on a positive picture taken earlier: parts that have moved or changed show up clearly (black or white), but static parts cancel out and disappear.

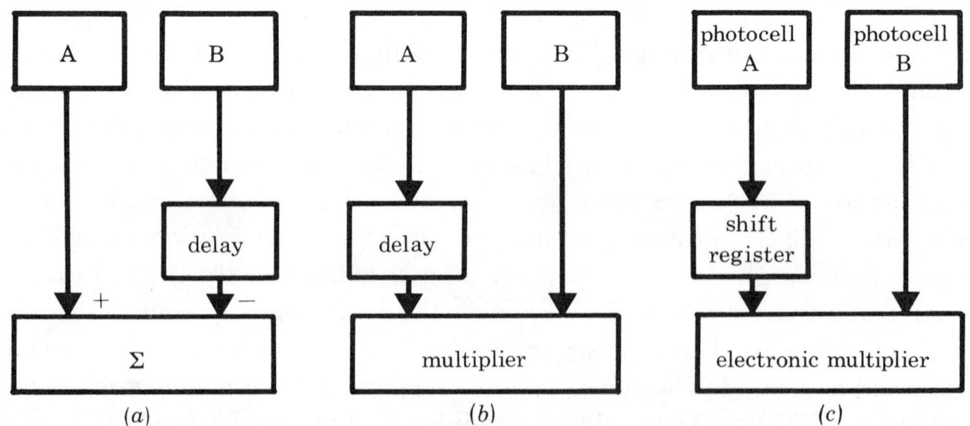

FIGURE 2. Models of physiological motion detectors. (a) After Barlow & Levick (1965). Receptors A and B sample adjacent retinal regions. B's output is delayed and subtracted from A's output. Device gives an output when stimulus moves from A to B. (b) After Reichardt (1961) (greatly simplified). As (a), but B's delayed output is multiplied into A's output, not subtracted from it. (c) Working model which is an electronic form of (b). Attempts to use this device as a model for human motion perception succeeded for perception of point-by-point random-dot motions (system 1), but failed for perception of moving texture edges or cyclopean edges (system 2).

passes first across B and then across A, with a stimulus transit time equal to B's internal delay time.

With R. Hansen, I constructed a simplified electronic version of Reichardt's model (see figure 2c). A randomly sectored black and white wheel rotated clockwise or anticlockwise past two photocells A and B, which were mounted side by side so that each contour moved past first one photocell and then the other. To sense motion from A to B, A's output was delayed for a fixed time interval by a shift register, and then multiplied into B's output by an electronic multiplier. To sense motion from B to A, B's output was delayed and multiplied by A's output by a second multiplier. The output voltage from one multiplier was subtracted from that of the other to give a final output voltage which deflected the needle of a centre-zero voltmeter. The meter needle deflected to the left for motion to the left (from B to A) and deflected to the right for motion to the right (from A to B). This device responded to velocity, not to position, and its output was zero whenever the stimulus wheel was stationary. Also, like Reichardt's model, it was tuned to a preferred velocity, giving the maximum output when the transit time of the stimulus from A to B was equal to the dealy time of the shift registers. The output voltage was reduced for velocities above or below the preferred velocity. It was arranged that the internal delay time of the shift registers could be manually switched to a longer time constant, which gave a slower optimal velocity. Further options could be built in if desired; for instance, it would be possible to make the delay times different for A and B, which would give optimal velocities which were asymetrical for the two directions A–B and B–A. Negative feedback might be used to adjust the internal delays on the model so that it would automatically match its optimum velocity to whatever stimulus velocity was applied to it over a period of time.

All of these models – optical, electronic and physiological – are variations on a theme. They all belong to a class of detectors that compare the luminance distributions seen at position A and time t_1 with that seen at position B and time t_2. The comparision is achieved by addition, subtraction or correlation, and despite minor differences between the models the performance of all the devices depends upon the *cross-correlation* between the patterns at (A, t_1) and (B, t_2).

3. APPLICABILITY OF THE MODEL: TWO SYSTEMS IN HUMAN MOTION PERCEPTION

The comparator model, which physiologists have found in retinae and which I have built in electronic form, is perfectly adequate as a model for the detection of apparent movement of a single spot such as Wertheimer studied. But with more complex stimuli such as pictures, the correspondence problem arises. Can a comparator solve the correspondence problem or do we need a new model?

There are two logically possible ways in which a visual system, natural or artificial, could see apparent movement, and they are illustrated in figure 3. Suppose that a human, or a machine, is watching a cine film of a clock with a sweep second hand. In the first frame the hand is vertical, and in the next frame it is rotated a few degrees clockwise. There are two quite different strategies by which he, she or it could detect the movement (Anstis 1970). The first strategy would be to detect each black point in the first picture, and see it as moving to the nearest black point in the second picture (figure 3a). This point-by-point strategy could be implemented by a population of the motion detectors which we have been describing. It requires only local comparisons between pictures, and demands no prior analysis of patterns within each picture. One important distinguishing feature of such a system is that the extraction of motion information from the pictures could *precede* the extraction of edges within each picture; indeed, the motion information might in principle be used to define those edges. An alternative strategy would be to segregate those black points within each picture that in some sense 'belong together' as a hand, and only after that to detect hand-to-hand motion between the two pictures (figure 3b). On this strategy, edge extraction would necessarily precede motion detection between pictures. It is clear that this process cannot be modelled by the simple

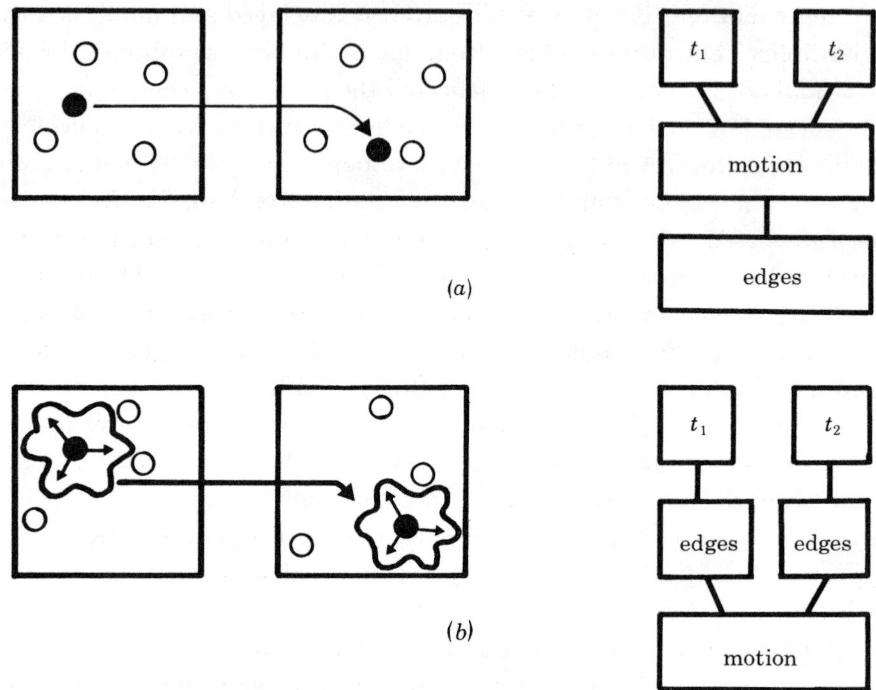

FIGURE 3. Two possible strategies for seeing apparent movement. Left: Two pictures exposed at times t_1, t_2. Though drawn side by side, pictures are really superimposed. Right: Hypothetical perceptual processes. (*a*) Visual system might compare pictures point-by-point (left), for instance, when viewing random-dot stereograms flashed in alternation. A.m. is seen, showing that motion between pictures is seen prior to any extraction of edges within each picture (right). This is system 1 (left column of table 1). (*b*) Visual system might extract edges (e.g. texture edges or cyclopean edges) to segregate zones or regions, and then look for motion between these regions. In this case, edge extraction must precede motion perception (right). This is system 2 (right column of table 1). (Anstis 1970, 1978.)

luminance comparators described earlier, since they do not have the capacity to extract edges. Does the human visual system employ simply the first strategy, for which we have an acceptable working model, or does it employ – either instead or in addition – the second strategy, for which the model cannot give an account?

With most cine film frames or pairs of pictures, there is no way of knowing which strategy is used by the visual system. However, it has proved possible to manipulate the nature of the similarity between pairs of pictures in different ways so that the visual system would be forced to use one strategy in some cases and the other strategy in other cases, if it did indeed have alternative strategies available to it. Pictures such as random-dot stereograms, which when considered separately contain no visible edges, but which considered as a pair show high point-by-point correlations, will signal apparent movement to a detector array and also to a human observer, who must be using the first strategy. As we shall show, however, other pictures can be devised with more subtle correspondences, such as those in which each picture contains subjective contours but there is *zero* point-by-point correlation between them. Here a detector array would be blind to the apparent movement which would nevertheless be clearly visible to a human observer, who must, therefore, be using the second, global strategy. So the comparator device is a successful model for the first type of human motion perception, but not for the second. We conclude, from the demonstration described above and from others described later, that these alternative strategies are not merely logical possibilities; there is good evidence that both strategies are used by the visual systen to perceive motion. Table 1 lists the characteristics of the two supposed visual processes. The table is based on accounts by Braddick (1974), Ramachandran (1978) and Anstis (1978).

TABLE 1. TWO SYSTEMS FOR MOTION PERCEPTION

system 1: peripheral apparent motion	system 2: cognitive apparent motion
can be modelled by comparator device	cannot be modelled by comparator device
short spatial range (up to 15′) (Braddick 1974)	long spatial range (up to tens of degrees)
based on simple point-by-point cross-correlations between pictures as in Julesz random-dot stereograms	subtler correspondences, e.g. cyclopean edges, texture edges, stereo edges
stimulates neural motion detectors (Grusser & Grusser-Cornehls 1973)	does not stimulate motion detectors, which cannot resolve cyclopean contours
adapts neural motion detectors to give motion after-effects	little or no motion after-effects
contrast reversal leads to reversal of a.m. (Anstis 1970)	contrast reversal does not affect perceived direction of motion
colour is not an adequate input for motion perception (Ramachandran & Gregory 1978)	
motion perception between pictures precedes edge extraction within pictures	edge extraction within pictures precedes motion perception between pictures

4. SYSTEM 1

(a) *Julesz random-dot stereograms*

Julesz (1971) has devised random-dot stereo pairs, in which each picture consists of computer-generated random dot patterns looking not unlike photographs of sandpaper. The two pictures in such a stereo pair are identical except that one picture contains a square central region which is slightly shifted to the right. It is important to note that the central square is not visible, indeed does not logically exist, within either picture considered on its own. (The first picture is random and the second picture is obtained by modifying the first. This is like switching some of the columns around in a random number table: the result is merely a second random number table. In the same way, the second picture is also random, and the central square exists only as a correlation between the two pictures.) If the pictures are presented one to each eye in a stereoscope, then binocular fusion gives the percept of a central square floating in depth in front of the surround. If, instead, the pictures are now presented in alternation to one eye only, with the surround regions in register, then the central square is perceived as moving to and fro from left to right (Anstis 1970; Julesz 1971; Lappin & Bell 1972; Braddick 1974). This central square does not exist until *after* the two pictures have been compared and motion perceived, but the edges of the square are clearly seen and are defined by the motion. Clearly, the edge information defining the boundaries of the central square exists only as a relation between the two pictures; it is an emergent property of their juxtaposition and is not a property of either picture taken alone. This fact implies that the perception of the motion between the pictures must be preceding the extraction of edges within each picture (figure 3 *a*).

(*b*) *Reversed apparent movement during contrast reversals*

Two identical pictures exposed in sequence, overlapping but with a small spatial shift between them, show apparent motion, which is of course in the direction of the physical displacement. Anstis (1970) and Anstis & Rogers (1975) reported a new effect: if a black and white slide is dissolved to its own photographic negative, overlapping but shifted out of perfect registration by a few arc minutes, then strong and compelling a.m. was reported toward the earlier stimulus, i.e. in the direction *opposite* to the physical displacement. This reversed apparent movement is probably caused by neural blurring or spatial summation which shifts the effective position of superimposed positive–negative contours (Rogers & Anstis 1975). Related effects occur if the positive and negative are held at fixed contrast levels, but the positive makes to and fro real movements, of a few arc minutes, through the in-register position over the stationary negative. Real movements of the positive are apparently enhanced if the negative is dim, but apparently reversed if the negative is bright. Anstis & Rogers (unpublished results) have found that these different effects can be combined into a repetitive four-stroke stimulus cycle, in which a positive picture is initially placed almost in register with an unchanging negative, and then jumps a few arc minutes to the left, grows dimmer, jumps back to the right, grows brighter again, and so on repetitively. This oscillating stimulus creates a compelling illusion of a pattern which drifts continually to the left without ever 'getting anywhere'. The effect is hard to describe but easy to see in films that we have made. The illusion is a form of 'aliasing': it can be shown that some of the low spatial frequency components of the pictures are in fact shifting continually to the left, even though the actual figure contours are not moving through more than a few arc minutes.

Reversed a.m. is probably a system 1 effect occurring early in the visual system. Blakemore & Anstis (unpublished) projected reversed a.m. dissolves on a screen in front of a cat while recording from some of its cortical motion detectors. The cortical units reported reversed motion whenever the human observers perceived it on the screen. In humans, reversed a.m. products motion after-effects in a direction appropriate to the illusory reversed movement, not to the physical displacement.

(*c*) *Colour not important for apparent movement*

In the preceding section, reversed apparent movement arose during contrast reversals, when the black parts of one picture were replaced by the white parts of a succeeding picture and vice versa. The situation is very different, however, during colour reversal, when coloured parts of one picture are replaced by complementary colours in a second picture. It is not satisfactory to use ordinary colour slides and their negatives, because such photographic negatives reverse both the colours and the brightness of their originals.

Anstis (1970) produced apparent movement between a Julesz random-dot pattern with green dots on a red ground which was followed by a second correlated pattern having red dots on a green ground. The luminances of all the colours could be adjusted independently. He found the the direction of the apparent movement was determined by luminance, not by colour. Thus, a red dot on a green ground followed by a geen dot on a red ground showed normal forward a.m. if both dots were lighter (or darker) than their respective backgrounds and they showed reversed a.m. if one dot was lighter than its background and the other dot was darker than its own background. If the dots in each pattern were matched in brightness to their respective backgrounds to give isoluminant coloured dots, then the apparent motion simply disappeared. This loss of apparent movement at isoluminance has been confirmed by Ramachandran & Gregory (1978). So colour does not provide a significant input to human motion perception. This is consistent with Zeki's (1977) finding that 'cells of the movement area [in the monkey cortex] are not concerned with colour'.

(d) Motion after-effects from apparent movement

The hypothesis that apparent movement in random-dot patterns is sensed by neural motion detectors is supported by the fact that inspection of such a.m. readily produces motion after-effects. Motion after-effects are almost certainly caused by adaptation of such neural units (Barlow & Hill 1963). Moreover, Braddick found that a.m. was not seen in such random-dot patterns if the spatial jumps exceeded 15'. He summarized evidence that 15' was the maximum spatial range for 'short-range' (system 1) motion perception. It is true that a.m. can still be seen for larger jumps if the stimuli are isolated lines instead of random-dot patterns, but such a.m. no longer gives motion after-effects, so it may be mediated by a different mechanism (system 2). Banks & Kane (1972) found that adaptation to a.m. produced by collapsing circles gave motion after effects only if the spatial jumps were less than about 12.5'.

As we shall describe later, inspection of a.m. produced by shifting texture edges gives slight or no motion after-effects. We suggest that system 1 motion perception is mediated by neural motion detectors, but system 2 is not.

5. System 2
(a) Texture edges and cyclopean edges

The edges on which system 1 operates are luminance edges. But Ramachandran *et al.* (1973) successfully obtained apparent movement from edges that were defined not by luminance but by texture. The existence of such edges was demonstrated by Pickett (1970), who showed that it was easy to discriminate abutting zones of texture when one zone contained random black and white dots while the other contained random horizontal dashes. Both zones contained 50 % black and 50 % white points, so they had the same mean luminance and the same first order of probability.

Ramachandran *et al.* used textured patterns that looked deceptively similar to Julesz patterns, but whose structure was in fact crucially different from that of the classical random-dot stereogram. Ramachandran *et al.* used two pictures in which the surrounds contained *uncorrelated* 'noise' or random dots, but with a central square zone that was shifted *en bloc*, being displaced slightly to the right in one picture (figure 4). This square zone was filled with horizontal dashes in one picture, and with vertical dashes in the other. The dashed zones were *not* correlated with each other. When the two pictures were superimposed and exposed in alternation, subjects reported a central square jumping to and fro. Note that there was *no* point-by-point correlation between the two pictures, as there is in the conventional Julesz stereogram pair. The important inference to be drawn from this observation is that in this instance motion perception could *not* be based upon point-by-point matching of images exciting the retina in succession. Instead, the recognition of visual texture, and of a square contour bounding it, must have been visually processed *before* motion was perceived (see figure 3*b*). This is exactly the reverse of the condition described under (*a*) above, and is an example of motion perception by system 2 (see table 1).

Virtually any form of texture edge, provided it is clearly discriminable when at rest, will also give a system 2 apparent movement when abruptly shifted. Figure 5 shows examples of edges based on vernier offset or spatial phase, and on magnification of spatial frequency components Stereoscopic depth edges are also effective. Steinbach & Anstis (1976) generated moving stereo gratings by using dynamic random-dot visual noise. Each eye on its own saw a randomly twinkling snowstorm, like the noise on a detuned t.v. receiver, but when the two monocular

FIGURE 4. (*a*) A zone of horizontal (or vertical) dashes against a background of random dots can be clearly perceived as a texture boundary, even though both zones have the same space-averated luminance (Pickett 1970). (*b*) When the pictures are switched on and off in alternation, the visual system analyses the square contour within each picture, then sees motion between the squares (system 2). Note that there is no point-by-point correlation between the two pictures. (Ramachandran *et al.* 1973.)

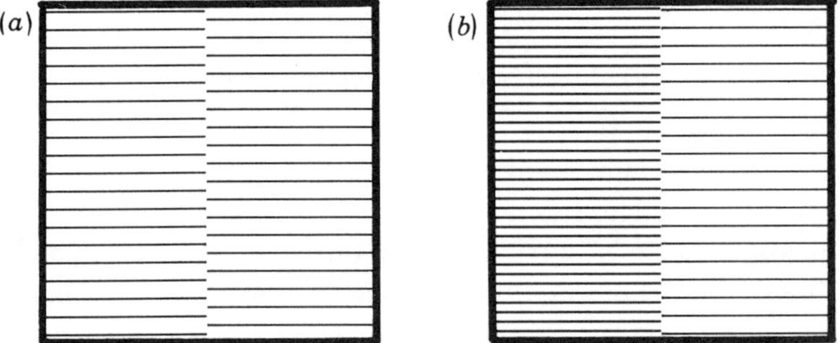

FIGURE 5. Examples of texture edges defined by vernier offset (spatial phase) and by spatial frequency.

views were binocularly fused in a stereoscope, a set of horizontal corrugations in depth were seen, and these bars were made to drift slowly downwards. The downward motion was clearly visible; it was found that the drifting bars could easily be tracked with smooth voluntary eye movements: there was no need for any real movement to brush across the retina to drive the eye movements. The display was not compelling enough to drive involuntary optokinetic nystagmus, but it did generate a very brief movement after-effect (see the next section).

What, then, is the nature of these 'texture edges' to which system 2 is sensitive? It would be misleading to call them 'subjective contours', because there is a physical difference on the two sides of the edge. 'Cyclopean edges' is a better term (Julesz 1971). The difference is not usually in the space-average luminance, but it can be in spatial frequency components, spatial phase, binocular disparity, etc. A difference in physical luminance must be translated into some difference in the response of a population of neurons, and so must difference in texture. Very little is known about the visual processing that extracts edges, but computer algorithms for edge extraction and zone segregation are well established (see Rosenfeld & Kak (1976), ch. 8). For instance, a zone of black and white random dots can easily be segregated from a mid-grey background by measuring the contour richness or 'digital gradient'. Presumably, analogous processing occurs in the visual system. With the displays described in this section, such processing must occur in system 2 *before* motion is perceived.

(b) Little or no motion after-effects from cyclopean edges

Whereas motion after-effects are easy to produce with short-range a.m. from luminance edges (system 1), they are hard to produce with moving cyclopean edges (sytem 2). Either they are very brief or they do not occur at all. Drifting stereo gratings gave motion after-effects (Papert 1964; Steinbach & Anstis 1976) but they lasted for only 1 s or less. The same was true for dichoptic motion produced by widely separate points (Anstis & Moulden 1970). All these motion after-effects must lie central to the point of binocular fusion, and they were all very brief. The drifting kinetic gratings which are described later (§7*b*) gave no motion after-effects, and there appear to be no reports of after-effects from shifting texture boundaries. It seems likely that neural motion detectors adapt readily, but the mechanisms which report the shift of 'computed' or cyclopean edges are stiff systems which show very little adaptation.

6. Patterns that can stimulate either system 1 or system 2

There are some pairs of patterns that give apparent movement in one direction when superimposed and exposed in alternation, but when the timing is slightly altered the apparent movement is radically changed in direction and perceptual organization. Pantle (1973) reported a.m. between two uncorrelated patterns, each containing a square cluster of red spots against a background of green sports (figure 6). The spots in each picture were in uncorrelated random positions. When the patterns were switched on and off alternately at about 0.5 Hz, subjects reported a cluster of red spots moving to and fro *in toto*. However, if one pattern dissolves into the other, with one pattern fading down as the other fades up, the apparent motion is entirely different. There is a random, incoherent movement, with each spot in one picture moving to the nearest spot in the other picture, independent of its colour. Instead of a disciplined square squad of spots jumping globally to and fro, a random rabble of spots swim about locally in all directions. This local incoherent motion between nearest neighbours is signalled by system 1, operating on a point-by-point comparison. The perceived motion of a cluster of elements is signalled by system 2, since it uses the global information about the property (redness) distributed across a number of spots to extract a subjective square contour, which is then seen to move. Anstis (1970) exposed in alternation two gratings that were tilted a few degrees away from vertical, one clockwise and one anticlockwise (figure 7). When they were switched on and off alternately at about 0.5 Hz, subjects reported a single striped field oscillating to and fro in a rotary manner. But when the alternation rate was raised to 5–10 Hz, or if the fields dissolved into each other instead of switching, then the perceived motion broke up into local, relatively incoherent motion, with horizontal strips of the field rotating independently, and shearing off from other strips along the lines of the moiré fringes. Again the local motion can be attributed to system 1, and the global motion of the whole field to system 2.

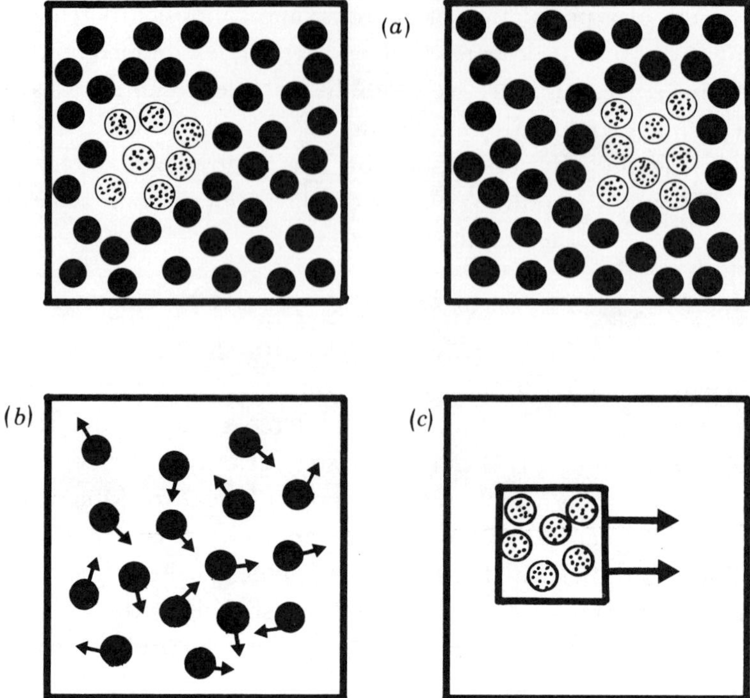

FIGURE 6. (*a*) Each picture contains a square cluster of red spots against a background of green spots (Pantle 1973).
(*b*) With the two pictures superimposed, during slow dissolves, incoherent local motion is seen, with each
spot moving to its nearest neighbour irrespective of colour (system 1). (*c*) If the pictures are switched sharply
on and off in alternation, the visual system extracts a subjective outline of a square in each pattern and then
(as in figure 4) sees motion between two squares (system 2).

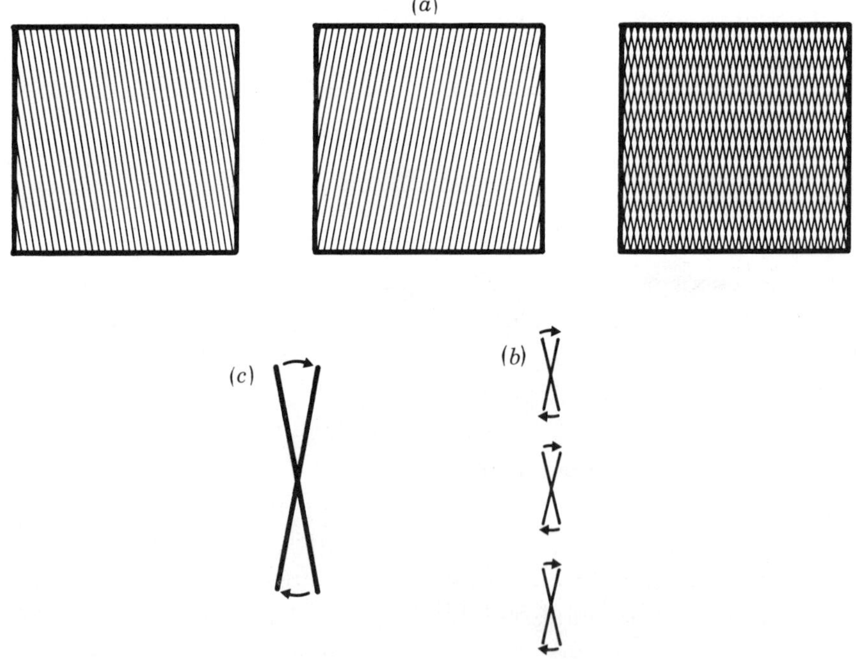

FIGURE 7. (*a*) Two superimposed gratings give horizontal moiré fringes when both gratings are on continuously.
(*b*) During dissolves from one grating to the other the picture appears to split up along the moiré fringes into
horizontal strips. Each strip shows local rocking movement (system 1). (*c*) When the gratings are sharply
switched on and off in alternation, a single rocking grating is seen (system 2). (Anstis 1970.)

V. Zemon has been independently studying this phenomenon of the crossed gratings (personal communication).

7. PATTERNS THAT DO STIMULATE BOTH SYSTEM 1 AND SYSTEM 2

We have seen that short-range luminance edges are handled by system 1, and most other kinds of edge – cyclopean and the like – are handled by system 2. But there are two special kinds of edge, flicker edges and kinetic edges, that seem to stimulate both systems. Flicker edges stimulate systems 1 and 2 in parallel, whereas kinetic edges stimulate them in series.

(a) Flicker edges

Consider a vertical edge that alternates in polarity between black–white and white–black at a rate of about 5–10 Hz. Suppose the edge makes a succession of small jumps to the right, each jump being 5–10′ in extent, with a polarity change synchronized to each jump. Thus a black–white edge is replaced by a white–black edge shifted to the right, which in turn is replaced by a black–white edge shifted further to the right, and so on. After an excursion of a degree or so, the edge jumps back to the left and the cycle repeats.

I have found (Anstis 1980) that observers unambiguously perceived a flickering edge moving (somewhat jerkily) to the right. This movement to the right was easy to see, and easy to track with the eyes. If the observers fixated on a stationary point and adapted to the rightward motion of 30–60 s, then they reported a motion after-effect afterwards, as might have been expected. What was quite unexpected, however, was that the direction of the after-effect was to the *right*, i.e. in the *same* direction as the stimulus motion, not in the opposite direction as one would normally expect.

We interpret this as follows. The jumps to the right were picked up by system 2, irrespective of the sign or polarity of the edge which reversed on each jump. Stimulation of system 2 gives a percept of motion, but no after-effect of motion. At the same time, system 1 was also being stimulated: note that the jumps were only 5–10′ in amplitude, well within the spatial range of system 1. But to system 1 each jump produces a *reversed* apparent movement, apparently to the left, as described earlier. It is the adaptation to the apparent leftwards motion that gives rise to a motion after-effect to the right. An interesting feature is that the leftward reversed apparent movement is never consciously perceived in this situation; the edge is perceived as jumping to the right, not to the left. So this is an example of a perceptually invisible motion giving rise to a visible after-effect. We know of no earlier reports of this example, although visible coloured after-images from sub-threshold coloured stimuli have been reported (see review by Anstis *et al.* 1978).

(b) Kinetic edges and wave motion

Imagine that the fingers of two hands are randomly speckled with luminous paint; suppose the fingers are interlaced and held vertically with one hand higher than the other. In a dark room one would be unable to discern the fingers: one would simply see a random speckle of luminous dots. But suppose the fingers were then slid vertically together and apart: one would immediately be able to distinguish the separate fingers by virtue of their vertical motion or 'common fate'. Thus when the fingers of the left hand move upwards and those of the right hand downwards, the (stationary) vertical edges between the moving fingers would be readily visible as a kind of standing wave.

Now suppose that the fingers are unlaced and the fingers of one hand are drummed on the table top. Each finger moves only up and down as before, never sideways. But a beetle on the table would perceive a thunderous creeping barrage of fingertips apparently advancing horizontally across the table. What moves horizontally is not, of course, the fingers themselves, but a *sequence* of fingers or a phase velocity, in other words a travelling transverse wave.

According to the approach outlined here, the sequence of visual events is as follows. The up and down movements of the fingers are picked up by system 1. The common motions seen by system 1 serve to segregate the edges of the fingers. Since these edges are defined by motion information without any luminance cues, we shall call these 'kinetic edges'. When the moving fingers are interlaced they define stationary kinetic edges, but when they are drumming they define travelling kinetic edges, which move at right angles to the fingers' motions. The displacements of the kinetic edges, i.e. the transverse waves, are picked up by system 2. We have produced travelling kinetic edges and waves both mechanically (Steinbach & Anstis 1976) and electronically (K. Nakayama, C. W. Tyler & S. M. Anstis, unpublished).

The mechanical display consisted of 50 long thin metal rods held in a frame and arranged in a vertical sheet somewhat like the teeth of a giant comb. Each rod was free to move independently of its neighbours along its own length but in no other direction. The bottom of each rod rested on a helicoidal barley-sugar twist Jacobean table leg, which lay with its long axis horizontal at the bottom of the sheet of rods. When this table leg was rotated about its own axis by means of a handle, it imparted a sinusoidal up and down motion to each rod; moreover, each rod had a slight phase lead over its right-hand neighbour. The resulting display was like 50 long thin metal fingers drumming on a table top. Each rod was randomly banded in black and white so that its vertical motions could be clearly seen. The travelling waves moving to the right defined a drifting kinetic grating. The wave motion to the right was easily perceptible, and provided an adequate stimulus for smooth tracking eye movements (Steinbach & Anstis 1976). If the eyes fixated a stationary point on the frame while an observer adapted to 60 s of wave motion to the right, then *no* motion after-effect could be seen thereafter.

In the electronic display, a static pattern of about 200×200 static random dots was set up on a television raster. Then, by means of a sinusoidal signal applied to the X (horizontal) inputs, it was arranged that each horizontal line of the raster moved horizontally to and fro, slightly lagging the line above it. All of the dots on the screen were moving to and fro horizontally, but the percept was a series of sinusoidal waves or ripples running downwards across the screen; in other words, a drifting kinetic grating. The stimulus was like the mechanical display just described laid on its side. Once again, the downward drift of the kinetic grating was easy to perceive, even though no dots or luminance borders were moving downwards. The downward motion gave an adequate stimulus for smooth pursuit eye movements, but it could not be used to generate a motion after-effect.

We conclude that system 1 responds to the horizontal motion of the dots, and that system 2, operating at a later level in the visual system, responds to the wave motion.

References (Anstis)

Anstis, S. M. 1970 Phi movement as a subtraction process. *Vision Res.* **10**, 1411–1430.

Anstis, S. M. 1978 Apparent movement. In *Handbook of sensory physiology* (ed. R. Held, H. W. Leibowitz & H.-L. Teuber), pp. 655–673. New York: Springer-Verlag.

Anstis, S. M. 1980 Direction of apparent movement of a moving flicker edge. (In preparation.)

Anstis, S. M. & Moulden, B. P. 1970 Aftereffect of seen movement: evidence for peripheral and central components. *Q. Jl exp. Psychol.* **22**, 222–229.

Anstis, S. M. & Rogers, B. J. 1975 Illusory reversal of visual depth and movement during changes of contrast. *Vision Res.* **15**, 957–961.

Anstis, S. M., Rogers, B. J. & Henry, J. 1978 Interactions between simultaneous contrast and coloured after-images. *Vision Res.* **18**, 899–911.

Banks, W. P. & Kane, D. A. 1972 Discontinuity of seen motion reduces the visual motion aftereffect. *Percept. Psychophys.* **12**, 69–72.

Barlow, H. B. & Hill, R. M. 1963 Evidence for a physiological explanation of the waterfall phenomenon. *Nature, Lond.* **200**, 1345–1347.

Barlow, H. B. & Levick, W. R. 1965 The mechanism of directionally selective units in rabbit's retina. *J. Physiol., Lond.* **178**, 477–504.

Braddick, O. 1974 A short range process in apparent motion. *Vision Res.* **14**, 519–528.

Grüsser, O. J. & Grüsser-Cornehls, U. 1973 Neuronal mechanisms of visual movement perception and some psychophysical and behavioral correlations. In *Handbook of sensory physiology*, vol. 7 (3 a): *Central processing of information* (ed. R. Jung), pp. 333–430.

Julesz, B. 1971 *Foundations of cyclopean perception*. Chicago: University of Chicago Press.

Korte, A. 1915 Kinematoscopische Untersuchungen. *Z. Psychol.* **72**, 193–206.

Lappin, J. S. & Bell, H. H. 1972 Perceptual differentiation of sequential visual patterns. *Percept. Psychophys.* **12**, 129–134.

Mackay, R. S. 1959 Display of moving parts of a scene. *Science, N.Y.* **130**, 223–224.

Pantle, A. J. 1973 Stroboscopic movement based upon global information in successively presented visual patterns. *J. opt. Soc. Am.* **63**, 1280A.

Papert, S. 1964 *M.I.T. Quarterly Progress Report.*

Pickett, R. M. 1970 Visual analyses of texture in the detection and recognition of objects. In *Picture processing and psychopictorics* (ed. B. S. Lipkin & A. Rosenfeld). New York: Academic Press.

Ramachandran, V. S. 1978 Studies in binocular vision. Ph.D. thesis, University of Cambridge.

Ramachandran, V. S. & Gregory, R. L. 1978 Does colour provide an input to human motion perception? *Nature, Lond.* **275**, 55–56.

Ramachandran, V. S., Rao, V. M. & Vidyasagar, T. R. 1973 Apparent movement with subjective contours. *Vision Res.* **13**, 1399–1401.

Reichardt, W. 1961 Autocorrelation: a principle in motion perception. In *Sensory communication* (ed. W. Rosenblith), pp. 303–317. New York: Wiley.

Rogers, B. J. & Anstis, S. M. 1975 Reversed apparent depth from positive and negative stereograms. *Perception* **4**, 193–201.

Rosenfeld, A. & Kak, A. 1976 *Digital picture processing.* New York: Academic Press.

Steinbach, M. J. & Anstis, S. M. 1976 Paper presented to the Annual Conference of the Association for Research in Vision and Ophthalmology, Sarasota, Florida.

Walls, G. 1942 *The vertebrate eye and its adaptive radiation.* Michigan: Cranbrook Press.

Wertheimer, M. 1912 Experimentelle Studien über das Sehen von Bewegung. *Z. Psychol.* **61**, 161–278. (Excerpted and transl. in *Classics in psychology* (ed. T. Shipley). New York: Philosophical Library 1961.)

Zeki, S. M. 1977 Colour coding in the superior temporal sulcus of rhesus monkey visual cortex. *Proc. R. Soc. Lond.* B **197**, 195–223.

Discussion

D. M. MacKay (*Department of Communication and Neuroscience, University of Keele, Keele, Staffordshire ST5 5BG, U.K.*). I should like to append some further evidence indicating that we must expect motion to be represented in more than one neural subsystem.

In the first place, there is an additional mode of motion perception, not so far mentioned, in which the retinal image is not displaced at all. During 'smooth pursuit' of a moving target, for example, there is a compelling perception of motion even when neither of the two subsystems mentioned by Dr Braddick is activated.

Secondly, the existence of separate subsystems for signalling *continuous drift* and *discontinuous displacement* is suggested by the fact that, for small enough displacements of the retinal image, a continuously illuminated target in a stroboscopically lit surround can be seen to move while the surround appears to remain at rest (MacKay 1976) came across a striking illusion that seems to show the possibility of rivalry between these two subsystems. The subject views an electronically generated field of dynamic visual noise with a movable rectangular 'window' (electronically) cut out of it so as to reveal a stationary under-layer of random texture. When the window is moved smoothly across the dynamic noise field, it seems to move in a succession of jerks which increase in size with eccentricity. The reason seems to be that the texture seen through the moving window is at rest relative to the fixated frame, and therefore gives rise to signals indicating zero drift, whereas the moving edge of the window itself generates signals indicating displacement. The conflict between the two sets of signals issues in a jerky succession of revisions of the perceived location of the window.

When we come to look for physiological candidates for these various functions the position becomes still more complex. My colleague P. Hammond and I have recently been using the same electronic display to generate textured stimuli for investigating the response characteristics of simple and complex cells in area 17 of cat (Hammond & MacKay 1975, 1977; Groos et al. 1976). As Gibson (1951) has particularly emphasized, textured bars camouflaged against similarly textured backgrounds become clearly perceptible when moving over the background. We have found no simple cells, however, which respond to such moving stimuli. Somewhat to our surprise, the cells that do respond are complex (presumably receiving an input independent of simple cells); but even these show no specific sensitivity to the shape or orientation of the textured bars. To make matters worse, the polar diagrams of responsiveness to a moving textured field generally have maxima in different directions from those for a moving black or white bar (Groos et al. 1976). Thus although the firing of such complex cells may serve to indicate motion, it cannot of itself represent either the shape or the velocity vector of the moving stimulus.

More recently, we have found that although the simple cells do not respond to texture motion, they are not uninfluenced by it (Hammond & MacKay 1978). A black bar on a textured background generally evokes a weaker response if the background moves with it. When only a small exploratory patch of texture is moved synchronously with the bar, its effect varies with its location relative to the conventionally defined receptive field, and can be significant far outside its boundaries. Along the axis parallel to the preferred bar orientation, the effect can in some cases vary from suppression (at the field centre) to facilitation (well outside the receptive field).

Even at this relatively peripheral level, then, it would seem that motion finds a diversity of representations in terms of neural activity, and that none of these is adequate to signify all forms of commonly perceived motion, let alone those generated in illusions. Certainly any hope of identifying one class of cell as *the* 'detector of motion' now seems illusory.

References

Groos, G. A., Hammond, P. & MacKay, D. M. 1976 Polar responsiveness of complex cells in cat striate cortex to motion of bars and of textured patterns. *J. Physiol., Lond.* **260**, 47P–48P.

Gibson, J. J. 1951 *The perception of the visual world*. Boston: Houghton Mifflin.

Hammond, P. & MacKay, D. M. 1975 Differential responses of cat visual cortical cells to textural stimuli. *Expl Brain Res.* **22**, 427–430.

Hammond, P. & MacKay, D. M. 1977 Differential responsiveness of simple and complex cells in cat striate cortex to visual texture. *Expl Brain Res.* **30**, 275–269.

Hammond, P. & MacKay, D. M. 1978 Modulation of simple cell activity in cat by moving textured backgrounds. *J. Physiol., Lond.* **284**, 117P.

MacKay, D. M. 1976 Perceptual conflict between visual motion and change of location. *Vision Res.* **16**, 557–558.

Phil. Trans. R. Soc. Lond. B **290**, 169–179 (1980)

Printed in Great Britain

The optic flow field: the foundation of vision

By D. N. Lee

Department of Psychology, University of Edinburgh, 7 George Square, Edinburgh EH8 9JZ, U.K.

As a basis for understanding the visual system, we need to consider the functions that vision has to perform, which are pre-eminently in the service of activity, and the circumstances in which it normally operates, namely when the head is moving. The fundamental ecological stimulus for vision is not a camera-like time-frozen image but a constantly changing optic array or flow field, the description of which must be in spatio-temporal terms. A mathematical analysis of the optic flow field is presented, revealing the information that it affords for controlling activity – information both about the topography of the environment and about the movement of the organism relative to the environment. Results of human behavioural experiments are also reported. It is suggested that the optic flow field should be the starting point in attempting to discover the physiological workings of the visual system.

1. Introduction

An animal is constantly active when awake, moving around its environment, interacting with objects and other organisms, and so on. Even when simply sitting or standing still and looking at something, the body is always swaying slightly and the sway has to be actively kept in check. The result of this continual activity is that the head is always moving relative to the environment and so the animal's view of the world is constantly changing. This means that the ecological stimulus for vision is a globally changing optic array or optic flow field. In other words, the ecological stimulus is inherently spatio-temporal.

Activity is also spatio-temporal. It occurs in space-time. The guidance of activity therefore requires that spatio-temporal information be obtainable through the perceptual systems. This paper is about how the optic flow field affords information for controlling activity.

2. Perceptuo-motor coordination

Over 40 years ago, Bernstein (cited in Bernstein 1967) offered two significant insights into how body movements are coordinated and regulated. First, from his empirical studies of rhythmical movements such as walking, which revealed a high homogeneity of movement of a form that could not be attributed to simple mechanical factors, he argued that there must exist in the central nervous system exact 'formulae of movement' which contain the whole course of the movement over time. Lashley (1951) had basically the same idea, arguing that all skilled activity involves the problem of serial ordering of units of action and so there must exist internalized 'schemata' which direct the sequencing of these units.

What form do these formulae of movement take? The answer might seem obvious: specific temporal patterns of efference to the muscles. This was the classical view. However, Bernstein's second insight was that this cannot be. For since the effect of the efference will necessarily vary, e.g. with the prevailing external forces on the limbs, which are never completely predictable, there cannot exist an unequivocal relation between the efference and the form of the movement.

Also, basically the same movement can be made by using quite different muscle systems (e.g. signing one's name on paper and on a blackboard). Bernstein therefore concluded that movements must be directed in terms of an internalized motor image or program corresponding to the intended form of the movement, and that continual perceptual regulation of the program was necessary.

Bernstein, like most present researchers (see, for example, Stelmach (ed), 1976), was mainly concerned with the control of movements involving minimal interaction with the environment. Consequently, his and most current theories lack sufficient regard for the important role that must be played by the perceptual systems, particularly vision, in the control of normal everyday activities like locomotion through an obstacle-laden environment.

A comprehensive theory of perceptuo-motor coordination must address the question: What types of information are required in controlling movement relative to the environment? Gibson (1966) postulated that there are two basic types of information needed: *exterospecific* information about the layout of the surfaces in the environment and about external objects and events, and *propriospecific* information about the animal's own bodily movements. Such a binary conception, however, tends to obscure the fact that the animal is in interaction with its environment. To control this interaction, the animal needs information about the position, orientation and movement of its body as a whole or part of its body relative to the environment. Lee (1978) proposed the term *expropriospecific* in an attempt to capture the relativistic nature of the information.

How does expropriospecific information fit into the scheme of motor control? Let us consider, for example, the control of locomotion. Given that locomotor acitivity must be directed by a motor program and that the program has to be continually regulated to correct for deviations of the activity from its intended course, the question arises as to how it is regulated. Since it is only the yet-to-run sections of the motor program that can be adjusted, it seems clear that what is required is expropriospecific information that is *predictive*, in the sense that it is of such a form that it can be integrated with the current motor program to yield a prediction of the potential future course of the locomotion were the program left to run, and that it is on this basis that upcoming sections of the motor program are regulated. In the following section I shall show how such predictive information is available in the optic flow field.

3. The optic flow field

What information is available in the light at the eye for controlling activity? Gibson (1950, 1958, 1966) was the first to tackle this problem and the following analysis owes much to his insights. Only an outline of the analysis will be given; for more details see Lee (1974, 1976) and Lee & Lishman (1977).

The environment consists of material substances bounded by surfaces. It is by means of the light reflected from the surfaces that visual perception is possible. Now a surface does not reflect light uniformly, unless it is mirror-like. It contains facets, patches of differing pigmentation and so on. In short, a surface may be considered to be densely covered with *texture elements* which reflect light differently from their neighbours. Thus the light reflected from the surfaces in the environment forms a densely structured optic array at a point of observation. The optic array may be thought of as a bundle of narrow cones of light with their apices at the point of observation; each cone has as its base a distinct environmental texture element and is thus optically differentiable from its neighbours in terms of the intensity and/or spectral composition of the light it contains.

At each point of observation there is a unique optic array. Consequently, when the head is moving relative to the environment, as it normally is, the optic array at the eye is never the same from one moment to the next. The array changes continuously over time, giving rise to an *optic flow field*. A convenient way of describing the optic flow field is in terms of the changing pattern of light incident on a projection surface that intercepts the time-varying optic array. Since the description of the optic flow field in terms of its projection on one surface can be uniquely transformed into a description for any other surface, the choice of a projection surface is simply a matter of convenience. For clarity of exposition, we shall here consider the projection of the optic flow field onto a plane surface behind the point of observation, like the image plane of a camera.

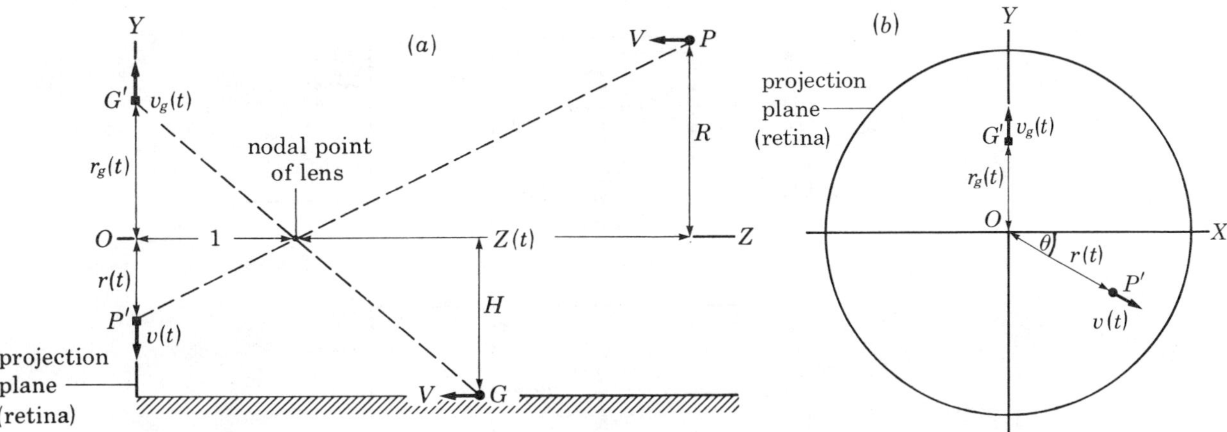

FIGURE 1. Showing how rectilinear movement of the point of observation relative to the environment generates an optic flow field. The schematic eye is considered to be stationary and the environment moving towards it with velocity V in the direction Z to O. P and G denote texture elements on surfaces in the environment, G being on the ground surface. Light reflected from the moving environmental texture elements passes through the nodal point of the lens giving rise to the moving optic texture elements P' and G' on the 'retina'. The densely textured environment gives rise to a densely textured optic flow field wherein all optic texture elements move outwards along radial flow lines emanating from O. How the optic flow field affords information about the environment and about an animal's movement relative to it is explained in the text. (Modified from Lee (1974).)

Let us start by determining the general structure of the rectilinear optic flow field that results when the point of observation is moving along a straight path through a rigid environment. It is equivalent geometrically to consider the point of observation to be stationary and the environment moving relative to it. In figure 1 the environment is moving with velocity V towards the point of observation in a direction perpendicular to the projection plane. P and G denote environmental texture elements; P' and G' denote the corresponding optic texture elements. It is clear that whatever the layout of the surfaces in the environment the optic flow field has the following invariant property: all optic texture elements move outwards along radial flow lines emanating from O, the centre of the projection plane (see figure 1, also figure 3 a, b).

There is a second important invariant property of the optic flow field relating to the fact that during movement of the point of observation surfaces go out of view and come into view as they are progressively occluded and disoccluded by nearer surfaces. The reflexion of this fact in the optic flow field is that when an optic texture element moving along a radial flow line catches up with a slower moving element, it 'occludes' or replaces it. This is because the faster moving optic element corresponds to a nearer environmental texture element (see equation (2), §3c).

It has been shown that the above two invariant properties of the optic flow field geometrically specify that the point of observation is moving rectilinearly relative to a rigid environment (Lee 1974). In other words, there is available in the optic flow field information about the physical state of affairs. To test whether this information is actually picked up by the visual system, and, if so, how potent the information is, human subjects were given visual information about how they were moving relative to the environment which conflicted with the information available through their other senses. This was done by moving their visible surroundings – a floorless 4m × 2m × 2m suspended 'room' – in such a way as to produce optic flow fields at their eyes that corresponded to forward and backward movement of themselves.

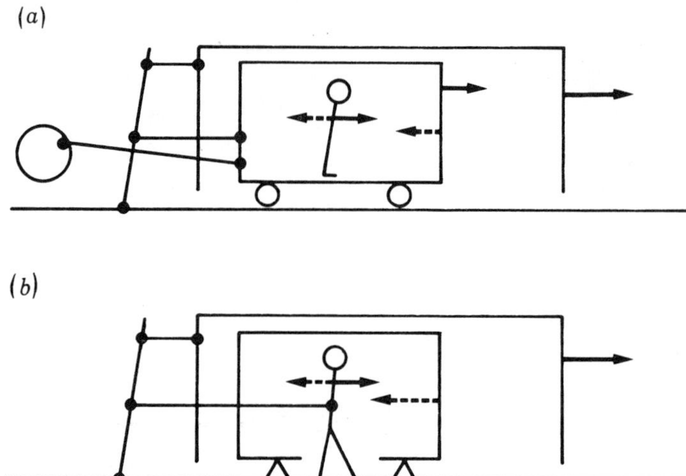

FIGURE 2. Experiments on visual perception of ego movement. (a) Passive movement: crank moves subject on trolley and surrounding 'room' (at twice the speed) forwards and backwards. (b) Active movement: with trolley floor removed, subject steps forward and back on laboratory floor moving the 'room' with him at twice his speed. Only one direction of movement is illustrated. Solid arrows indicate the movement relative to the laboratory floor. Broken arrows indicate the visually specified movement – the movement relative to the 'room'. The lengths of the arrows are proportional to speed. In each experiment, 13 out of 16 subjects reported that they and the trolley were moving in the visually specified way shown; they perceived the 'room' to be stationary. The remaining subjects' reports were confused: none apprehended what was actually happening. (Modified from Lishman & Lee (1973).)

(a) *Visual perception of ego movement*

In one set of experiments (Lishman & Lee 1973), the subject was in a trolley inside the experimental room. Several combinations of room and trolley movement were used in two subsets of experiments. In the passive movement experiments, the subject stood on the trolley floor while the room and trolley were moved by the experimenter. In the active movement experiments, the subject himself moved the trolley and room by holding a bar connected to a lever system and walking back and forth either on the trolley floor or, with that removed, on the real floor beneath the trolley. Figure 2 shows two of the twelve experimental conflict situations. In the great majority of cases, vision dominated the conflict. The movement of the self experienced was not the movement relative to the Earth but the visually specified movement relative to the experimental room, which was perceived to be stationary. This might seem particularly strange in the active movement cases (see, for example, figure 2*b*). Surely the subjects knew when they were stepping forward and when they were stepping back. The experiments, in fact, bring to light the distinction between propriospecific and expropriospecific information, between sensing one's bodily actions and sensing how one is moving relative to the environment as a result of those actions. Swimming in a current illustrates this point well; without vision, the swimmer cannot tell how he is moving relative to the shore. For further evidence on the power of vision in specifying movement relative to the environment see Johansson (1977), Turvey & Remez (1978), Warren (1976) and Wehrhahn & Reichardt (1975).

(b) The role of vision in balance control

Maintaining stance is a fundamental motor skill. It requires expropriospecific information about the orientation and sway of the body relative to the environment. The classical view, still current in many textbooks, was that the information is obtained primarily through the vestibular system and the mechano-receptors in the feet and ankles. The experiments described in § 3*a*, however, lead to the suspicion that vision plays a major role in balance control.

In a series of experiments with the use of the moveable room to simulate the visual effects of body-sway, this suspicion was confirmed (Lee & Aronson 1974; Lee & Lishman 1975). The main conclusion drawn from the experiments was that vision generally affords the most sensitive and reliable information for balance and is an integral component of the control system. For example, oscillating the experimental room through as little as 6 mm caused adult subjects to sway approximately in phase with this movement. The subjects were like puppets visually hooked to their surroundings and were unaware of the real cause of their disturbance. Vision was found to be especially important, often crucial for balance control (*a*) when the support surface is compliant, unsteady or narrow, which renders unreliable the information obtainable through the feet, and (*b*) when learning a new stance, which requires attunement to unfamiliar afference from the feet and ankles. Toddlers and adults in unpractised stances could readily be knocked off balance by movement of the experimental room. However, while balance is often impossible without vision when first learning a new stance, with practice vision often becomes non-critical, suggesting that visually guided practice facilitates attunement to information available through the feet. This is supported by experiments with blind people who were found to sway twice as much as sighted people with their eyes closed (Edwards 1946). Recent neurophysiological work by Glickstein & Gibson (1976) and Thoden *et al.* (1977) has suggested possible anatomical mechanisms whereby visual information is incorporated into balance control.

(c) Visual information about the relative layout of the environment

Let us now examine in more detail the structure of the rectilinear optic flow field to determine what other information it contains for controlling activity. What we are seeking are properties of the optic flow field that afford information about the geometrical layout of the surfaces in the environment and about the animal's movement relative to its environment.

The position of an environmental texture element P relative to the eye may conveniently be defined by the distance coordinates $Z(t)$ and R shown in figure 1, together with the angle between the OZP and OZX planes. This angle is specified in the optic flow field by the angular coordinate θ of the optic texture element P'. But are the distance coordinates $Z(t)$ and R optically specified? From similar triangles,

$$Z(t)/R = 1/r(t).\tag{1}$$

This equation is an expression of the well known problem of the missing depth dimension which arises when the visual stimulus is treated as an image, a time-independent spatial structure. The problem is that the *position* of an optic texture element specifies only the direction in which an environmental texture element lies, not its distance away. This problem of the missing depth dimension has puzzled theorists for a century or more and has led to the view that there must be embodied in the visual system quite detailed 'assumptions' about what is being viewed for three-dimensional perception to be possible. However, if we examine the spatio-temporal structure of the visual stimulus, we find that the depth dimension is not in fact missing.

Differentiating equation (1) with respect to time we obtain

$$R/V = r(t)^2/v(t), \tag{2}$$

where $V = -\mathrm{d}Z(t)/\mathrm{d}t$ is the velocity of the environmental texture element P and $v(t) = \mathrm{d}r(t)/\mathrm{d}t$ is the velocity of the corresponding optic texture element P' (see figure 1). Eliminating R between (1) and (2),

$$Z(t)/V = r(t)/v(t). \tag{3}$$

These equations, (2) and (3), mean that the distance coordinates $(R, Z(t))$ of all visible texture elements are optically specified to within a scale factor of V. In other words, there is information available in the optic flow field about the relative distances, sizes and orientations of surfaces and objects in the environment (see also Koenderink & van Doorn 1977; Nakayama & Loomis 1974).

In § 3*e* we shall examine how this spatial information might be body-scaled for use in controlling activity, but first let us consider another important type of information given in the optic flow field, namely temporal information.

(d) Visual information about time-to-contact

In (3), $Z(t)/V$ is the time that will elapse before the point of observation is level with the surface texture element P. The equation states that the time is optically specified by the value of $r(t)/v(t)$. This higher-order optic variable $r(t)/v(t)$ – which gives rise to the experience of an obstacle 'looming up' – is an important one, for it affords information for timing actions relative to the environment. For example, if the texture element P lies on a surface directly ahead, the optic variable specifies the time-to-contact with that surface. This is the type of information that a bird, for instance, needs in preparing to land.

In the following sections it will be shown how the optic variable $r(t)/v(t)$ affords information for controlling various types of locomotor activity. The variable appears to be a particularly informative one. I shall designate it by the symbol $\tau(t)$, thus

$$\tau(t) = r(t)/v(t), \tag{4}$$

and treat $\tau(t)$ as the basic variable associated with an optic texture element rather than its velocity $v(t)$. Thus, by using (4), (2) and (3) may be written as

$$R/V = r(t)\,\tau(t) \tag{5}$$

and

$$Z(t)/V = \tau(t). \tag{6}$$

(e) *Visual body-scaled information*

In §3c we showed that there is available in the optic flow field information about the relative sizes and distances of objects and surfaces in the environment. This purely exterospecific information is, however, of little functional value to an animal. What it basically needs is information that is relevant to controlling its activity, e.g. that a hurdle is a certain fraction of its own height, so many strides away and so on. That is, an animal needs body-scaled information about its environment. The following are two ways that body-scaled information might be obtained from the optic flow field.

Consider an animal running straight over a level stretch of ground. Suppose at a particular time t its speed is V. One bodily yardstick it could use is the height H of its eye above the ground, which will be more or less constant. Since H is the R-coordinate of any texture element on the ground over which the animal's eye will pass, applying (5) to the ground texture element G depicted in figure 1,

$$H/V = r_g(t)\, \tau_g(t), \tag{7}$$

and eliminating V between (5), (6) and (7),

$$R/H = r(t)\, \tau(t)/(r_g(t)\, \tau_g(t)) \tag{8}$$

and

$$Z(t)/H = \tau(t)/(r_g(t)\, \tau_g(t)). \tag{9}$$

In other words, there is a particular relation between the optic flow from the line of ground ahead and the optic flow from other environmental texture elements which specifies the distances and sizes of surfaces and objects in the environment in units of the animal's eye height. A horse, for instance, presumably needs such information when preparing to leap a fence.

Another bodily yardstick is stride length or stride duration. Consider a long jumper approaching the take-off board. The athlete not only has to strike the board but has to do so in the right posture for take-off. The last few strides to the board are critical in setting up the right posture. Now a skilled athlete can, after sprinting 40 m, strike the take-off board with a standard error of about 10 cm. How is such accuracy achieved? Since no adjustments to the stride pattern are normally apparent, many coaches and athletes believe that it is all a matter of developing a standard run-up. However, a recent film analysis of athletes showed that their run-ups were nowhere near as standard as they thought (Lee *et al.* 1977). The standard errors of their footfall positions increased considerably down the track, reaching a peak of 35 cm for one Olympic athlete. Over the last three strides, however, the standard error decreased dramatically to about 8 cm at the take-off board, the length of each stride being highly correlated with the athlete's distance from the board.

The athletes were clearly visually adjusting the lengths of their last three strides to zero-in on the take-off board. Furthermore, since the total duration of these three strides was only about 0.7 s, it is likely that they were programming these strides as a unit. What visual information could the athletes have been using? One possibility is information about time to reach the board (specified by the value of the optic variable $\tau(t)$ corresponding to the board), for the task of zeroing-in on the board may be conceived of as programming the durations of the forthcoming strides to just fill the time remaining to reach the board. This temporal conception of the task is probably more appropriate than a spatial one (i.e. programming stride lengths), since the athlete has direct control over the duration of his strides by how hard he thrusts on the ground, whereas the length of his strides are a function also of his speed of travel.

(f) Visual information for controlling braking

Consider a driver approaching an obstacle in the road. How does he manage to stop safely? He not only has to start braking early enough but he also has to adjust his deceleration to an adequate level during the stop (if, for instance, he brakes too lightly to begin with he will run out of braking power). In other words, a driver can get himself into a 'crash state' (i.e. when his current speed is too high in relation to his distance from the obstacle) well before he actually hits the obstacle.

How does a driver avoid getting into a 'crash state' while he is braking? He clearly needs visual expropriospecific information about how he is closing on the obstacle so that he can appropriately adjust his braking. It might seem that he needs to obtain information about his distance from the obstacle, his closing velocity and deceleration, and then perform complicated mental calculations. However, this is not necessary: the value of the time derivative of the optic variable $\tau(t)$ corresponding to the obstacle affords him sufficient information.

Suppose that at a time t the driver is a distance $Z(t)$ from the obstacle, his instantaneous velocity is $V(t)$ and he is braking with a deceleration D. Then his deceleration D is adequate if and only if the distance that it will take him to stop with that deceleration is less than or equal to his current distance from the obstacle, i.e. if and only if

$$V(t)^2/2D \leqslant Z(t),$$

or

$$Z(t)\,D/V(t)^2 \geqslant 0.5. \tag{10}$$

Now $Z(t)/V(t)$ is specified by the value of the optic variable $\tau(t)$ for the obstacle (see equation (6)), i.e.

$$Z(t)/V(t) = \tau(t); \tag{11}$$

differentiating this equation with respect to time we obtain

$$Z(t)\,D/V(t)^2 = 1 + \mathrm{d}\tau(t)/\mathrm{d}t. \tag{12}$$

Hence, from (10) and (12), the value of the time derivative of the optic variable $\tau(t)$ specifies whether the driver's current deceleration is adequate or not. It is adequate if and only if

$$\mathrm{d}\tau(t)/\mathrm{d}t \geqslant -0.5. \tag{13}$$

In other words, the driver has available visual exropriospecific information about his potential future course were he to maintain his current braking level. A safe braking strategy would consist in the driver adjusting his braking so that $\mathrm{d}\tau(t)/\mathrm{d}t$ remained as a safe value. The deceleration profiles produced by this hypothetical braking strategy (Lee 1976) in fact matched quite closely those of test drivers recorded by Spurr (1969), the only data on visually controlled braking found in the literature.

(g) Visual information for controlling steering

How does a driver control his steering? As with braking, the driver can get himself into a 'crash state' well before he actually runs off the road. This can occur not only if he takes a bend too fast but also if he does not adjust his steering early enough on a bend and so gets into the situation where he needs to steer an impossibly tight curve. What the driver needs is visual exropriospecific information not so much about his current position on the road but about his potential future course were he to maintain his current steering angle. This is, in fact, specified in the optic flow field at his eye (see figure 3). McLean & Hoffmann's (1973) investigations of straight-lane driving indicated that drivers do use such visual information. They found that steering adjustments were made primarily on the basis of heading angle (corresponding to potential future course) rather than current lateral position on the road.

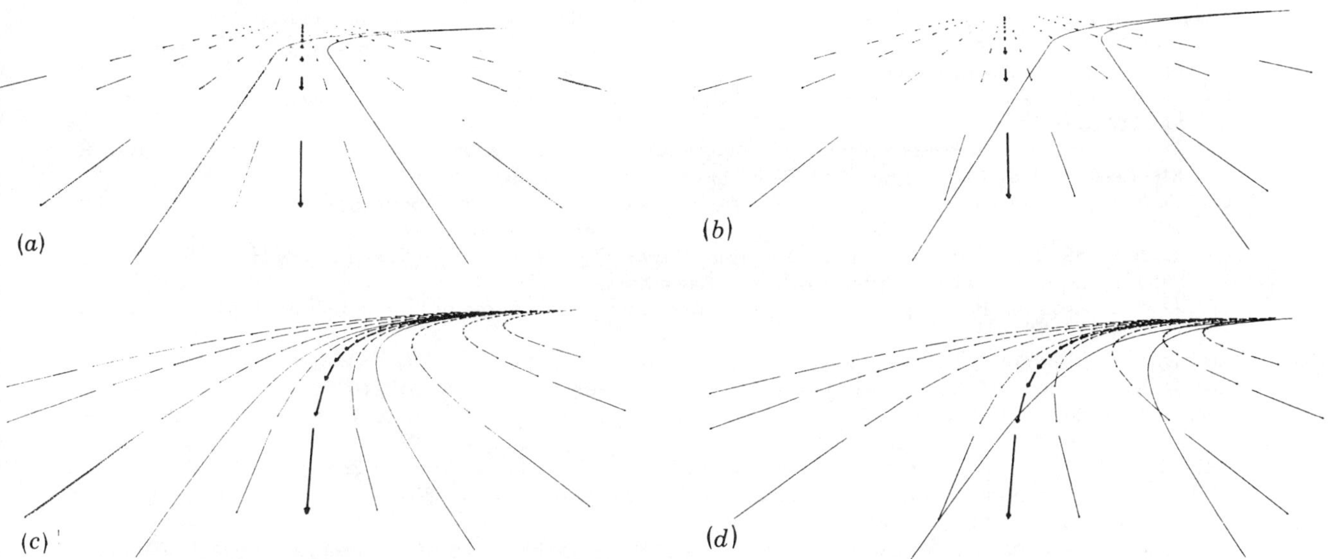

FIGURE 3. The optic flow field, projected onto a plane as in figure 1, when driving down a road. The solid lines represent the edges of the road, the broken ones the optic flow lines. The central heavily drawn flow line is the 'locomotor flow line': it specifies the potential future course of the vehicle were the current steering angle to be maintained. (a) Steering straight towards a bend on course. (b) Steering straight but off course. (c) Steering a bend of uniform curvature on course. (d) The same but off course. To see how the optic flow fields are generated, consider the vehicle to be stationary and the ground moving under it. In (a) and (b), points on the ground are moving along parallel straight paths: the radiating optic flow lines are the projections of these paths. In (c) and (d), points on the ground are moving along concentric circular paths, the centre corresponding to the centre of curvature of the vehicle's path: the hyperbolic optic flow lines are the projections of these paths. (Modified from Lee & Lishman (1977).)

4. CONCLUDING REMARKS

As Neisser (1977) has pointed out, any account of visual perception must entail as a logical primitive an adequate description of what is available to the eye. Equally importantly, a theory of visual perception must take into account the functions performed by vision. In this paper we have been concerned with the fundamental function of vision which, it is argued, is the obtaining of information in the service of activity, and with formulating a description of the input to the eye that takes cognisance of the fact that the input is constantly varying over time. It is suggested that it is with this type of analysis that one needs to start in seeking to discover the actual mechanisms of vision.

The work reported here was supported by the Medical Research Council under grant G 974/294/C and by the Science Research Council under grant B/RG/0631 1.

References (Lee)

Bernstein, N. 1967 *The coordination and regulation of movements*. Oxford: Pergamon Press.

Edwards, A. S. 1946 Body sway and vision. *J. exp. Psychol.* **36**, 526–535.

Gibson, J. J. 1950 *The perception of the visual world*. Boston: Houghton Mifflin,

Gibson, J. J. 1958 Visually controlled locomotion and visual orientation in animals. *Br. J. Psychol.* **49**, 182–194.

Gibson, J. J. 1966 *The senses considered as perceptual systems*. Boston: Houghton Mifflin.

Glickstein, M. & Gibson, A. R. 1976 Visual cells in the pons of the brain. *Scient. Am.* **235** (5), 90.

Johansson, G. 1977 Studies on visual perception of locomotion. *Perception* **6**, 365–376.

Koenderink, J. J. & van Doorn, A. J. 1977 How an ambulant observer can construct a model of the environment from the geometrical structure of the visual inflow. In *Kybernetik* 1977 (ed. G. Hauske & E. Butenandt), pp. 224–247. Munich: Oldenburg.

Lashley, K. 1951 The problem of serial order in behavior. In *Cerebral mechanisms in behavior* (ed. L. A. Jeffress), pp. 112–136. New York: John Wiley.

Lee, D. N. 1974 Visual information during locomotion. In *Perception: essays in honor of James J. Gibson* (ed. R. B. MacLeod & H. L. Pick Jr), pp. 250–267. Ithaca: Cornell University Press.

Lee, D. N. 1976 A theory of visual control of braking based on information about time to collision. *Perception* **5**, 437–459.

Lee, D. N. 1978 The functions of vision. In *Modes of perceiving and processing information* (ed. H. L. Pick Jr & E. Saltzman), pp. 159–170. Hillsdale: Erlbaum Associates.

Lee, D. N. & Aronson, E. 1974 Visual proprioceptive control of standing in human infants. *Percept. Psychophys.* **15**, 529–532.

Lee, D. N. & Lishman, J. R. 1975 Visual proprioceptive control of stance. *J. hum. Movemt. Stud.* **1**, 87–95.

Lee, D. N. & Lishman, J. R. 1977 Visual control of locomotion. *Scand. J. Psychol.*, **18**, 224–230.

Lee, D. N., Lishman, J. R. & Thomson, J. 1977 Visual guidance in the long jump. *Athletics Coach*, **11**, 26–30; **12**, 17–23.

Lishman, J. R. & Lee, D. N. 1973 The autonomy of visual kinaesthesis. *Perception* **2**, 287–294.

McLean, J. R. & Hoffman, E. R. 1973 The effects of restricted preview on driver steering control and performance. *Hum. Factors* **15**, 421–430.

Nakayama, K. & Loomis, J. M. 1974 Optical velocity patterns, velocity sensitive neurons and space perception: a hypothesis. *Perception* **3**, 63–80.

Neisser, U. 1977 Gibson's ecological optics: consequences of a different stimulus description. *J. theory soc. behav.* **7**, 17–28.

Spurr, R. T. 1969 Subjective aspects of braking. *Automobile Engr.* **59**, 58–61.

Stelmach, G. (ed.) 1976 *Motor control: issues and trends*. New York: Academic Press.

Thoden, U., Dichgans, J. & Savidis, T. 1977 Direction-specific optokinetic modulation of monosynaptic hind limb reflexes in cats. *Exp. Brain Res.* **30**, 155–160.

Turvey, M. T. & Remez, R. 1978 Visual control of locomotion: an overview. In *Proceedings of Conference on Interrelations of the Communicative Senses*, Asilomar, California Sept.–Oct. 1978. (In the press.)

Warren, R. 1976 The perception of egomotion. *J. exp. Psychol. hum. Percept. Perform.* **2**, 448–456.

Wehrhahn, C. & Reichardt, W. 1975 Visually induced height orientation of the fly *Musca domestica*. *Biol. Cybernet.* **20**, 37–50.

Discussion

H. Kalmus (*Galton Laboratory, University College, Gower Street, London, WC1, U.K.*). Some of Dr Lee's ideas concerning the optical flow field can be expanded and synthesized into a mathematical theory by considering results from work on optomotor reactions of insects, performed long ago (Kalmus 1948).

Insects, for instance flies, are more suitable than man for studying visual movement in large areas, because they have a wider visual field, lack a vestibular system and possess a smaller array of possible reactions.

Developing Dr Lee's remarks that visual perception and locomotion form one system which performs 'sensory motor skills', it can be stated that just as any movement or dislocation of a rigid body can be described as a sum of translation and rotation, so a class of coherent contour movements in the environment can – in insects at least – be partitioned into a translational and a rotational component, which correspond to the momentum and angular momentum in dynamics. The integrals representing these quasi-vectors have been calculated in the quoted paper.

The translational component of the moving contours induces the animal to move against it, while the rotational component induces it to turn with it. In most natural situations the latter reaction serves to control the position of the animal in space.

A fly constrained mechanically either to move on a straight path or to turn on the spot can be used as an instrument for extracting the translational and rotational quasi-vectors from a complex moving contour system.

It is reasonable to assume that the human visual system also is capable of similar computations and that these serve the control of movement and position. Against the integrated flow of visual signals, representing the physical environment at large, systematically deviating local contour movements are recognized as separate objects, which if they possess biological importance may elicit special motor reactions.

Reference

Kalmus, H. 1948 Optomotor responses in *Drosophila* and *Musca. Physiologia comp. oecol.* **1**, 127–147.

Phil. Trans. R. Soc. Lond. B **290**, 181–197 (1980)

Printed in Great Britain

Perceptions as hypotheses

By R. L. Gregory

Brain and Perception Laboratory, Department of Anatomy, The Medical School,
University Walk, Bristol BS8 1TD, U.K.

Perceptions may be compared with hypotheses in science. The methods of acquiring scientific knowledge provide a working paradigm for investigating processes of perception.

Much as the information channels of instruments, such as radio telescopes, transmit signals which are processed according to various assumptions to give useful data, so neural signals are processed to give data for perception. To understand perception, the signal codes and the stored knowledge or assumptions used for deriving perceptual hypotheses must be discovered. Systematic perceptual errors are important clues for appreciating signal channel limitations, and for discovering hypothesis-generating procedures. Although this distinction between 'physiological' and 'cognitive' aspects of perception may be logically clear, it is in practice surprisingly difficult to establish which are responsible even for clearly established phenomena such as the classical distortion illusions.

Experimental results are presented, aimed at distinguishing between and dis-covering what happens when there is mismatch with the neural signal channel, and when neural signals are processed inappropriately for the current situation. This leads us to make some distinctions between perceptual and scientific hypotheses, which raise in a new form the problem: What are 'objects'?

1. Introduction

Are perceptions like hypotheses of science? This is the question that I propose to examine; but there is an immediate difficulty, for there is no general agreement on the nature of scientific hypotheses. It may be said that hypotheses *structure* our accepted reality. More specifically, it may be said that hypotheses allow limited data to be used with remarkable effect, by allowing interpolations through data-gaps, and extrapolations to be made to new situations for which data are not available. These include the future. (They also include inventions and indeed the whole of applied science, which apart from cases of pure trial and error, are surely created by the predictive power of hypotheses.)

I shall hold that all of these statements are true, and that they apply to perception. In addition, both the hypotheses of science and the perceptual processes of the nervous system allow recog-nition of familiar situations or objects from strictly inadequate clues, as signalled by the trans-ducer-instruments of science and the transducer-senses of organisms. This is at least true for typical situations: in atypical situations the hypotheses of both science and perception may be dangerously and systematically misleading. Errors and illusions can be highly revealing for appreciating the similarities – and the differences – between perceptions and the conceptual hypotheses of science.

It is not always allowed that hypotheses are predictive, or have all or even any of the powers that I have credited them with. I take Sir Karl Popper to hold that hypotheses do not have predictive power, and that they do not have *a priori* probabilities. This is part of his rejection of induction as a way of gaining knowledge. Here I shall not follow Popper's notion of 'objective knowledge' (Popper 1972), for my theme is what happens to observers when they observe and when they learn. On this account much of learning is induction and behaviour is set very largely by probabilities based on past experience and so is predictive. Probable objects are more readily seen than improbable objects, so 'subjective' probability seems to apply, both for selecting perceptions and for perceptions to have the predictive power evident in much behaviour and all skills.

To suggest that perceptions are like hypotheses is to suppose that the instruments and the procedures of science parallel essential characteristics of the sense organs and their neural channels, regarded as transducers transmitting coded data; and the data-handling procedures of science may be essentially the same as cognitive procedures carried out by perceptual neural processes of the brain. There will clearly be surface differences detween science and perception, and we may expect some deeper differences, but for the suggestion to be interesting there should be more than overall *similarities*: there should be significant conceptual *identities*.

I shall start by setting out three claims, which I hope to justify, and no doubt qualify.

Claims:

(1) that perceptions are essentially like predictive hypotheses in science;

(2) that the procedures of science are a guide for discovering processes of perception;

(3) that many perceptual illusions correspond to and may receive explanations from understanding systematic errors occurring in science.

It is hoped that by exploring this analogy (or perhaps deep identity) between science and perception, we may develop an effective epistemology related to how the brain works. I shall attempt to indicate concepts and processes that seem important for the opening moves towards the end play of this understanding.

The approach is based on regarding perception and science as *constructing hypotheses* by 'fiction-generators' which may hit upon truth by producing symbolic structures matching physical reality.

2. Steps to perception

In the first place we regard the sense organs (eyes, ears, touch receptors, and so on) as transducers essentially like photocells, microphones and strain guages. The important similarity, indeed identity, is that the sense organs and detecting instruments convert patterns of received energy into signals, which may be read according to a code. As a signal, the neural activity is fully described in physical terms and measurable in physical units; but the code must be known in order to use or appreciate it as data. We suppose that the coded data are – in perception and science – used for generating hypotheses. For perception we may call them 'perceptual hypotheses'. These are what are usually called 'perceptions'. Here are the three stages of perception, in these terms.

(a) Signals

Patterns of neural events, related to input stimulus patterns according to the transducer characteristics of sense organs.

For the eye, for example, there is a roughly logarithmic relation between intensity of light and the firing rate of the action potentials at the initial stage of the visual channel. Colour is coded by the proportion of rates of firing from the three spectrally distinct kinds of cone receptor cell, and so on. These transducer characteristics must be understood before the physiologist can appreciate what is going on. He can then (with other knowledge or assumptions) describe the neural signals as data representing states of affairs.

(b) Data

Neural events are accepted as *representing* variables or states, according to a code which must be known for signals to be read or appreciated as data.

This necessity of knowing the code is surely clear from examples such as signals conveying data in Morse code. The dots and dashes have no significance, and may not even be recognized as signals conveying data when the code is not known. The same holds for the words on this page: we must know the rules of the English language, and a great deal more, to see them as more than patterns of ink on paper.

It is generally true that a lot more than the code must be known before signals can be read as data. For a detecting instrument (such as a radio-telescope, magnetometer, or voltmeter) it is essential to know something of the source, whether it is a star, a given region of the Earth, or just which part of the circuit a voltmeter is connected to. The outputs of some instruments (such as optical telescopes, microscopes, and X-ray machines as used in medicine) may give sufficient structure for the source to be identified without extra information. This is especially so when the structure of the output matches our normal perceptual inputs. This is, however, somewhat rare for instruments. A voltmeter provides no such structured output by which we can recognize its source of signals without collateral knowlege. Some sense organs (especially the eye) provide highly structured signals allowing identification of the source; but visual and any other sensory data can be ambiguous (including touch, hence the game of trying to identify by touch objects in a bag), and indeed all sensory and instrumental data are, strictly speaking, ambiguous. The fact that vision is usually sufficient for immediate object identification distracts us from realizing the immense importance of contextual knowledge for reading data from signals. Scientific data from instruments are almost always presented with explicit collateral information, on how the instrument was used, what source it was directed to, its calibration corrections and scale settings. The gain setting of oscilloscopes and the magnification scale of photographs and optical instruments of all kinds are essential for scientific use. If the scale is given incorrectly, serious misinterpretation can result, even to confusing the surface of a planet with biological structures. So, not only the signal code must be known, but also a great deal of context knowledge is required for signals to be read as data. This holds for perception as it does for the use of scientific instruments, though for perception the context knowledge is generally implicit and so its contribution may not be recognized.

It is important to note that signals can be fully described and measured with physical concepts and physical units, but this is not so for data. Data are highly peculiar, being (it is not too fanciful to say) in this way outside the physical world, though essential for describing the physical world.

The codes necessary for reading signals as data are not laws of physics. They are, rather, essentially arbitrary and held conventionally. Some may be more convenient or efficient than others, but in no case are they part of the physical world as laws of physics are, or reflect, 'deep structures' of reality. Further, data are used to select between *hypothetical* possibilities, only one of which (if indeed any) exists. The greater the number of alternatives available for the selection (or rather the greater their combined probability) the greater the quantity of information in the data (Shannon & Weaver 1949). The information content thus depends not only on what *is* but on the hypothetical stored alternatives of what *may be*. But these are not in the (physical) reality of the situation, so data cannot be equated with what (physically) *is*; neither can they be equated with signals, for data are *read from* signals by following the conventional rules (which are not physical laws) of a code.

(c) *Hypotheses*

There is, unfortunately, no general agreement as to just what hypotheses are or what characterizes them. This, it must be confessed, is a weakness in our position. If there is no agreement on what are hypotheses, how can it be argued cogently that perceptions are hypotheses? Just what is being claimed? With the present lack of agreement, one must either be vague or stick out for a particular account, which may be arbitrary, of the nature of hypotheses. Current accounts range from Popper's view that they have no prior probabilities and no predictive power (and that they cannot be confirmed but only disconfirmed) to very different accounts, such as that they can be in part predicted; that they can be used for prediction; and that they can be confirmed (though not with certainty) as well as disconfirmed by observations. I shall not entirely follow Popper's account of hypotheses (Popper 1972), but hold, rather, an alternative account: that they have *predictive power*, and that they can be suggested by observation and induction, and can be confirmed or disconfirmed though not with logical certainty.

It may be objected here that if perceptions are themselves hypotheses, they cannot be evoked to confirm or disconfirm the explicit hypotheses of science. This is, however, no objection, for it is common experience that a perception can confirm or disconfirm other perceptions. And one scientific hypothesis may (it is usually held) confirm or disconfirm other hypotheses in science. So there is no clear distinction between hypotheses and perception here to make my argument invalid.

There is, however, this problem of the lack of agreement of what constitutes hypothesis. The notion of hypothesis has grown in importance with the rejection of hopes of certainty in science like the supposed certainty of geometrical knowledge before non-Euclidian geometries, and with Kuhn's (1962) paradigms. Perhaps all scientific knowledge is now regarded as hypothesis. But if Popper is right, would we have any wish to associate perception with hypotheses? For in his view they have none of the power we attribute to perception. What, then, are hypothesis?

I suggest that *hypotheses are selections of signalled and postulated data organized to be effective in typical (and some novel) situations*. Hypotheses are effective in having powers to predict future events, unsensed characteristics, and further hypotheses. They may also predict what is *not* true. I shall assume that we accept that these are important characteristics of scientific hypotheses and perception.

To amplify this, we may now consider in some detail similarities – and also differences, for there clearly *are* differences – between hypotheses and perceptions. We shall look first at similarities when perceptions and scientific hypotheses are appropriate. We shall then go on to compare them when they are inappropriate, or 'false', and finally we shall consider ways in which perceptions clearly differ from hypotheses of science.

3. Perception and scientific hypotheses compared

(a) *Results of appropriate uses of perception and science*

(1) *Interpolation across gaps in signals or data*

This allows continuous behaviour and control with only intermittent signals, which is typical of organisms and important in science, though rare in machines.

Interpolations may be little more than inertial or may be highly sophisticated and daring constructs. Let us first consider interpolation in a graph, such as figure 1. The curve is derived according to two very different kinds of processes. It is generated from the readings by following procedures, which are easy to state and to carry out automatically without particular external considerations. The most common procedure here is fitting by least squares. The curve may not touch any of the points representing the readings and yet it is accepted as the 'best' curve. It is an idealization – a hypothesis of what should occur in the absence of irrelevant disturbances and an infinite set of readings with no gaps.

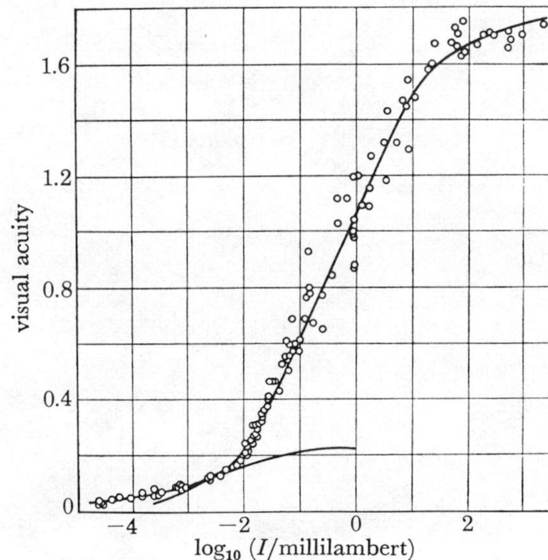

FIGURE 1. A typical graph of experimental readings with a fitted curve. The fitting may be done both 'upwards', by a routine procedure such as by 'least-mean' squares; and 'downwards', from which (generally theoretical) function is most likely. The fitted curve may be regarded as a predictive hypothesis. Contour perception seems similar.

Any graph of experimental or observational data has some *scatter* in the readings through which the curve is drawn. The scatter may de due to random disturbances of the measuring device, or to variation in what is being measured, such as quantal fluctuations. These kinds of scatter have very different statuses, though for some purposes they may be treated alike and there may be a mixture of the two. In any case the curve may not touch any of the points indicating the readings. So it is a kind of fiction, accepted as the fact of the situation.

The second kind of procedure for obtaining the curve and for gap-filling is selecting a *preferred* curve, on theoretical or other general grounds, which may be aesthetic. The first kind of procedure is 'bottom-upwards' from the readings, by following procedures without reference to contextual considerations; the second is 'top-downwards', from stored knowledge or assumptions suggesting what is a likely curve. This may be set by a general preference (or prejudice) for example for a linear, or a logarithmic, or some other favoured type of function; or it may be set by particular considerations. Both have their dangers: the first biases towards the accepted, and the second tends to perpetuate false theories by bending the data in their direction.

The example of a graph illustrates that hypotheses – for the accepted curve or function may *be* a predictive hypothesis – can be *non-propositional*. Perhaps hypotheses are generally thought of as sets of propositions, but there seems no reason to restrict hypotheses to propositions as expressed in language. An equation such as $E = \frac{1}{2}mv^2$ is a hypothesis, in this case concerning quite abstract concepts (energy, mass and velocity), believed to represent something of the deep structure of physics, but it is not propositional in form. It could be written in language as a set of sentences expressing propositions but this would be relatively clumsy. It could also be expressed as a graph, and this could be adequate for some purposes. Analogue computers, indeed, work from this kind of non-propositional representation.

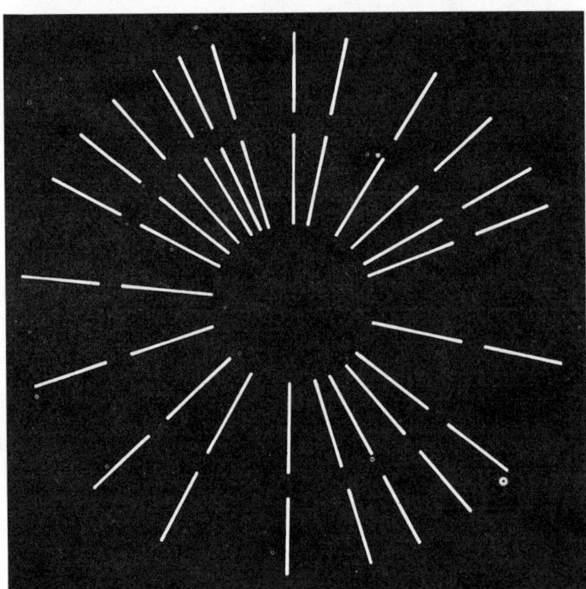

FIGURE 2. Illusory contours and regions of modified brightness seem to be postulates of nearer eclipsing objects, to 'explain' unlikely gaps. It seems that an essentially Bayesian strategy is responsible.

There seems no reason to hold that 'perceptual hypotheses' require a propositional brain language, underlying spoken and written language, though this might be so. The merits of this notion need not be considered here, as we are free to regard hypotheses as not *necessarily* being in propositional form.

Perhaps interpolations are generally regarded as gap-filling in situations for which we do not have complete or strictly adequate readings, but interpolation can be far more elaborate than this, for example postulating unknown species to fill gaps in evolutionary sequences. For a visual example, consider figure 2. Perhaps 'illusory contours' are edges of objects postulated to account for gaps in available sensory signals or data. They take more or less ideal forms, and they are (generally useful) fictions joining data. This indeed defines interpolation in perception and science.

2. *Extrapolation from signals and data, to future states and unsensed features*

Extrapolation allows hypotheses to take off from what is given or accepted, into the unknown. Going beyond accepted data is not very different from filling gaps, except that interpolations are limited to the next accepted data point; extrapolations, however, have no endpoint in what is known or assumed, so extrapolations may be infinitely daring, and so may be dramatically wrong.

Extrapolation beyond the end of graphs of functions supported by data is sometimes essential (as for determining 'absolute zero' temperature by extrapolating beyond the range through which measures can, even in principle, be made). Extrapolations can leap from spectral lines to stars, and from past to future. With interpolation and extrapolation, data become stepping stones and springboards for science and perception. This is to say that perceptions are not confined to stimuli, just as science is not limited to signals or available data; neither, of course, is confined to fact.

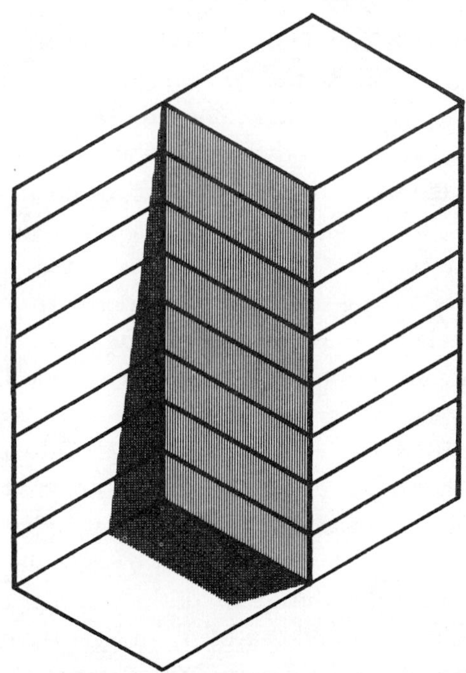

FIGURE 3. In this depth-ambiguous figure the grey rectangular region changes in brightness for most observers according to whether this area is a probable shadow. The systematic brightness change with depth-reversal is, clearly, centrally initiated and is a 'downwards' effect.

(3) *Discovery and creation of objects, in perceptual and conceptual space*

The perceptual selection of sensed characteristics may create *objects*. There is also strong evidence for creating visual *characteristics* from what is accepted as objects (cf. figure 3).

We know too little about the criteria for *assigning* data to objects, and *creating* object-hypotheses from data. What science describes as an object may or may not correspond to what appears to the senses as an object; different instruments reveal the world as differently structured. Further, general theories change what are regarded as objects. There is evidently a complex multi-way traffic here by which the world is parcelled out into objects; it seems that here again we have 'upwards' and 'downwards' procedures operating. The various rules of 'closure', 'common fate' and so on, emphasized by the Gestalt psychologists such as Wertheimer (1923), reflect features typical of the vast majority of objects as we see them. Most objects are closed in form, and their parts move together. These common object characteristics become identifying principles – and may structure random patterns to *create* object forms, even from noise. More recently, the work in artificial intelligence on object recognition makes use of typical features – especially the intersections of lines at corners of various kinds – to describe objects and their forms in depth (Guzman 1968). The effectiveness of these classifications and rules depends on what objects are generally like (cf. Guzman 1971). For exceptional objects, the rules mislead, as we see in the Ames demonstrations (Ittelson 1952) and in distortion figures (Gregory 1968). The object-recognizing and object-creating rules are applied *upwards* to filter and structure the input. (It is, however, interesting to note that they may have been *developed* downwards, by generalized experience of what are, through the development of perception, taken as objects. For the Gestalt writers this is largely innate; but our similar experience and needs might well generate common object-criteria through experience.)

Knowledge can work downwards to parcel signals and data into objects; as knowledge changes, the parcelling into objects may change, both for science and perception, We see this most clearly when examining machines: the criteria for recognizing and naming the various features as separate depend very much on our knowledge of functions. Thus the pallets on the anchor of a clock escapement are seen and described as objects in their own right once the mechanism is understood, though they are but shapes in one piece of metal, which happens also to look like an anchor. So we see here again the importance of *upward* and *downward* processing in perception and science – the complex interplay of signals, data and hypotheses. Unravelling this is surely essential for understanding the strategies and procedures of perception and science. It is also important for appreciating the status of objects. How far are objects *recognized* and how much are they *created* by perception and science? This is a deep question at the heart of empiricism.

What may be a profound difference between perceptual and conceptual objects is that perceptual objects are always, as Frege put it (Dummett 1978) *concrete objects*, while the conceptual objects of science may be *abstract objects*. The point is that objects as perceived have spatial extension, and may change in time, while conceptual objects (such as numbers, the centre of gravity of concrete objects, and the deep structure of the world as described by laws of physics) cannot be sensed, may be unchanging and spaceless, and yet have the status of objects in that they are *public* though not sensed. We all agree that the number 13 is a prime number, that it is greater than 12 and less than 14, that it is odd and not even, and that *all* prime numbers except 2 are odd numbers. This kind of agreement is characteristic of the agreement and public ownership of objects as known by the senses (tables, stones, and so on), yet numbers cannot be sensed, though they are as 'public' as tables and stones.

This situation is rendered even more difficult by the consideration that, clearly, *concrete* objects have some features that are abstract, as we believe especially from scientific knowledge. Take, as an example, centre of gravity: stones have centres of gravity, which is useful as a scientific concept, and are indeed what Newton took to be the 'objects' of the solar system for his astronomy. Centres of gravity may indeed lie not *in* but *between* concrete objects, such as between Earth and Sun, or between binary stars. Does the centre of gravity exist, as stones and stars exist? Or is it a useful fiction created as a tool for scientific description?

Even within what is clearly perception, we can be uncertain of what is 'concrete' and what is 'abstract'. We see that a triangle has three sides, and yet number is regarded, at least by Frege, as 'abstract'. Are shadows 'concrete objects'? The trouble here is that they are known by only one sense (if we except differences of sensed temperature) and they have few causal properties. Also, they are always attached to what is clearly a concrete object (which may be the ground) and by contrast they seem far less concrete, almost abstract though we see them.

These are exceedingly difficult issues, which can hardly be resolved without deeper understanding of hypothesis-generation, and further analysis of the similarities and differences between perceptual and conceptual hypotheses.

If we consider such 'objects' as electrons, which are clearly inferred indirectly from observational evidence, how do they compare with concrete objects of perception? If we believe that normal perception of concrete objects such as tables and stones requires a great deal of inference ('unconscious inference', to use Helmholtz's term), then the difference may not be great. The more perception depends on inference the more similar we may suppose is the status of perceptual and conceptual objects.

We shall now consider inappropriate or 'false' hypotheses and perceptions. Here I describe certain phenomena of perception, such as various kinds of illusions, as our actually *seeing* what are *described* when occurring in science as errors; various kinds of ambiguities, distortions, paradoxes and fictitious features. The claim is that these categories, which are normally applied to arguments and descriptions, appear in perceptions as experiences of recognizable kinds, which can be investigated much as the phenomena of physics can be investigated; though for some of these perceptual phenomena rather different kinds of explanations from those of physics may be required.

(b) Results of inappropriate uses of perception and science

(1) Ambiguity, sometimes with spontaneous alternations and disagreements

The point here is that alternative hypotheses can be elicited by the same signals. There are many examples of visual ambiguity in which a figure (or sometimes an object) is seen to switch from one orientation to another, or transform into another design or object. This has been attributed to bi-stable (or multi-stable) brain circuits (Attneave 1971) and, very differently, to putative hypotheses in rivalry for acceptance when their probabilities on the available evidence are nearly equal. The first would be an account in terms of *signals*, the second in terms of *data*. Inspection suggests strongly that the second is what is going on in most cases, for the stimulus pattern can be immensely varied, but what it *represents* matters a great deal. There are, however, many examples of the first kind: retinal rivalry, from different colours presented to the eyes producing spontaneous alternations, and lines of different orientation presented binocularly, producing rivalry. Here it is purely the stimulus characteristics that matter. On the other hand, figures such as the Necker cube, the Schroeder staircase or the Boring wife–mistress figure, present equal evidence for example for two very different faces, which gives the ambiguity. For the Necker cube there is no evidence favouring either of two or more orientations. For both figures the ambiguity no doubt depends on our knowledge of faces and cubes. (We studied the case of a man blind from infancy and allowed to see by corneal graft when in his fifties: when we showed him ambiguous figures such as Necker cubes he saw no depth and no reversals. He made nothing of pictures of faces (Gregory & Wallace 1963).) It is likely that different experience might change the bias of ambiguous alternations in cases such as the Boring figure.

That science can be ambiguous is shown by the frequent changes of opinion and the occasional disputes which give it light and heat. For a current example of scientific ambiguity: are quasars astronomically near objects with abnormal red shifts, perhaps due to their powerful gravitational fields (and thus not obeying the Hubble law of increasing red shift with distance), or are they very distant, but of enormous intrinsic brightness? Here is a clear case of an important ambiguity which is not yet quite resolved. It might de resolved by further data derived by instrumental signals, or by a change in the general theoretical position, for which this is a central question. In short, the change that resolves the paradox might be 'upwards' or 'downwards' – both in science and in perception.

(2) *Distortion, especially spatial distortions*

Distortions can occur at the *signal* level by loss of calibration (as by sensory adaptation), by inappropriate calibration corrections, by mismatch of the instrument or sense organ 'transducer' to the input (or affecting the input, as by loading with a voltmeter of low internal resistance, or detecting temperature by touch of thin metal, which rapidly adopts the skin temperature).

Distortions may also occur in the *data* and stored knowledge level, as when knowledge is transferred inappropriately to the current situation, so that signals are misread.

Signal errors are to be understood through physics and physiology; data errors (which are cognitive errors) are understood by appreciating what knowledge or strategies are being brought to bear, and in what ways they are inappropriate to the current problem or situation.

Visual distortions can occur with: (i) mirrors, mirages, sticks bent in water, or astigmatic lenses giving optical distortion of the input; (ii) astigmatic lenses of the eyes (physiological optical distortion); (iii) inappropriate neural correction of optical astigmatism (a calibration correction error); (iv) neural signal distortion (which may be pathological or may be due to other signals interfering by cross-talk, or neural lateral inhibition, or some such); (v) signals being misread as data (especially by 'negative transfer' of knowledge: generally from typical to similar but atypical situations).

I shall not expand on these, except the last, and that only briefly. Here again we find the distinction between processing *upwards* and *downwards* important. To take an example of misreading data that has received a great deal of attention, though explanations are still controversial, we may consider visual distortion illustions.

Since the perceived size of things is ambiguously represented by retinal image size, size must be *scaled*. Visual scale is set by what I have called (Gregory 1970) 'constancy scaling'. It seems that scaling can set *upwards*, from stimulus patterns normally accepted as data for distances (especially converging lines and corners normally indicating depth by perspective). When these stimulus shapes occur without their normal depth – as when perspective is presented on a picture plane – they may be accepted as though they correctly represented depth, there to set the scaling inappropriately. Features represented as distant on a picture plane are perceptually expanded, for normally expansion with increased object distance is required to compensate for the shrinking of retinal images with object distance; but this is not appropriate for the flat-perspective drawings. Scale-setting is essential for maintaining perceived size independently of object distance (giving 'size constancy'), but when scale-setting by perspective features occurs other than by the retinal projection of parallel lines, etc., lying in the three dimensions of normal space, then the scale is set inappropriately, to generate distortion 'upwards' from the misleading perspective features.

'Downwards' distortions occur when an incorrect depth hypothesis is adopted. This is clear from depth-ambiguous objects, such as wire cubes, which change shape with each depth reversal, though the retinal input and neural signals from the eye remain unchanged. Ambiguous objects and figures are extremely useful in this way for separating upward from downward perceptual processes (Gregory 1968, 1970).

Astronomy is rich in examples of scales set *upwards* from instrumental readings (with fewest assumptions by heliocentric parallax) and also *downwards* from considerations such as the mass–luminosity relation applied to a certain class of variable star, so that their observed periodicity can be used, together with their apparent luminosity, to infer distance. This involves a great deal of stored knowledge and associated assumptions. When these change, the Universe may be rescaled.

There seems to be a remarkable similarity in the setting of scale for perceptual and for scientific hypotheses. Perceptual space is not, however, Euclidian, except for near objects. Consider the perception of an engine driver: the rails appear parallel only for a few hundred metres, then they converge alarmingly. The driver can use his *perceptual* Euclidian near-space, in which parallel lines never meet, with confidence; but for greater distances he must reject his non-Euclidian perceptual space in favour of his Euclidian *conceptual* space, to drive his train further without a certainty of disaster. If, now, the driver reads Einstein in his spare time, he will adopt still another space: then what he relies upon professionally will become for him a parochialism, adequate for the job but not for fuller understanding. Each view – perceptual or conceptual – which seems undistorted will appear distorted from the spaces of his other views.

(3) *Paradoxes, especially spatial paradoxes*

Paradoxes can be generated by conflicting inputs, or by generating hypotheses from false or inappropriate assumptions. A well known conflicting-input perceptual paradox is given by adapting one hand to hot water and the other to cold, and then placing both hands in a dish of warm water. To one hand this will be cold and to the other hot. The adaptation has produced (or rather *is*) mis-calibration, which gives incompatible signals to produce a paradox, since we do not allow that an object can be both hot and cold at the same time.

In recent science there has been a relaxing of the strictures of paradox, such that what now seems paradoxical to common sense may, sometimes, be accepted as scientifically true. An example is light accepted as both waves and particles. Also, what *appears* paradoxical may be *understood* as non-paradoxical – as indeed for the 'impossible triangle' object or drawing (figures 4 and 5). Here we discover that conceptual understanding is sometimes powerless to correct or modify even clearly bizarre perceptions. We can, at the same time, hold incompatible perceptual and conceptual hypotheses: so we can *see* a paradox.

The 'impossible triangle' is clearly a cognitive illusion, for there is nothing special about this as a *stimulus* to disturb the physiology or signals of the visual channel. By making a model (figure 5), it may be seen and understood that this occurs with a special view of a normal object. When viewed from the critical position, the perceptual system assumes that two ends of what appear to be sides of a triangle are joined and lie at the same distance, though they are separated in distance. Even when we know this we still experience the visual paradox. It is very interesting that this false visual assumption – that the ends are at the same distance though they are separated – can generate a perception which is clearly extremely unlikely, and recognized as unlikely or even impossible. This shows convincingly that perceptions are built up by following rules from assumptions. Since perceptions can be extremely improbable and even impossible, it follows that perceiving is not *merely* a matter of accepting the most likely hypotheses. Figures and objects of this kind present useful opportunities for discovering perceptual assumptions and rules by which perceptual hypotheses that may conflict with high level knowledge are generated 'upwards' from assumptions by rule-following.

Our ability to generate and accept extremely unlikely perceptions must be imporant for survival, for occasionally highly unlikely events and situations do occur and need to be appreci-

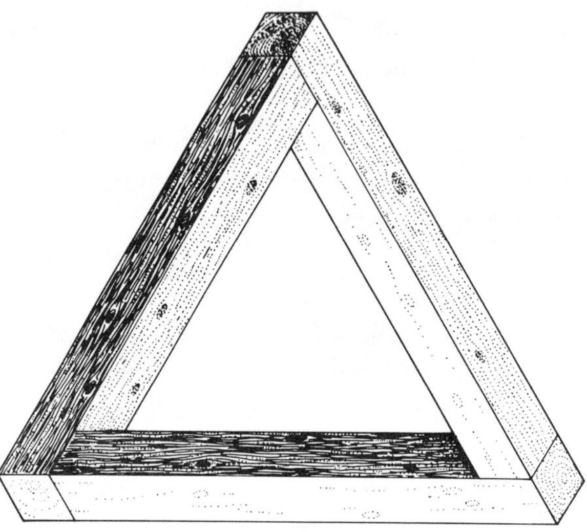

FIGURE 4. The Penrose 'impossible triangle' drawing. This appears paradoxical; but it can be an object lying in normal three-dimensional space as viewed from a critical position, as shown in figure 5.

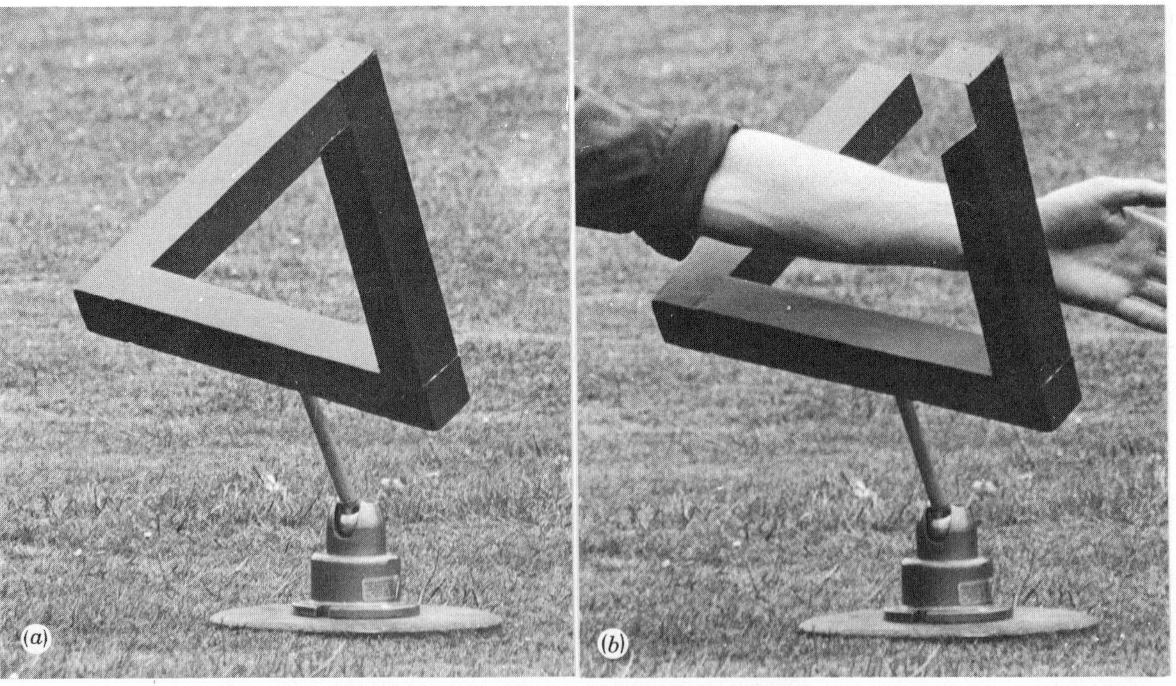

FIGURE 5. This wooden object appears paradoxical when viewed from a critical position. This is as true of the object itself as of the photograph.

ated. Indeed, perceptual learning would be impossible if only the probable were accepted. At the same time, though, there is marked probability biasing in favour of the likely against the unlikely; as in the difficulty, indeed the impossibility, of seeing a hollow mask as hollow, without full stereoscopic vision (figure 6). So there are, again, the two opposed principles – processing upwards and downwards – the first generating hypotheses which may be highly unlikely and even clearly impossible, the second offering checks 'downwards' from stored knowledge, and filling gaps which may be fictional and false.

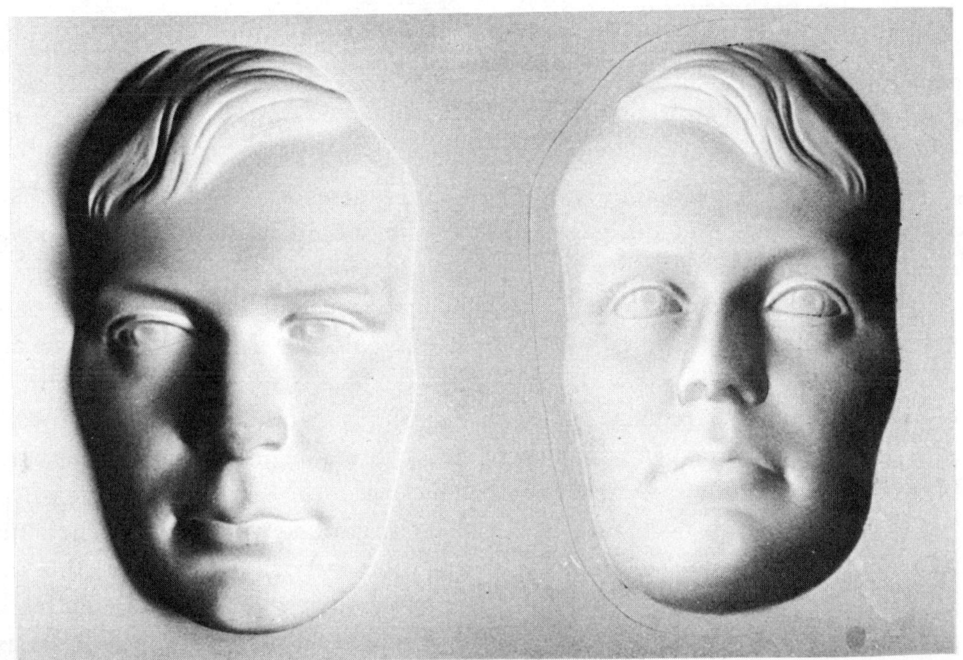

FIGURE 6. The 'face' on the right is in fact the hollow mould of the face on the left. Though hollow, the mould appears as a normal face. Texture and even stereoscopic counter-information are rejected to maintain this highly probable (but incorrect) hypothesis.

(4) *Fictions, sometimes to fit and sometimes to depart from fact*

We can see perceptual fictions in phenomena such as the illusory contours (figure 2). These were described by Schuman (1904) and have recently become well known with the beautiful examples due to Kanizsa (1966). If we are right in thinking (Gregory 1972) that they are postulated masking objects to 'explain' the surprising gaps in these figures, we at once assign to them a cognitive status. Related examples are shadows of writing: letters that would cast such shadows are seen though there is no stimulus pattern of letters. The letters are evidently fictions to 'explain' what are accepted as shadows by postulating letter-shaped objects (Gombrich 1960).

It is resonable to suppose that a very great deal of perception is in this sense fictional: generally useful but occasionally clearly wrong, when it can be an extremely powerful deception. No doubt this holds also for science.

It is particularly interesting that the *absence* of signals can be accepted as data. This is so for the discovery of the van Allen radiation belts, when the space probes' sensors were overloaded so that they failed to provide signals; and the gaps of the illusory contours figures which provide data for an eclipsing (though non-existent) object. These examples indicate ways by which the hypotheses of science and perception become richer than signalled data. They show also that we cannot equate neural signals with experience.

(5) *Causes and inferences link hypotheses and perception to the world*

Hypotheses of science and perceptions are, I believe, linked to reality very indirectly. What kind of relations do they have? There are two important questions here: (*a*) Are they *causally* linked? (*b*) Are they linked by *inference*? We should allow the possibilities that either or both may be true or false. Let us consider these.

(*a*) That hypotheses are *causally* linked to reality would be held, if there are what we have called *signal* links between reality and hypotheses. We accept this for transducers and signal channels, but what of the signals when read as *data*? There can be gaps in signals. These are often filled by interpolating processes(§3.*a*.1), so here science and perception clearly maintain hypotheses (and maintain continuous control from hypotheses) through signal gaps. Nevertheless, we do not want to say that this gap-filling requires processes outside causal explanation. Part of the aim of theories of perception and accounts of science is indeed to explain gap-filling, and these explanations, if they are to be like most explanations, should preferably be causal. We may, however, expect to find some deep conceptual difficulties over *data*, though not signals, as causes.

What of *data* distortions? Are they breaks in causal sequences? One can see cases of data errors (rather than signal errors) in which there clearly are no causal breaks in the signals, and it is possible to understand why the signals are read as misleading data. This occurs when signals are read normally as though occurring in a typical situation, when in fact the situation is atypical. Particular perceptual examples are, on this account, many of the distortion illusions (cf. Gregory 1963). Here the scaling is supposed to be set quite normally by signalled features, but these features do not have their usual significance in these figures. For example, converging lines on a picture plane are read as perspective, as though the convergence were produced as in normal three-dimensional space when parallel lines lying in depth are imaged on the retina. Picture perspective misleads not by distorting neural signals, but by providing signals that are read as depth data although the picture is flat. There is no break in the usual causation of perception, but there is marked distortion, and the distortion is of data, not of signals.

To understand why this happens we always need to know what knowledge (in this case that convergence of lines is associated with depth) has been transferred to the current situation, and why in this situation it is inappropriate.

What of paradoxical hypotheses? Since we do not accept that reality can be paradoxical, we cannot accept that paradoxical hypotheses or perceptions can match or represent reality. There is therefore some kind of gap – but is this a causal gap? We can think of signal distortion paradoxes where there clearly is no causal gap, for example the hands sensing hot and cold for the same bowl of water, when one hand has been adapted to hot and the other to cold. Here we have incompatible signals owing to adaptation of one of more channels, combining to form a paradox – but without any causal break.

Figures such as the Penrose impossible triangle drawing (figure 4) or our impossible model (figure 5) are very different from signal distortions. We attribute these perceptual paradoxes not to signal errors, but to false assumptions. So these are top-down errors.

The question is: Do top-down injections of data or assumptions produce causal gaps in signal processing? They certainly introduce considerations that may be very far removed from the current situation, and for quite displaced assumptions it may be very difficult indeed to see how they have come into play. If we give them a 'mental' status, then we may be tempted to say that they are caused mentally; it seems better, however, to say that the situation is something like a filing card index, in that references are sought by criteria of relevance and so on, as formulated within a physical search system. This may go wrong by misreading of signals or by indexing errors, and it may also produce misleading data because what is generally relevant is not appropriate in the particular situation. These mistakes are very different, but they can be explained in terms of the logic of the procedures plus the mechanical steps used to carry out the procedures.

(*b*) If probabilities can affect reasoning and acceptance or rejection of hypotheses, then just how can we hold that signals though not data are causal? To maintain a causal account we must allow that assessed probabilities have causal effects. We may, however, translate this into: *Signals have causal effects according to the significance in the situation of the data that they convey.*

If the distinction between signals and data is seen as a dualism, at least this dualism does not apply uniquely to mind and brain. As argued earlier, it applies with equal force in the case of instruments supplying signals and data for science. So the activity of science becomes a test-tube – indeed a laboratory – for appreciating the mind–brain problem.

We may now consider some *differences* between scientific and perceptual hypotheses.

(*c*) *Differences between scientific and perceptual hypotheses, when they are appropriate or inappropriate*

(1) *Perceptions are from one vantage-point and run in real time; science is not based on an observer's view*

Perceptions differ from conceptions by being related to events in real time from a local region of space, while conceptions have no locale and are essentially timeless. They not only lack any locale in the three-dimensional space of the physical world, but they may express variables and relations in all manner of conceptual spaces, which are not claimed to exist though they are useful fictions for descriptive purposes.

So perception is far more limited in range and application than conception. The basis of empiricism is that all conception depends upon perception. But conception can break away from perception, to create new worlds – though perhaps always using as building blocks the objects of perception.

(2) *Perceptions are of instances; science is of generalizations*

We perceive individual objects, but we can conceive, also, generalizations and abstractions. Thus we can see *a* triangle, but we can conceive general properties of *all* triangles – triangularity. Is this difference absolute or, rather, a matter of degree? A chess player may claim that he *sees* the situation rather than the pieces; and when reading, one is more aware of the meaning of the words than their form, and this can hold when the words express generalizations. This is a tricky issue requiring investigation. I incline to think that there is not a sharp distinction here between perceiving and conceiving.

(3) *Perceptions are limited to 'concrete objects'; science has also 'abstract objects'*

This distinction is due to the logician Frege, and is discussed above (§3.*a*.3). Again, this is a tricky issue, closely bound up with the deepest problems of perception and epistemology. The distinction is not clear-cut.

Concrete objects are what are (or are believed to be) sensed. They may be simple or complex. Thus a magnetic field may be simple and a table is complex. It is not, however, at all clear that sensing is *ever* free from inference: for example, perceiving a table is far more than sensing various parts, and sensing a magnetic field requires all manner of inferences about the transducer and how it is placed and used. The contribution of inferences and assumptions to sensing even simple objects makes the distincion between concrete and abstract objects difficult and perhaps impossible to make clearly, for abstract objects – such as numbers and centres of gravity – are or at least may be known via sense experience, and perhaps nothing is sensed 'directly'. If nothing is sensed or perceived directly – if *all* perception and all scientific observation, however instrumented, involve inference – then it seems that there are no purely concrete objects. This is indeed a major conclusion from the thesis that perceptions are hypotheses. This conclusion applies equally to perception and to science.

(4) *Perceptions are not explanations, but conceptions can be explanatory*

Scientific hypotheses are closely linked to explanation: it is an explanation that the tides are caused by the pull of the Moon. Perceptions certainly have far less explanatory power, but perhaps they do have some. One understands social situations, or mechanisms, through looking: is this understanding part of the *perception*? I incline to think that it is. This difference is rather of degree than kind.

(5) *Perception includes awareness; the physical sciences exclude awareness*

This is by far the most striking difference between hypotheses of science and perceptions: sensations are involved in perception (though not all perceptions) but awareness, or consciousness, has no place in the hypotheses of physics.

The scientist may be aware that he is working on a hypothesis; but the hypothesis is not itself aware – or so we assume! On the other hand, we do want to say that awareness is an integral part of many perceptual hypotheses, so here we have a clear distinction between scientific hypotheses and some perceptions.

Returning to our distinctions between signals and data: a traditional view was that perceptions are made up of sensations, but this we have rejected. It must, however, be confessed that the role, if any, of awareness or consciousness in perception is totally mysterious. Much of human behaviour controlled by perception can occur without awareness: consciousness is seldom, if ever, necessary. Perhaps consciousness is particularly associated with mismatch between expectation and signalled events; but if this is so, its purpose remains obscure, because it is not clearly causal.

Popper & Eccles (1977) argue from phenomena of visual ambiguity – especially maintaining or changing visual orientations by will – that mind, as associated with consciousness, has some control over brain. This argument was also suggested by William James (1890), but, as he points out, it could be *other brain processes* affecting reversal rates, or whatever. There seems no good reason to suppose that consciousness, at least in this situation, is causal.

Is consciousness so difficult to understand and describe, just because it is *not* part of scientific hypotheses about the physical world? It is these, only, that provide conceptual understanding? If so, we must be careful with our suggestion that perceptions are hypotheses: for if *all* we can know are hypotheses of physics, then perceptions are *bound* to look like hypotheses of physics. This is an impasse for which I have no ready answer. I can only hope that further consideration will unravel or cut these Gordian knots of knowing.

We may conclude that, all in all, there are marked similarities and important identities between hypotheses of science and perceptions. It is these that justify calling perceptions 'hypotheses'. The differences are, however, extremely interesting, and I fear that I have not done them justice. This is not through any desire to minimize them, but rather that I do not know what to add. Possibly this is because we think in terms of the hypotheses of science so that when something crops up that departs from them drastically, we are lost. We are lost for consciousness. It is very curious that we can think conceptually with such effect 'outwards' but not 'inwards'. It may be that developments in artificial intelligence will provide concepts by which we shall see ourselves.

References (Gregory)

Attneave, F. 1971 Multistability in perception. *Scient. Am.* **225** (6), 62–71.

Dummett, M. 1978 *Frege.* London: Duckworth.

Gibson, J. J. 1950 *Perception of the visual world.* London: Allen & Unwin.

Gregory, R. L. 1963 Distortion of visual space as inappropriate constancy scaling. *Nature, Lond.* **119**, 678.

Gregory, R. L. 1968 Perceptual illusions and brain models. *Proc. R. Soc. Lond.* B **171**, 279–296.

Gregory, R. L. 1970 *The intelligent eye.* London and New York: Weidenfeld & Nicolson.

Gregory, R. L. 1972 Cognitive contours. *Nature, Lond.* **238**, 51–52.

Gregory, R. L. & Wallace, J. G. 1963 Recovery from early blindness: a case study. *Monogr. Suppl.* no. 2, *Q. Jl exp. Psychol.* Cambridge: Heffers. (Reprinted in Gregory, R. L. 1974 *Concepts and mechanisms of perception.* London: Duckworth).

Gombrich, E. H. 1960 *Art and illusion.* London: Phaidon.

Guzman, A. 1968 Decomposition of a visual scene into three-dimensional bodies. In *Proc. of the Fall Joint Computer Conference*, pp. 291–304.

Guzman, A. 1971 Analysis of curved line drawings using context and global information. In *Machine intelligence*, vol. 6 (ed. B. Meltzer & D. Michie), pp. 325–375. University of Edinburgh Press.

Ittelson, W. H. 1952 *The Ames demonstrations in perception.* Princeton University Press.

James, W. 1890 *Principles of psychology.* Macmillan.

Kanizsa, G. 1966 Margini quasi-percettivi in campi con stimulazioni omogenea. *Riv. Psicol.* **49**, 7.

Kuhn, T. 1962 *The structure of scientific revolutions.* University of Chicago Press.

Penrose, L. S. & Penrose, R. 1958 Impossible objects: a special type of illusion. *Br. J. Psychol.* **49**, 31.

Popper, K. R. 1972 *Objective knowledge: an evolutionary approach.* Oxford: Clarendon Press.

Popper, K. R. & Eccles, J. C. 1977 *The self and its brain.* Springer International.

Shannon, C. E. & Weaver, W. 1949 *The mathematical theory of communication.* Urbana: University of Illinois Press.

Schumann, F. 1904 Einige Beobachtungen uber die Zusammenfassung von Gesichtseindrucken zu Einheiten. *Psychol. Stud., Lpz.* **1**, 1.

Wertheimer, M. 1938 Laws of organisation of perceptual forms. In *Source book of Gestalt psychology* (ed. W. H. Ellis), pp. 71–88. New York: Routledge Kegan Paul.

Phil. Trans. R. Soc. Lond. B **290**, 199–218 (1980)

Printed in Great Britain

Visual information processing: the structure and creation of visual representations

By D. Marr

M.I.T. Artificial Intelligence Laboratory and Department of Psychology,
545 Technology Square, Cambridge, Massachusetts 02139, U.S.A.

For human vision to be explained by a computational theory, the first question is plain: What are the problems that the brain solves when we see? It is argued that vision is the construction of efficient symbolic descriptions from images of the world. An important aspect of vision is therefore the choice of representations for the different kinds of information in a visual scene. An overall framework is suggested for extracting shape information from images, in which the analysis proceeds through three representations: (1) the primal sketch, which makes explicit the intensity changes and local two-dimensional geometry of an image; (2) the $2\frac{1}{2}$-D sketch, which is a viewer-centred representation of the depth, orientation and discontinuities of the visible surfaces; and (3) the 3-D model representation, which allows an object-centred description of the three-dimensional structure and organization of a viewed shape. The critical act in formulating computational theories for processes capable of constructing these representations is the discovery of valid constraints on the way the world behaves, that provide sufficient additional information to allow recovery of the desired characteristic. Finally, once a computational theory for a process has been formulated, algorithms for implementing it may be designed, and their performance compared with that of the human visual processor.

Introduction

Modern neurophysiology has learned much about the operation of the individual nerve cell, but disconcertingly little about the meaning of the circuits that they compose in the brain. The reason for this can be attributed, at least in part, to a failure to recognize what it means to understand a complex information-processing system; for a complex system cannot be understood as a simple extrapolation from the properties of its elementary components. One does not formulate, for example, a description of thermodynamical effects by using a large set of equations one for each of the particles involved. One describes such effects at their own level, that of an enormous collection of particles, and tries to show that in principle, the microscopic and macroscopic descriptions are consistent with one another.

The core of the problem is that a system as complex as a nervous system or a developing embryo must be analysed and understood at several different levels. Indeed, in a system that solves an information-processing problem, we may distinguish four important levels of description (Marr & Poggio 1977; Marr 1977*a*). At the lowest level, there is basic component and circuit analysis: how do transistors (or neurons) or diodes (or synapses) work? The second level is the study of particular mechanisms: adders, multipliers and memories, these being assemblies made from basic components. The third level is that of the algorithm, the scheme for a computation; and the top level contains the *theory* of the computation. A theory of addition, for example, would encompass the meaning of that operation, quite independent of the representation of the numbers to be added, i.e., whether they are, say arabic or roman. But it would also include the realization that the first of these representations is the more suitable of the two. An algorithm, on the other hand, is a particular method by which to add numbers. It therefore applies to a particular representation, since plainly an algorithm that adds arabic numerals would be useless for roman. At still a further level down, one comes upon a mechanism for addition – say a pocket calculator – which simply implements a particular algorithm. As a second example, take the case of Fourier analysis. Here the computational theory of the Fourier transform – the decomposition of an arbitrary mathematical curve into a sum of sine waves of differing frequencies – is well understood, and is expressed independently of the particular way in which it might be computed. One level down, there are several algorithms for computing a Fourier transform, among them the so-called fast Fourier transform, which comprises a sequence of mathematical operations, and the so-called spatial algorithm, a single, global operation that is based on the mechanisms of laser optics. All such algorithms produce the same result, so the choice of which one to use depends upon the particular mechanisms that are available. If one has fast digitial memory, adders and multipliers, one will use the fast Fourier transform, and if one has a laser and photographic plates, one will use an 'optical' method.

Now each of the four levels of description will have its place in the eventual understanding of perceptual information processing, and of course there are logical and causal relations among them. But the important point is that the four levels of description are only loosely related. Too often in attempts to relate psychophysical problems to physiology there is confusion about the level at which a problem arises: is it related, for instance, mainly to the physical mechanisms of vision (like the after-images such as the one seen after staring at a light bulb) or mainly to the computational theory of vision (like the ambiguity of the Necker cube)? More disturbingly, although the top level is the most neglected, it is also the most important. This is because the nature of computations that underlie perception depend more upon the computational *problems* that have to be solved than upon the particular hardware in which their solutions are implemented. To phrase the matter another way, an algorithm is likely to be understood more readily by understanding the nature of the problem that it deals with than by examining the mechanism (and the hardware) by which it is embodied. There is, after all, an analogue to all of this in physics, where a thermodynamical approach represented, at least historically, the first stage in the study of matter: it succeeded in producing a theory of gross properties such as temperature. A description in terms of mechanisms or elementary components – in this case atoms and molecules – appeared some decades afterwards.

Our main point, therefore, is that the topmost of our four levels, that at which the necessary structure of computation is defined, is a crucial but neglected one. Its study is separate from the study of particular algorithms, mechanisms or hardware, and the techniques needed to pursue it are new. In the rest of this article, I summarize some examples of vision theories at the uppermost level.

Conventional approaches

The problems of visual perception have attracted the curiosity of scientists for many centuries. Important early contributions were made by Newton (1704), who laid the foundations for modern work on colour vision, and Helmholtz (1910), whose treatise on physiological optics maintains its interest even today. Early in this century, Wertheimer (1938) noticed the apparent motion not of individual dots but instead of wholes, or 'fields', in images presented sequentially, as if in a cine film. In much the same way do we perceive the migration across the sky of a

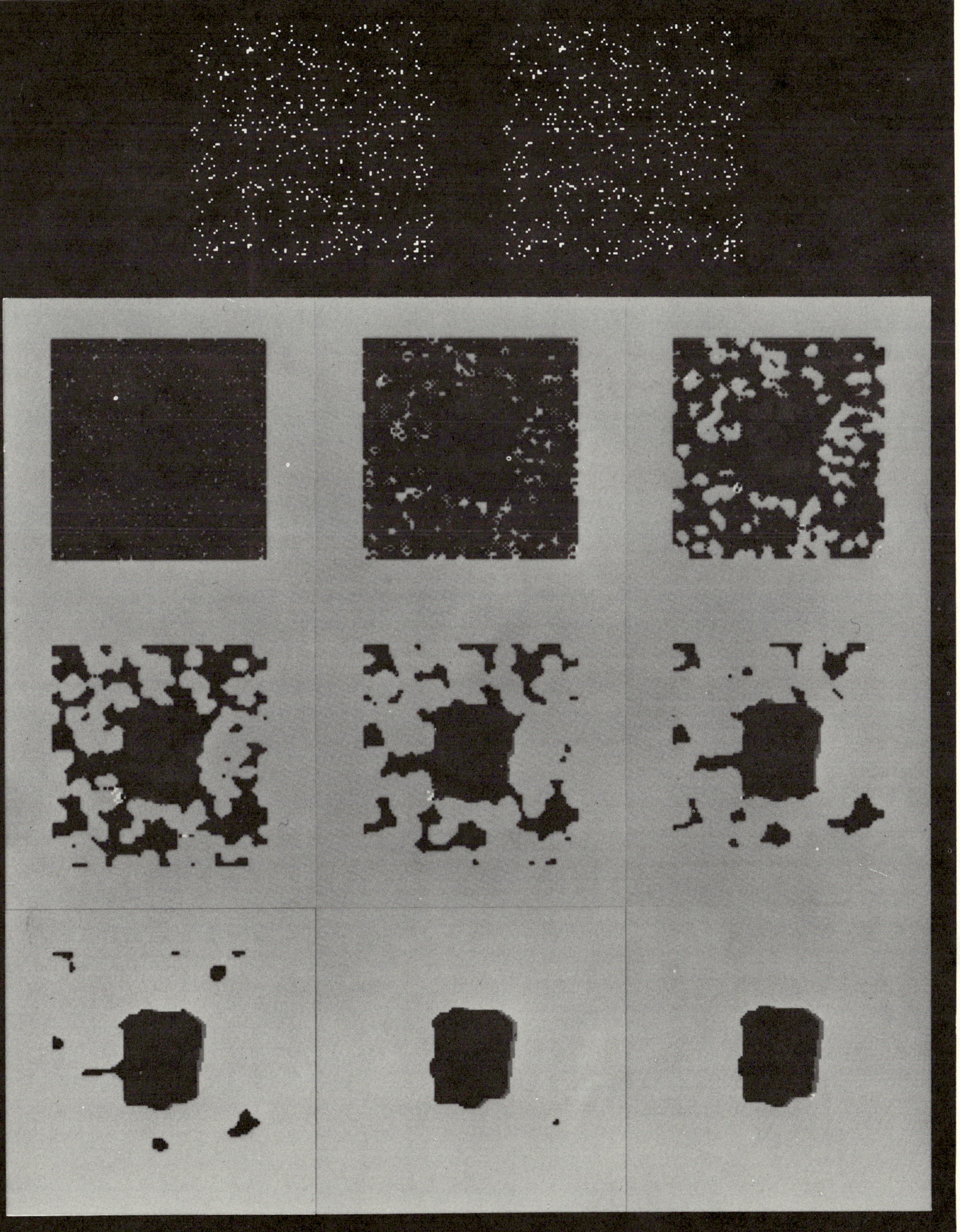

FIGURE 1. A sparse random-dot stereogram (the top two images), and its decoding by Marr & Poggio's (1976) cooperative algorithm. The initial state contains all possible matches within a given disparity range, and the algorithm embodies the constraints of uniqueness and continuity to eliminate false targets. Shades of grey are used to signify matches at different disparities. The figure shows the initial state, and the states after 1, 2, 3, 4, 5, 6, 8 and 14 iterations. The algorithm progressively reveals a square hovering in depth. This algorithm is not the one used by the human visual system.

flock of geese, the flock somehow constituting a single entity, and not individual birds. This observation started the Gestalt school of psychology, which was concerned with describing the qualities of wholes, including solidarity and distinctness, and trying to formulate the laws that governed their creation. The attempt failed for various reasons, and the Gestalt school dissolved into the fog of subjectivism. With the death of the school, many of its early and genuine insights were unfortunately lost to the mainstream of experimental psychology.

The next developments of importance were recent and technical. The advent of electrophysiology in the 1940s and 1950s made single-cell recording possible, and with Kuffler's (1953) study of retinal ganglion cells – the neurons of the eye that give rise to the optic nerve – a new approach to the problem was born. Its most renowned practitioners are Hubel & Wiesel (1962, 1968), who since 1959 have conducted an influential series of investigations on single cell responses at various points along the visual pathway in the cat and the monkey.

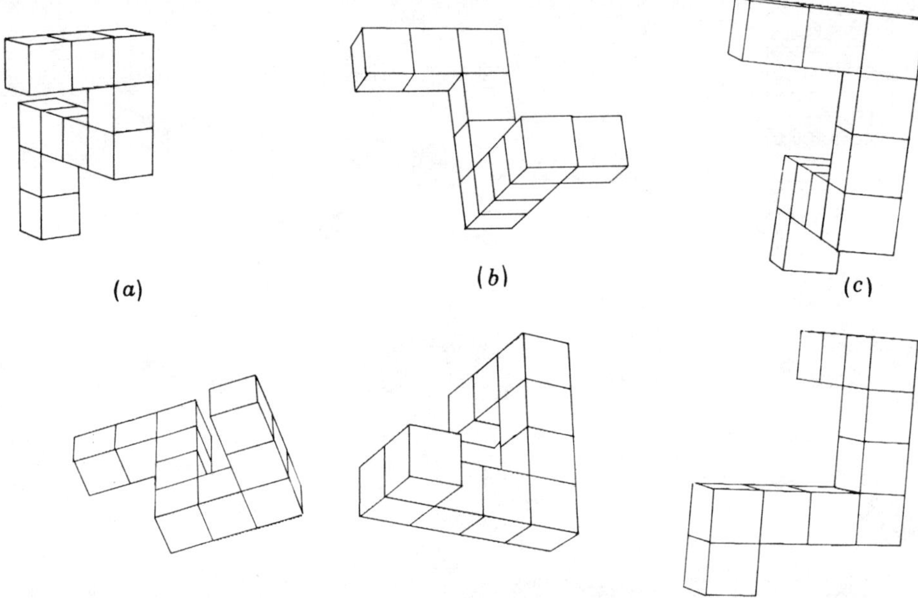

FIGURE 2. Some drawings similar to those used in Shepard & Metzler's (1971) experiments on mental rotation. Those shown in (a) and (b) are identical and the relative angle between the two is 80°. Those in (c) are not identical, and no rotation will bring them into congruence.

Students of the psychology of perception were also affected by a technological advance, the advent of the digital computer. Most notably, it allowed Bela Julesz in 1959 to devise random-dot stereograms (see Julesz 1971), which are image pairs constructed of dot patterns that appear random when viewed monocularly, but which fuse when viewed one through each eye to give a percept of shapes and surfaces with a clear three-dimensional structure. An example is shown in figure 1. Here the image for the left eye is a matrix of black and white squares generated at random by a computer program. The image for the right is made by copying the left image and then shifting a square-shaped region at its centre slightly to the left, providing a new random pattern to fill in the gap that the shift must create. If each of the eyes sees only one matrix, as if they were both in the same physical place, the result is the sensation of a square floating in space. Plainly such percepts are caused solely by the stereo disparity between matching elements in the images presented to each eye.

More recently, considerable interest has been attracted by a rather different approach. In 1971, Shepard & Metzler made line drawings of simple objects that differed from one another either by a three-dimensional rotation, or by a rotation plus a reflexion (see figure 2). They asked how long it took to decide whether two depicted objects differed by a rotation and a reflexion, or merely a rotation. They found that the time taken depended on the 3-D angle of rotation necessary to bring the two objects into correspondence. Indeed, it varied linearly with this angle. One is led thereby to the notion that a mental rotation of sorts is actually being performed: that a mental description of the first shape in a pair is being adjusted incrementally in orientation until it matches the second, such adjustment requiring greater time when greater angles are involved.

Interesting and important though these findings are, one must sometimes be allowed the luxury of pausing to reflect upon the overall trends that they represent, in order to take stock of the kind of knowledge that is accessible through these techniques. For we repeat: perhaps the most striking feature of neurophysiology and psychophysics at present is that they *describe* the behaviour of cells or of subjects, but do not *explain* it. What are the visual areas of the cerebral cortex actually doing? What are the problems in doing it that need explaining, and at what level of description should such explanations be sought?

A COMPUTATIONAL APPROACH TO VISION

In trying to come to grips with these problems, our group at the M.I.T. Artificial Intelligence Laboratory has adopted a point of view that regards visual perception as a problem primarily in information processing. The problem begins with a large, grey-level intensity array, which suffices to approximate an image such as the world might cast upon the retinas of the eyes, and it culminates in a *description* that depends on that array, and on the purpose that the viewer brings to it. Our particular concern in this article will be with the derivation of a description well suited for the recognition of three-dimensional shapes.

The primal sketch

It is a commonplace that a scene and a drawing of the scene appear very similar, despite the completely different grey-level images to which they give rise. This suggests that the artist's symbols correspond in some way to natural symbols that are computed out of the image during the normal course of its interpretation. Our theory therefore asserts that the first operation on an image is to transform it into a primitive but rich description of the way its intensities change over the visual field, as opposed to a description of its particular intensity values in and of themselves. This yields a description of markedly reduced size that still captures the important aspects required for image analysis. We call it a *primal sketch* (Marr 1976). Consider, for example, an intensity array of 1000 by 1000, or 10^6 points in all. Even if the possible intensity at any one point were merely black or white – two different brightnesses – the number of all possible arrays would still be 2^{10^6}. In a real image, however, there tend to be continuities of intensity – areas where brightness varies uniformly – and this tends to eliminate possibilities in which the black and white oscillate wildly. It also tends to simplify the array. Typically, therefore, a primal sketch need not include a set of values for every point in an image. As stored in a computer, it will instead constitute an array with numbers representing the directions, magnitudes, and spatial extents of intensity changes assigned to certain specific points in an image, points that

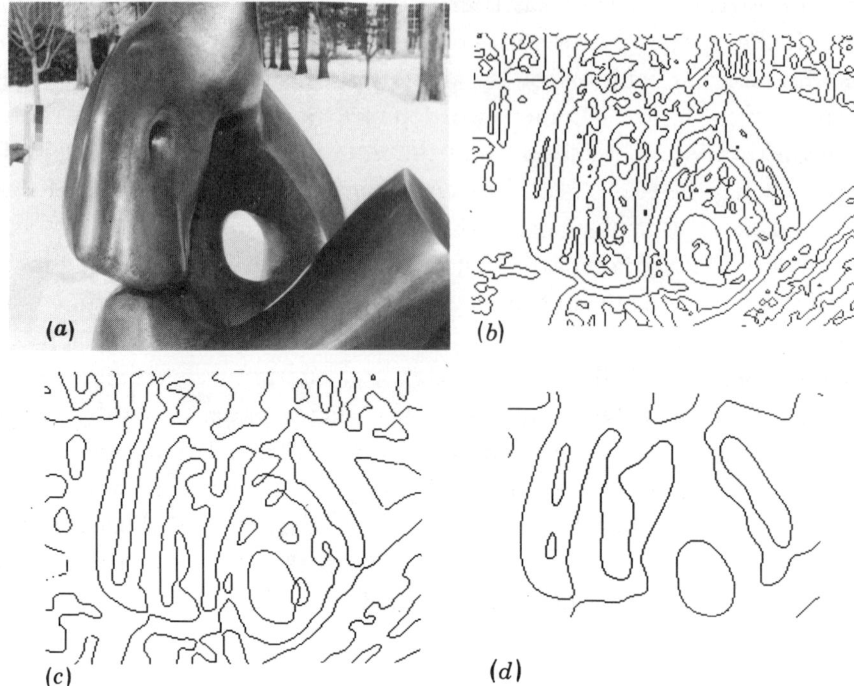

FIGURE 3. The image (a), which is 320 × 320 pixels, has been convolved with $\nabla^2 G$, a centre–surround operator with central excitatory region of width $2\sigma = 6$, 12 and 24 pixels. These filters span approximately the range of filters that operate in the human fovea. The zero-crossings of the filtered images are shown in (b), (c) and (d). These are the precursors of the raw primal sketch. (From Marr & Hildreth 1979, figure 6).

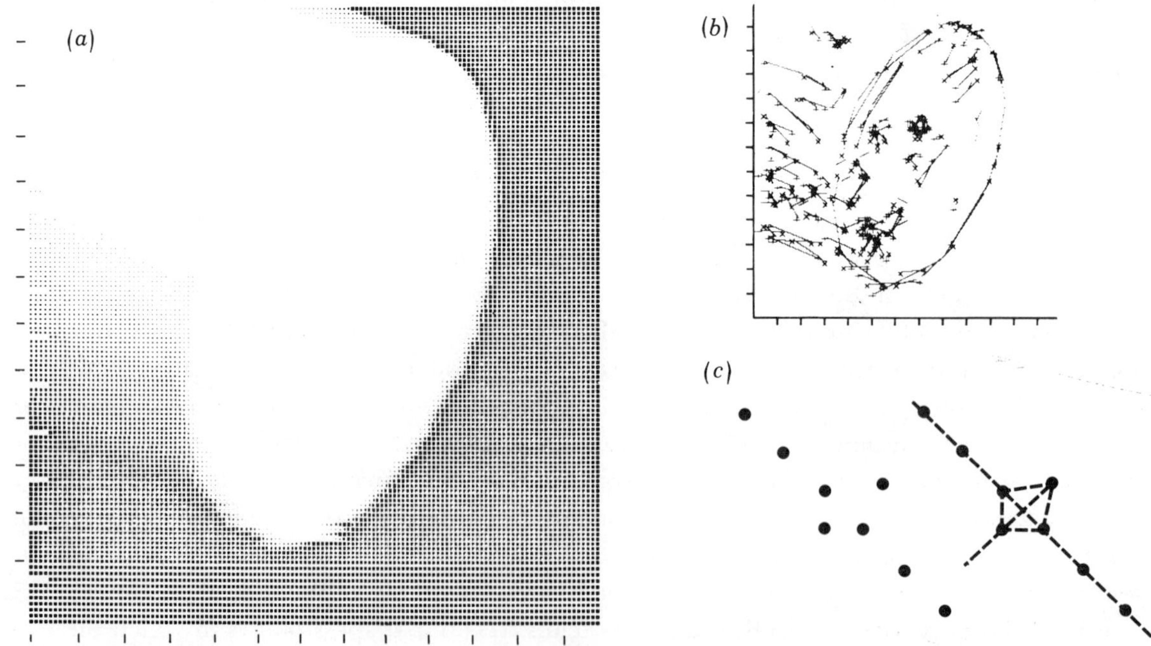

FIGURE 4. The primal sketch makes explicit information held in an intensity array (a). There are two kinds of information: one (b) concerns changes in intensity, represented by orientated edge, bar and blob primitives, together with associated parameters that measure the contrast and spatial extent of the intensity change; and the other (c) is the local geometry of significant places in the image. Such places are marked by place-tokens, which can be defined in a variety of ways, and the geometric relations between them are represented by virtual lines (Marr 1976, figures 7 and 12a).

tend to be places of locally high or low intensity. The positions of these points, particularly their arrangement among their immediate neighbours – that is to say, the local geometry of the image – must also be made explicit in the primal sketch, as it would otherwise be lost. (It was implicit, of course, in the 1000 by 1000 array, but we are no longer retaining data for each of those 10^6 places.) One way to do this is to specify 'virtual lines' – directions and distances – between neighbouring points of interest in the sketch.

The process of computing the primal sketch involves several steps. The first is the derivation of the *raw primal sketch* (see Marr & Hildreth 1979), which involves detecting and representing the intensity changes in the image. First, the image is filtered through a set of medium bandpass second differential operators $\nabla^2 G$, (where ∇^2 is the Laplacian and G is a Gaussian distribution), and the zero-crossings in the filtered images are found (see figure 3). This representation of the intensity changes is probably complete (Marr *et al.* 1979).

Although in general there is no reason why the zero-crossings found by the different channels should be related, in practice they will be. The reason is that most intensity changes in an image arise from physical phenomena that are spatially localized. This constraint allowed Marr & Hildreth to formulate the *spatial coincidence assumption* which states: If a zero-crossing is present in a set of independent $\nabla^2 G$ channels over a contiguous range of sizes, and it has the same position and orientation in each channel, then the set of such zero-crossings may be taken to indicate the presence of an intensity change in the image that is due to a single physical phenomenon (a change in reflectance, illumination, depth or surface orientation).

This assumption allows one to combine the zero-crossings from different channels into edge-segment descriptors, bars and blobs (see figure 4*b*), which constitute the raw primal sketch. To obtain the full primal sketch, these primitive elements are grouped, perhaps hierarchically, into units called place-tokens, which associate properties like length, width, brightness and so forth with positions in the image (Marr 1976). Virtual lines may then be used to represent the local geometry of these place-tokens (see figure 4*c* and Stevens 1978).

Recently, Marr & Ullman (1979) have extended the work of Marr & Hildreth to include the detection and use of directional selectivity. They have proposed specific roles for the X and Y channels found originally by Enroth-Cugell & Robson (1966), and in an explicit model for one class of cortical simple cell, they showed how to combine X and Y information to form a directionally selective unit.

Modules of early visual processing

The primal sketch of an image is typically a large and unwieldy collection of data, even despite its simplification relative to a grey-level array; for this is the unavoidable consequence of the irregularity and complexity of natural images. The next computational problem is thus its decoding. Now the traditional approach to machine vision assumes that the essence of such a decoding is a process called *segmentation*, whose purpose is to divide a primal sketch, or more generally an image, into regions that are meaningful, perhaps as physical objects. Tenenbaum & Barrow (1976), for example, applied knowledge about several different types of scene to the segmentation of images of landscapes, an office, a room, and a compressor. Freuder (1975) used a similar approach to identify a hammer in a simple scene. Upon finding a blob, his computer program would tentatively label it as the head of a hammer, and begin a search for confirmation in the form of an appended shaft. If this approach were correct, it would mean that a central problem for vision is arranging for the right piece of specialized knowledge to be made available at the appropriate time in the segmentation of an image. Freuder's work, for example, was almost entirely devoted to the design of a system that made this possible. But despite considerable efforts over a long period, the theory and practice of segmentation remain rather primitive, and here again we believe that the main reason lies in the failure to formulate precisely the goals of this stage of the processing – a failure, in other words, to work at the topmost level of visual theory. What, for example, is an object? Is a head an object? Is it still an object if it is attached to a body? What about a man on horseback?

Marr (1978) argued that the early stages of visual information processing ought instead to squeeze the last possible ounce of information from an image before taking recourse to the descending influence of 'high-level' knowledge about objects in the world. Let us turn, then, to a brief examination of the physics of the situation. As noted earlier, the visual process begins with arrays of intensities projected upon the retinas of the eyes. The principal factors that determine these intensities are (1) the illuminant, (2) the surface reflectance properties of the objects viewed, (3) the shapes of the visible surfaces of these objects, and (4) the vantage point of the viewer. Thus if the analysis of the input intensity arrays is to operate autonomously, at least in its early stages, it can only be expected to extract information about these four factors. In short, early visual processing must be limited to the recovery of localized physical properties of the visible *surfaces* of a viewed object, particularly local surface dispositions (orientation and depth) and surface material properties (colour, texture, shininess, and so on). More abstract matters such as a description of overall three-dimensional shape must come after this more basic analysis is complete.

An example of early processing is stereopsis. Imagine that images of a scene are available from two nearby points at the same horizontal level – the analogue of the images that play upon the retinas of your left and right eyes. The images are somewhat different, of course, in consequence of the slight difference in vantage point. Imagine further that a particular location on a surface in the scene is chosen from one image; that the corresponding location is identified in the other image; and that the relative positions of the two versions of that location are measured. This information will suffice for the calculation of depth – the distance of that location from the viewer. Notice that methods based on grey-level correlation between the pair of images fail to be suitable because a mere grey-level measurement does not reliably define a point on a physical surface. To put the matter plainly, numerous points in a surface might fortuitously be the same shade of grey, and differences in the vantage points of the observer's eyes could change the shade as well. The matching must evidently be based instead on objective markings that lie upon the surface, and so one had to use changes in reflectance. One way of doing this is to obtain a primitive description of the intensity changes that exist in each image (such as a primal sketch), and then to match these descriptions. After all, the line segments, edge segments, blobs, and edge termination points included in such a description correspond quite closely to boundaries and reflectance changes on physical surfaces. The stereo problem – the determination of depth given a stereo pair of images – may thus be reduced to that of matching two primitive descriptions, one from each eye; and to help in this task there are physical constraints that translate into two rules for how the left and right descriptions are combined.

Uniqueness

Each item from each image may be assigned at most one disparity value, that is to say, a unique position relative to its counterpart in the stereo pair. This condition rests on the premise that the items to be matched have a physical existence, and can be in only one place at a time.

Continuity

Disparity varies smoothly almost everywhere. This condition is a consequence of the cohesiveness of matter, and it states that only a relatively small fraction of the area of an image is composed of discontinuities in depth.

In the case of random-dot stereograms, the computational problem is rather well defined, essentially because of Julesz's demonstration that random-dot stereograms, containing no monocular information, still yield stereopsis. In 1976, Marr & Poggio developed a method for computing local disparities in a pair of random-dot stereograms by an iterative, parallel procedure known technically as cooperative algorithm (see figure 1 and Marr *et al.* 1977). This sort of algorithm has the property that it can be defined completely in terms of simple local interactions because at each of its iterations, each point is affected only by a calculation performed on its immediate neighbourhood. Yet all points are so affected during each successive iteration, so the

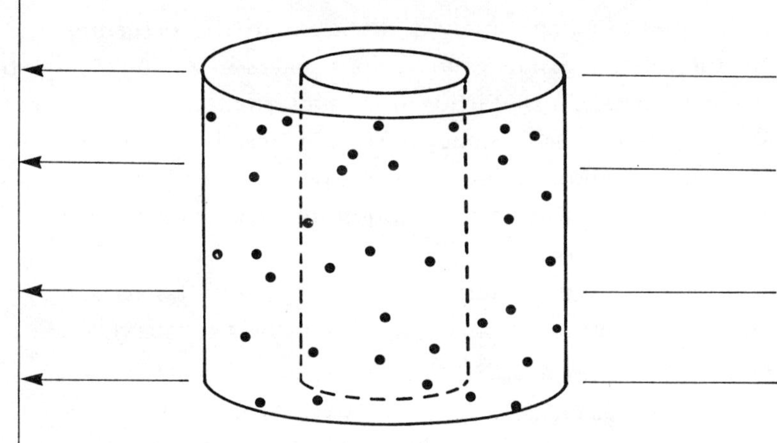

FIGURE 5. The motion analogue of the random-dot stereogram. Two transparent, concentric cylinders are rotated in opposite directions. Each has dots scattered on its surface. A cine camera photographs the scene from the side, and each frame contains only a pattern of random dots. When a human watches the film, however, he immediately perceives the two counter-rotating cylinders. (From Ullman 1979 *b*.)

transformations take on a complex global nature. Subsequent comparison of the algorithm's performance with psychophysical data showed that it did not hold up well as a model for human stereopsis. To be sure, it performed better than people do on the standard stereograms like that shown in figure 1; but it did not explain people's ability to see stereograms in which one of the two images is defocused slightly or enlarged slightly relative to the other. These observations led Marr & Poggio (1979) to devise another algorithm, based on the human use of spatial-frequency-tuned channels and vergence eye movements. This algorithm is consistent with all of the currently known psychophysical data.

A second example of early visual processing concerns the derivation of structure from motion. It has long been known that as an object moves relative to the viewer, the way its appearance changes provides information that we can use to determine its shape (Wallach & O'Connell 1953). The motion analogue of a random-dot stereogram is illustrated in figure 5, and as expected, humans can easily perceive shape from a succession of frames, each of which on its own is merely a set of random-dots. In various papers and a forthcoming book on the subject, Ullman (1979 *a*, *b*) decomposed the problem into two parts: matching the elements that occur in consecutive images, and deriving shape information from measurements of their changes in position. Ullman then showed that these problems can be solved mathematically. His basic idea is that, in general, nothing can be inferred about the shape of an object given only a set of sequential views of it; some extra assumptions have to be made. Accordingly, he formulates an assumption of rigidity, which states that if a set of moving points has a *unique* interpretation as a rigid body in motion, that interpretation is correct. (The assumption is based on a theorem, which he proves, stating that three distinct views of four non-coplanar points on a rigid body are sufficient to determine uniquely their three-dimensional arrangement in space.) From this he derives a method for computing structure from motion. The method gives results that are quantitatively superior to the ability of humans to determine shape from motion, and which fail in qualitatively similar circumstances. Ullman has also devised a set of simple algorithms by which the method may be implemented.

The $2\frac{1}{2}$-D sketch

Both of the techniques of image analysis discussed in the preceding paragraphs provide information about the relative distances to various places in an image. In stereopsis, it is the matching of points in a stereo pair that leads to such information. In structure from motion, it is the matching of points in successive images. More generally, however, we know that vision provides several sources of information about shapes in the visual world. The most direct, perhaps, are the aforementioned stereo and motion, but texture gradients in a single image are

TABLE 1. THE FORM IN WHICH VARIOUS EARLY VISUAL PROCESSES DELIVER
INFORMATION ABOUT THE CHANGES IN A SCENE

(r is depth; δr is small, local change in depth; Δr is large changes in depth; s is local surface orientation.)

information source	natural parameter
stereo	disparity, hence especially δr and Δr
motion	r, hence δr, Δr
shading	s
texture gradients	s
perspective cues	s
occlusion	Δr
contour	s

nearly as effective. Furthermore, the theatrical techniques of facial make-up reveal the sensitivity of perceived shapes to shading (see Horn 1975), and colour sometimes suggests the manner in which a surface reflects light. It often happens that different parts of a scene are open to inspection by different techniques. Yet different as the techniques are, they all have two important characteristics in common: they rely on information from the image rather than *a priori* knowledge about the shapes of the viewed objects, and the information that they specify concerns the depth or surface orientation at arbitrary points in an image, rather than the depth of orientation associated with particular objects (see table 1).

To make the most efficient use of different and often complementary channels of information deriving from stereopsis, from motion, from contours, from texture, from colour, from shading, they need to be combined in some way. The computational question that now arises is thus how best to do this, and the natural answer is to seek some representation of the visual scene that makes explicit just the information that these processes can deliver. We seek, in other words, a representation of surfaces in an image that makes explicit their shapes and orientations, much as the arabic rerpesentation of a number makes explicit its composition by powers of ten. It might be contrasted with the representation of a surface as a mathematical expression, in which the orientation is only implicit, and not at all apparent. We call such a representation the $2\frac{1}{2}$D sketch (Marr & Nishihara 1978; Marr 1978), and in the particular candidate for it shown in figure 6, surface orientation is represented by covering an image with needles. The length of each needle defines the dip of the surface at that point, so that zero length corresponds to a surface that is perpendicular to the vector from the viewer to the point, and increasing lengths denote surfaces that dip increasingly away from the viewer. The orientation of each needle defines the local direction of dip.

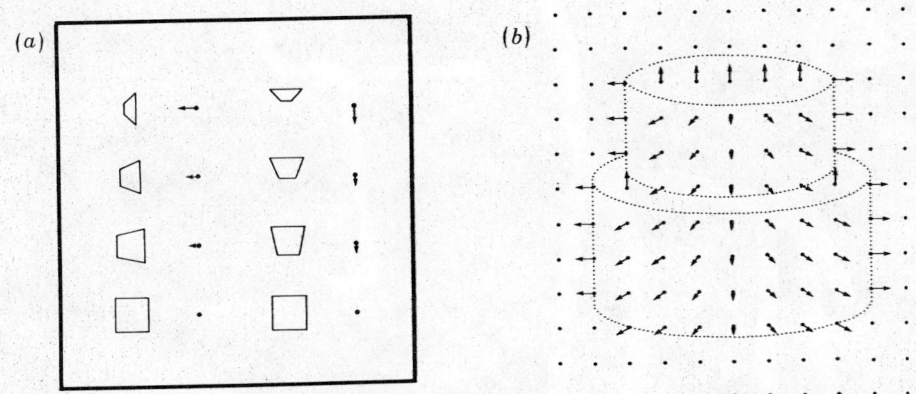

FIGURE 6. Illustration of the $2\frac{1}{2}$-dimensional sketch. In (a), the perspective views of small squares placed at various orientations to the viewer are shown. The dots with arrows show a way of representing the orientations of such surfaces symbolically. In (b), this representation is used to show the surface orientations of two cylindrical surfaces in front of a background orthogonal to the viewer. The full $2\frac{1}{2}$-dimensional sketch would include rough distances to the surfaces as well as their orientations, contours where surface orientation changes sharply, and contours where depth is discontinuous (subjective contours). A considerable amount of computation is required to maintain these quantities in states that are consistent with one another and with the structure of the outside world (see Marr 1978, §3). (From Marr & Nishihara 1978, figure 2.)

Our argument is that the $2\frac{1}{2}$-D sketch is useful because it makes explicit information about the image in a form that is closely matched to what image analysis can deliver. To put it another way, we can formulate the goals of this stage of visual processing as being primarily the construction of this representation, discovering, for example, what are the surface orientations in a scene, which of the contours in the primal sketch correspond to surface discontinuities and should therefore be represented in the $2\frac{1}{2}$-D sketch, and which contours are missing in the primal sketch and need to be inserted into the $2\frac{1}{2}$-D sketch to bring it into a state that is consistent with the nature of three-dimensional space. This formulation avoids the difficulties associated with the terms 'region' and 'object' – the difficulties inherent in the image segmentation approach; for the grey level intensity array, the primal sketch, the various modules of early visual processing, and finally the $2\frac{1}{2}$-D sketch itself deal only with discovering the properties of *surfaces* in an image. One is pleased about that, for we know of ourselves as perceivers that surface orientation can be associated with unfamiliar shapes, so its representation probably precedes the decomposition of the scene into objects. One is thus free to ask precise questions about the computational structure of the $2\frac{1}{2}$-D sketch and of processes to create and maintain it. We are currently much occupied with these matters.

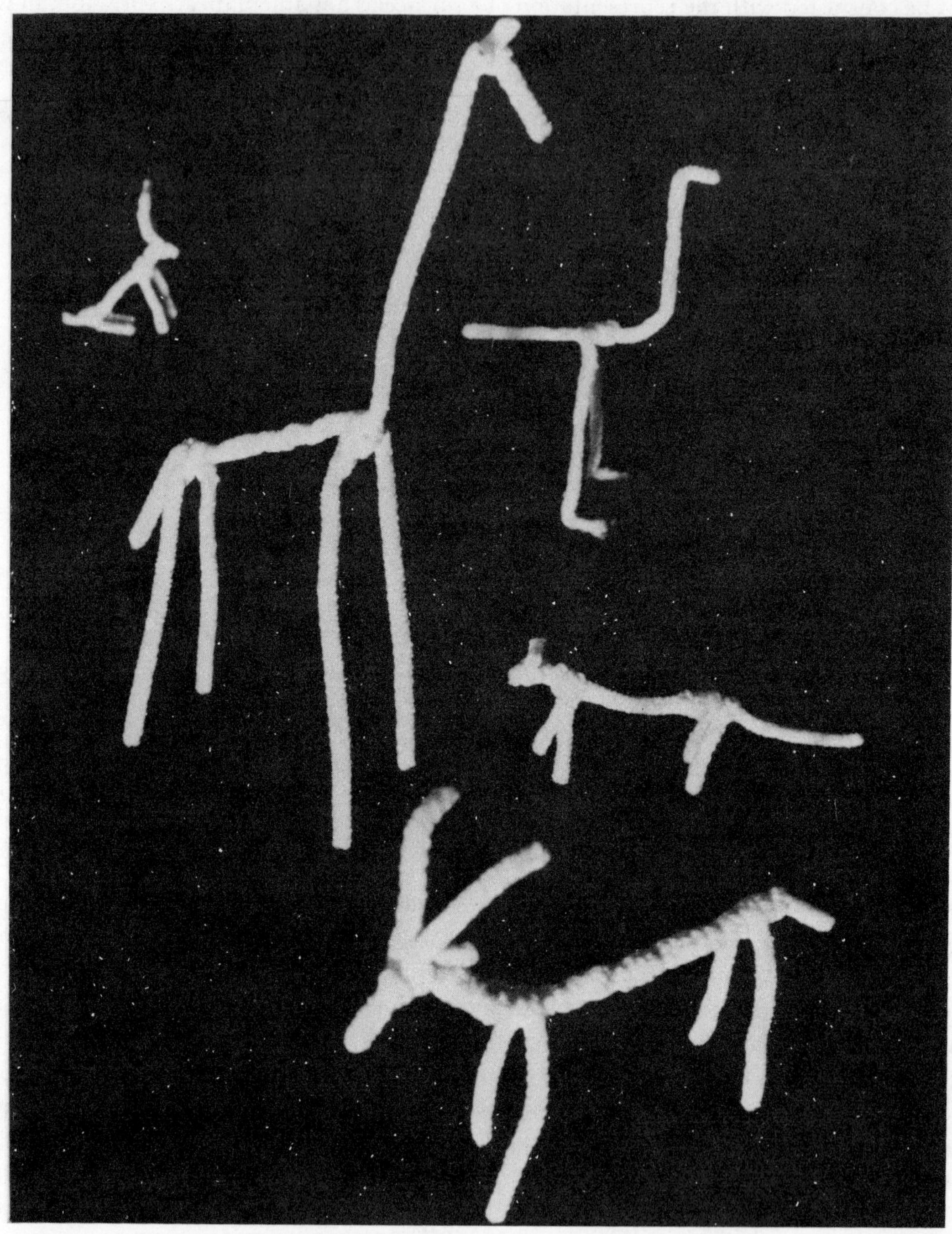

FIGURE 7. The portrayal of animals by a small number of pipe-cleaners serves to show that the representation of a three-dimensional shape need not make explicit its surface to describe it so well that it can easily be recognized. The success of the representation is due, one suspects, in large measure to the correspondence between the pipe-cleaners and the axes of the volumes that they stand for. (From Marr & Nishihara 1978, figure 1.)

LATER PROCESSING PROBLEMS

The final components of our visual processing theory concern the application of visually derived surface information for the representation of three-dimensional shapes in a way that is suitable specifically for recognition (Marr & Nishihara 1978). By this we mean the ability to recognize a shape as being the same as a shape seen earlier, and this in essence depends on being able to describe shapes consistently each time they are seen, whatever the circumstances of their positions relative to the viewer. The problem with local surface representations such as the 2½-D sketch is that the description depends as much on the viewpoint of the observer as it does on the structure of the shape. In order to factor out a description of a shape that depends on its structure alone, the representation must be based on readily identifible geometric features of the overall shape, and the dispositions of these features must de specified relative to the shape in itself. In brief, the coordinate system must be 'object-centred', not 'viewer-centred'. One aspect of this deals with the nature of the representation scheme that is to be used, and another with how to obtain it from the 2½-D sketch. We begin by discussing the first, and will then move on to the second.

The 3-D model representation

The most basic geometric properties of the volume occupied by a shape are (1) its average location (or centre of mass), (2) its overall size, as exemplified, for example, by its mean diameter or volume, and (3) its principal axis of elongation or symmetry, if one exists. A description

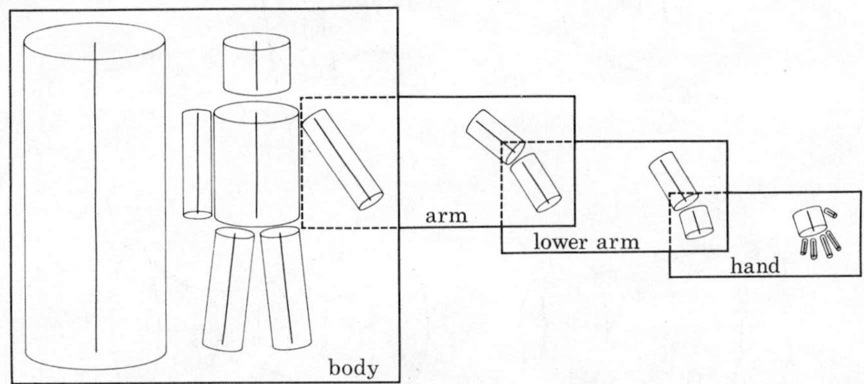

FIGURE 8. The arrangement of 3-D models into the representation of a human shape. First the overall form – the 'body' – is given an axis. This yields an object-centred coordinate system which can then be used to specify the arrangement of the 'arms', 'legs', 'torso' and 'head'. The position of each of these is specified by an axe is of its own, which in turn serves to define a coordinate system for specifying the arrangement of further subsidiary parts. This gives us a hierarchy of 3-D models, shown here extending downwards as far as the fingers. The shapes in the figure are drawn as if they were cylindrical, but that is purely for illustrative convenience. (From Marr & Nishihara 1978, figure 3.)

based on these qualities would certainly be inadequate for an application such as shape recognition; after all, one can tell little about the three-dimensional structure of a shape given only its position, size and orientation. But if a shape itself has a natural decomposition into components that can be so described, this volumetric scheme is an effective means for describing the relative spatial arrangement of those components. The illustration of figure 7 shows a familiar version of this type of description, the stick figure (see Blum 1973). The recognizability of the animal shapes depicted in the illustration is surprising considering the simplicity of representation used to describe them.

The reason that such a description works so well lies, we think, in (1) the volumetric (as opposed to surface-based) definition of the primitive elements – the sticks – used by the representation, (2) the relatively small number of elements used, and (3) the relation of elements to each other rather than to the viewer. In short, this type of shape representation is volumetric, modular, and can be based on object-centred coordinates. Figure 8 illustrates the scheme of representation that was developed from these ideas. Here the description of a shape is composed of a hierarchy of stick-figure specifications that we call 3-D models. In the simplest, a single axis element is used to specify the location, size and orientation of the entire shape; the human body displayed in the illustration will serve as an instance, This element is also used to define a coordinate system that will specify the dispositions of subsidiary axes, each of these specifying in turn a coordinate system for 3-D models of 'arm', 'hand', and so on. This hierarchical structure makes it possible to treat any component of a shape as a shape in itself. It also provides flexibility in the detail of a description.

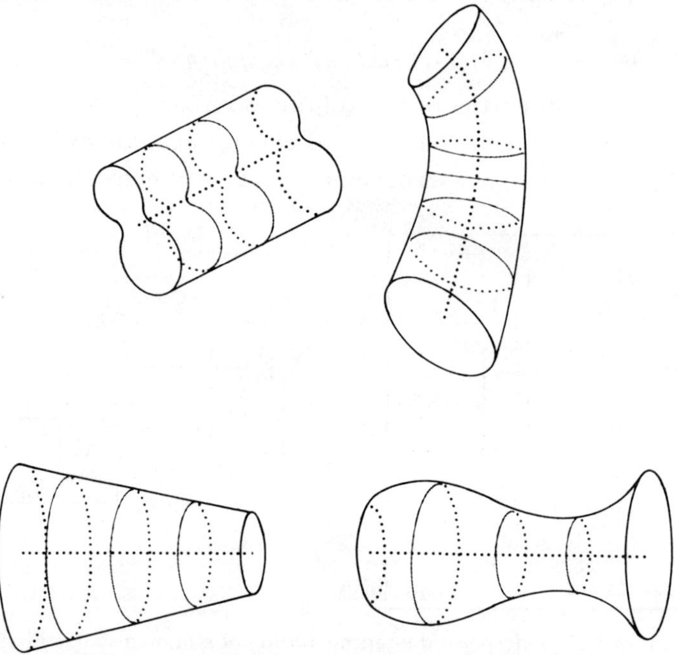

FIGURE 9. The definition of a generalized cone. It is the surface created by moving a cross-section along a given smooth axis. The cross section may vary smoothly in size, but its shape remains constant. Several examples are shown here. In each, the cross section is shown at several positions along the trajectory that spins out the construction.

Shapes admitting 3-D model descriptions

If the scheme for a given shape is to be uniquely defined and stable over unimportant variations such as viewpoint – if, in a word it is to be canonical – its definition must take advantage of any salient geometrical characteristics that the shape possesses inherently. If a shape has natural axes, then those should be used. The coordinate system for a sausage should take advantage of its major axis, and for a face, of its axis of symmetry.

Highly symmetrical objects, like a sphere, a square, or a circular disk, will inevitably lead to ambiguities in the choice of coordinate systems. For a shape as regular as a sphere this poses no great problem, because its description in all reasonable systems is the same. One can even allow other factors, like the direction of motion or spin, to influence the choice of coordinate frame. For other shapes, the existence of more than one possible choice probably means that one has to represent the object in several ways, but this is acceptable provided that their number is small. For example, there are four possible axes on which one might wish to base the coordinate system for representing a door, namely the midlines along its length, its width, and its thickness, and also the axis of its hinges. (This last would be especially useful to represent how the door opens.) For a typewriter, there are two reasonable choices, an axis parallel to its width, because that is usually its largest dimension, and the axis about which a typewriter is roughly symmetrical.

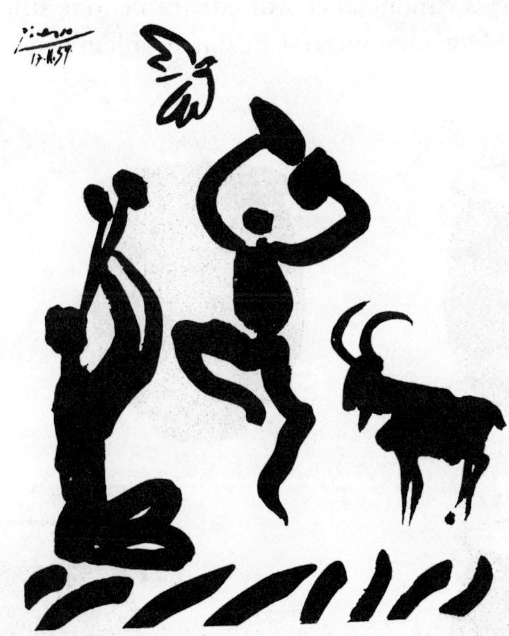

FIGURE 10. 'Rites of Spring' by Pablo Picasso. We immediately interpret such silhouettes in terms of particular three-dimensional surfaces – this despite the paucity of information in the image itself. In order to do this, we plainly must invoke certain *a priori* assumptions and constraints about the nature of the shapes.

In general, if an axis can be distinguished in a shape, it can be used as the basis for a local coordinate system. One approach to the problem of defining object-centred coordinates is therefore to examine the class of shapes having an axis as an integral part of their structure. Consider, accordingly, the class of so-called *generalized cones*, each of these being the surface swept out by moving a cross section of constant shape but smoothly varying size along an axis, as shown in figure 9. Binford (1971) has drawn attention to this class of constructions, suggesting that it might provide a convenient way of describing three-dimensional surfaces for the purposes of computer vision (see also Agin 1972; Nevatia 1974). We regard it as an important class not because the shapes themselves are easily describable, but because the presence of an axis allows one to define a canonical local coordinate system. Fortunately, many objects, especially those whose shape was achieved by growth, are described quite naturally in terms of one or more generalized cones. The animal shapes of figure 7 provide some examples; the individual sticks are simply the axes of generalized cones that approximate the shapes of parts of these creatures.

Many artefacts can also be described in this way – say a car (a small box sitting atop a longer one) or a building (a box with a vertical axis.)

It is important to remember, however, that there exist surfaces that cannot conveniently be approximated by generalized cones, for example a cake that has been transected at some arbitrary plane, or the surface formed by a crumpled newspaper. Cases like the cake could be dealt with by introducing a suitable surface primitive for describing the plane of the cut, in much the same way as an axis in the 3-D model representation is a primitive that describes a volumetric element. But the crumpled newspaper poses apparently intractable problems.

Finding the natural coordinate system

Even if a shape possesses a canonical coordinate frame, one still is faced with the problem of finding it from an image. Our own interest in this problem grew from the question of how to

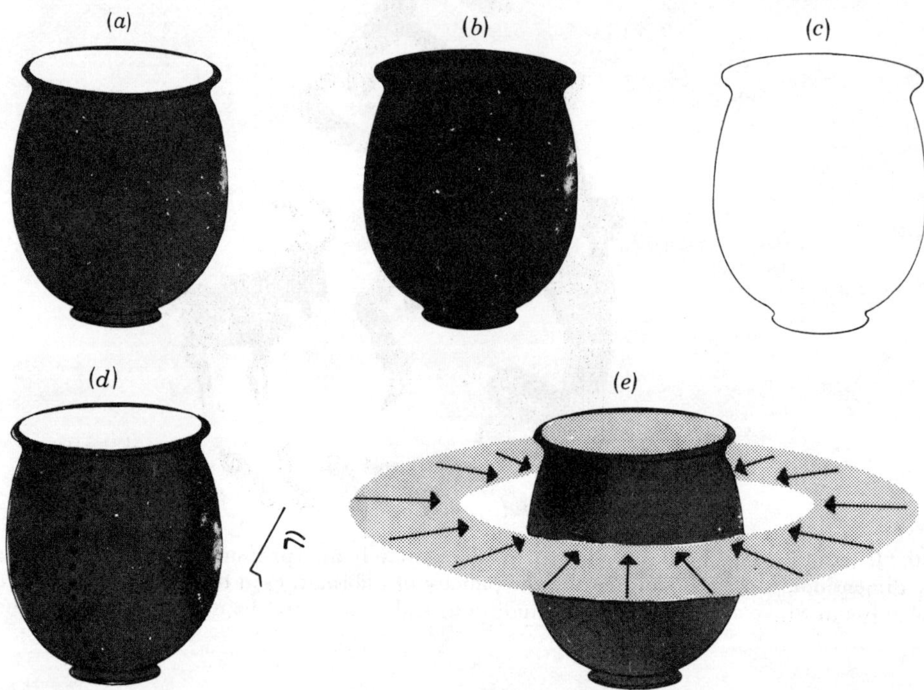

FIGURE 11. Four structures of importance in studying the *a priori* conditions mentioned in figure 10. (*a*) A three-dimensional surface Σ; (*b*) its silhouette, S_V, as seen from viewpoint V; (*c*) the contour C_V of S_V; (*d*) the set of points Γ_V on Σ that project onto the contour. Finally, (*e*) illustrates schematically the meaning of the phrase 'all distant viewing directions that lie in a plane'.

interpret the *outlines* of objects as seen in a two-dimensional image (Marr 1977*b*), and our starting point was the observation that when one looks at the silhouettes in Picasso's 'Rites of Spring' (reproduced here in figure 10), one perceives them in terms of very particular three-dimensional shapes, some familiar, some less so. This is quite remarkable, because the silhouettes could in theory have been generated by an infinite variety of three-dimensional shapes which, from other viewpoints, would have no descernible similarities to the shapes we perceive. One can perhaps attribute part of the phenomenon to a familiarity with the depicted shapes, but not all of it, because one can use the medium of a silhouette to convey a new shape, and because even with considerable effort it is difficult to imagine the more bizarre three-dimensional surfaces that could have given rise to the same silhouettes. The paradox, then, is that the bounding contours in Picasso's 'Rites' apparently tell us more than they should about the shape of the figures. For example, neighbouring points on such a contour could in general arise from widely separated points on the original surface, but our perceptual interpretation usually ignores this possibility.

The first observation to be made is that the contours that bound these silhouettes are contours of surface discontinuity, which are precisely the contours with which the $2\frac{1}{2}$-D sketch is concerned. Secondly, because we can interpret the silhouettes as three-dimensional shapes, then implicit in the way we interpret them must lie some *a priori* assumptions that allow us to infer a shape from an outline. If a surface violates these assumptions, our analysis will be wrong, in the sense that the shape that we assign to the contours will differ from the shape that actually caused them. An everyday example is the shadowgraph, where the appropriate arrangement of one's hands can, to the surprise and delight of a child, produce the shadow of a duck or a rabbit.

What assumptions is it reasonable to suppose that we make? To explain them, we need to define the four constructions that appear in figure 11. These are (1) a three-dimensional surface Σ, (2) its image or silhouette S_V as seen from a viewpoint V, (3) the bounding contour C_V of S_V, and (4) the set of points on the surface Σ that project onto the contour C_V. We shall call this last the *contour generator* of C_V, and we shall denote it by Γ_V.

Observe that the contour C_V, like the contours in the work of Picasso, imparts very little information about the three-dimensional surface that caused it. Indeed, the only obvious feature available in the contour is the distinction between convex and concave places – that is to say, the presence of inflexion points. In order that these inflections be 'reliable', one needs to make some assumptions about the way in which the contour was generated, and we choose the following restrictions (Marr 1977).

(1) Each point on the contour generator Γ_V projects to a different point on the contour C_V.

(2) Nearby points on the contour C_V arise from nearby points on the contour generator Γ_V.

(3) The contour generator Γ_V lies wholly in a single plane.

The first and second restrictions say that each point on the contour of the image comes from one point on the surface (which is an assumption that facilitates the analysis but is not of fundamental importance), and that where the surface looks continuous in the image, it really is continuous in three dimensions. The third restriction is simply the demand that the difference between convex and concave contour segments reflects properties of the surface, rather than of the imaging process.

It turns out to be a theorem that if the surface is smooth (for our purposes, if it is twice differentiable with continuous second derivative) and if restrictions 1–3 hold for all distant viewing positions in any one plane (as illustrated in figure 11), then the viewed surface is a generalized cone with straight axis. (The converse is also true: if the surface is a generalized cone with straight axis, then conditions 1–3 will be found to be true.)

This means that if the convexities and concavities of a bounding contour in an image are actual properties of a surface, then that surface is a generalized cone or is composed of several such cones. In brief, the theorem says that a natural link exists between generalized cones and the imaging process itself. The combination of these two must mean, we think, that generalized cones will play an initimate role in the development of vision theory.

Discussion

I have tried in this survey of visual information processing to make two principal points. The first is methodological: namely, that it is important to be very clear about the nature of the understanding that we seek. The results that we try to achieve should be precise ones, at the level of what we call a computational theory. The critical act in formulating computational theories turns out to be the discovery of valid constraints on the way the world is structured – constraints that provide sufficient information to allow the processing to succeed. Consider stereopsis, which presupposes continuity and uniqueness in the world, or structure from visual motion, which presupposes rigidity, or shape from contour, which presupposes the three restrictions just discussed, or even edge detection, which presupposes the assumption of spatial coincidence. The discovery of constraints that are valid and universal leads to results about vision that have the same quality of permanence as results in other branches of science.

The second point is that the critical issues for vision seem to me to revolve around the nature of the representations and the nature of the processes that create, maintain and eventually interpret them. I have suggested an overall framework for visual information processing (summarized in table 2) that includes three categories of representation upon which the processing is to operate. The first encompasses representations of intensity variations and their local geometry

TABLE 2. A FRAMEWORK FOR THE DERIVATION OF SHAPE INFORMATION FROM IMAGES

image(s)
$\downarrow$

primal sketch(es)	Describes the intensity changes present in an image, labels distinguished locations like termination points, and makes explicit local two-dimensional geometrical relations

$\downarrow$

$2\frac{1}{2}$-D sketch	Represents contours of surface discontinuity, and depth and orientation of visible surface elements, in a coordinate frame that is centred on the viewer

$\downarrow$

3-D model representation	Shape description that includes volumetric shape primitives of a variety of sizes, whose positions are defined by using an object-centred coordinate system. This representation imposes considerable modular organization on its descriptions

in the input to the visual system. One among these, the primal sketch, is expressly intended to be an efficient description of these variations which captures just that information required by the image analysis to follow. The second category encompasses the representations of visible surfaces – the descriptions, in other words, of the physical properties of the surfaces that caused the images in the first place. The nature of these representations, the $2\frac{1}{2}$-dimensional sketch in particular, is determined primarily by what information can be extracted by modules of image analysis such as stereopsis and structure from motion. Like the primal sketch of the previous category, the $2\frac{1}{2}$-dimensional sketch is intended to be a final or output representation: this is where the separate contributions from the various image-analysis modules can be combined into a unified description. The third category encompasses all representations that are subsequently constructed from information contained in the $2\frac{1}{2}$-D sketch. The designs of these tertiary representations are determined largely by the use to which they are to be put, as for the 3-D model representation, to be used for shape recognition. If one had wanted instead, for example, to represent a shape simply for later *reproduction*, say by the milling of a block of metal, then the $2\frac{1}{2}$-D sketch would itself have been sufficient, as the milling process depends explicitly on information about local depth and orientation, such as that sketch can provide.

Finally, a remark of a rather different nature. As we have seen, some aspects of human early visual processing, like stereopsis, have apparently been understood well enough to implement them in machines (Marr & Poggio 1979; Marr & Grimson 1979). The computational power required by these early processes is prohibitive, and until recently the prospects for real-time implementation of human-like early vision were remote. It now appears, however, that the emerging VLSI and CCD technologies will be able to supply the necessary processing power. This could make the next two decades very interesting.

I thank K. Nishihara and M. Feiertag for help in assembling this survey. I thank the Royal Society for permission to reproduce figures 3, 4, 6, 7 and 8, and the M.I.T. Press for figure 5. This work was conducted at the Artificial Intelligence Laboratory, a Massachusetts Institute of Technology research programme supported in part by the Advanced Research Projects Agency of the Department of Defense, and monitored by the Office of Naval Research under contract number N00014-75-C-0643, and in part by NSF contract number 77-07569-MCS.

References (Marr)

Agin, G. J. 1972 Representation and description of curved objects. *Stanford Artificial Intelligence Project*, memo AIM-173. Stanford University.

Binford, T. O. 1971 Visual perception by computer. Presented to the I.E.E.E. Conference on Systems and Control, Miami, December.

Blum, H. 1973 Biological shape and visual science, part 1. *J. theor. Biol.* **38**, 205–287.

Enroth-Cugell, C. & Robson, J. D. 1966 The contrast sensitivity of retinal ganglion cells of the cat. *J. Physiol., Lond.* **187**, 517–522.

Freuder, E. C. 1975 A computer vision system for visual recognition using active knowledge. *M.I.T. A.I. Lab. Tech. Rep.* no. 345.

Helmholtz, H. L. F. von 1910 *Treatise on physiological optics* (trans. J. P. Southall, 1925). N.Y.: Dover.

Horn, B. K. P. 1975 Obtaining shape from shading information. In *The psychology of computer vision* (ed. P. H. Winston), pp. 115–155. New York: McGraw-Hill.

Hubel, D. H. & Wiesel, T. N. 1962 Receptive fields, binocular interaction and functional architecture in the cat's visual cortex. *J. Physiol., Lond.* **160**, 106–154.

Hubel, D. H. & Wiesel, T. N. 1968 Receptive fields and functional architecture of monkey striate cortex. *J. Physiol., Lond.* **195**, 215–243.

Julesz, B. 1971 *Foundations of cyclopean perception.* Chicago: University of Chicago Press.

Kuffler, S. W. 1953 Discharge patterns and functional organization of mammalian retina. *J. Neurophysiol.* **16**, 37–68.

Marr, D. 1976 Early processing of visual information. *Phil. Trans. R. Soc. Lond.* B **275**, 483–524.

Marr, D. 1977*a* Artificial intelligence – a personal view. *Artificial Intelligence* **9**, 37–48.

Marr, D. 1977*b* Analysis of occluding contour. *Proc. R. Soc. Lond.* B **197**, 441–475.

Marr, D. 1978 Representing visual information. *Lectures on mathematics in the life sciences*, volume 10: *Some mathematical Questions in Biology*, pp. 101–180.

Marr, D. & Hildreth, E. 1979 Theory of edge detection. *Proc. R. Soc. Lond.* B. (In the press.)

Marr, D. & Nishihara, H. K. 1978 Representation and recognition of the spatial organization of three-dimensional shapes. *Proc. R. Soc. Lond.* B **200**, 269–294.

Marr, D. & Poggio, T. 1976 Cooperative computation of stereo disparity. *Science, N.Y.* **194**, 283–287.

Marr, D. & Poggio, T. 1977 From understanding computation to understanding neural circuitry. *Neurosci. Res. Prog. Bull.* **15**, 470–488.

Marr, D. & Poggio, T. 1979 A computational theory of human stereo vision. *Proc. R. Soc. Lond.* B **204**, 301–328.

Marr, D., Poggio, T. & Palm, G. 1977 Analysis of a cooperative stereo algorithm. *Biol. Cybernet.* **28**, 223–239.

Marr, D., Poggio, T. & Ullman, S. 1979 Bandpass channels, zero-crossings and early visual information processing. *J. opt. Soc. Am.* **69**, 914–916.

Marr, D. & Ullman, S. 1979 Directional selectivity and its use in early visual processing. (In preparation.)

Nevatia, R. 1974 Structured descriptions of complex curved objects for recognition and visual memory. *Stanford Artificial Intelligence Project*, memo AIM-250. Stanford University.

Newton, I. 1704 *Optics.* London.

Shepard, R. N. & Metzler, J. 1971 Mental rotation of three-dimensional objects. *Science, N.Y.* **171**, 701–703.

Stevens, K. A. 1978 Computation of locally parallel structure. *Biol. Cybernet.* **29**, 19–28.

Tenenbaum, J. M. & Barrow, H. G. 1976 Experiments in interpretation-guided segmentation. *Stanford Res. Inst. Tech. Note* no. 123.

Ullman, S. 1979*a* The interpretation of structure from motion. *Proc. R. Soc. Lond.* B **203**, 405–426.

Ullman, S. 1979*b* *The interpretation of visual motion.* M.I.T. Press.

Wallach, H. & O'Connell, D. N. 1953 The kinetic depth effect. *J. exp. Psychol.* **45**, 205–217.

Wertheimer, M. 1938 Principles of perceptual organizations. In *Source book of Gestalt psychology* (ed. W. H. Ellis), pp. 71–88. New York: Routledge Kegan Paul.

Discussion

S. Lal (*Department of Physiology, Chelsea College, London SW3 6LX, U.K.*). There seem to me to be two objections to the theory of early visual processing presented. The first relates to the well-known result that any differentiation process will magnify noise, i.e. it will decrease the signal: noise ratio. Since we know that random fluctuations of neural signals are common, it would be most disadvantageous (at least at low signal levels) to use differentiating operations to extract information about a visual scene. The second objection relates to the impossibility of deducing from local features alone the global characteristics of the intensity function. Yet some global description and analysis is a prerequisite for extracting relevant information from a visual scene.

D. Marr.

1. Noise is probably not so important under conditions of normal vision (to which my remarks apply). In low illumination after sufficient adaptation, of course, retinal receptive field properties do change – away from acting as differentiators and towards acting as photon collectors.

2. The general idea is that one starts with rather local descriptive elements and gradually computes more global constructs, but things can go the other way. In stereopsis, for example, the coarse results obtained from matching the larger channels are then used to control disjunctive eye-movements, which bring signals from the smaller channels into the 'relevant' disparity range (see Marr & Poggio 1979).

H. B. Barlow, F.R.S. (*Physiological Laboratory, Cambridge CB2 3EG, U.K.*). I am afraid that this is more commentary than question. For many years the kind of problems of early processing that Marr has been talking about were thought, at least by some, to be trivially easy. According to this view the problem of finding the position of an edge was not the sort of thing to which one should devote valuable computer time, nor the even more valuable artificial intelligencer's intelligence. That view was wrong, for it is a difficult task, and it is a crucial first step for further progress to understanding the nature of these difficulties. It is crucial not only to improve edge-finders in programmes, but even more to enable physiologists to understand neural mechanisms. I am sure many of us must come away from a talk like this with new ideas about what to look for when recording from cortical neurons and analysing how they achieve their selectivity.

Understanding the nature of the difficulties is also necessary when one wants to test whether a computer method of doing something is what really happens. The natural test to apply is to measure *how well* the computer method overcomes the difficulties and compare this with the human observer's performance under various conditions. This is what I was trying to do with symmetry detection, where the first step was to identify (I hope correctly) the natural difficulty in symmetry detection as the occurrence of spurious symmetry. The point here is that one can only begin to make such comparisons when the natural difficulty has been identified, and it seems to be the artificial intelligence approach that leads most directly to this information.